Straight Wire

The Concept and Appliance

Lawrence F. Andrews, D.D.S.

L.A. Wells

L.A. Wells Co.
2025 Chatsworth Boulevard
San Diego, CA 92107

Editorial Coordinator: Julie Olfe, La Jolla, CA 92037
Designer: Mike Kelly, K-W Publications, San Diego, CA 92126
Principal Illustrator: Lisa Schirmer, San Diego, CA 92106

ISBN 0-9616256-0-0

10 9 8 7 6 5 4 3 2 1

Printed in the United States of America

With love, respect, and gratitude, this work is dedicated
to
Mary Malinda (Williamson) Andrews
and Wilbur Alan Andrews,
my mother and father

Contents

Foreword

The future and scope of orthodontics depends on creative people, their conceptual focus and achievement of goals. This creative energy benefits our specialty and, in turn, the public's health, by cultivating history that is progressive rather than repetitious. Lawrence F. Andrews created some of this progressive momentum with the development of the straight-wire appliance for orthodontics.

The introduction of Dr. Andrews's philosophy and appliance in 1970 stirred the orthodontic specialty rather profoundly. A story unfolds here that should make every reader ponder how he or she has functioned without this vital understanding of concepts, treatment goals, and appliance design. This writing is not a wilted mixture of previously presented material. It is a crisp blend of the philosophy, objectives, and development of the straight-wire appliance. It is true that you don't have to be an aeronautical engineer to fly a plane. However, since our specialty includes biomechanics, we are both engineer and pilot. This juxtaposition welds our right to specialize and separates us from those less trained. The information contained in this book is fundamental to our care for patients; yet it has escaped many eyes until now.

It has been my privilege to know and learn from the author, Lawrence F. Andrews, for the past twenty-five years. Because of his unpretentious and unassuming nature, few know his background. He is a graduate of Ohio State University. Cloaked in scarlet and gray, Larry earned his varsity "O" and learned discipline and team play under the tutelage of Ohio State's legendary football coach, Woody Hayes. Larry Andrews completed dental school there in 1954 and orthodontic training in 1958. Since then he has participated in a cascade of postgraduate courses and societies, which helped sculpture his destiny. Included are the American Board of Orthodontics, the Angle Society, and the Tweed Foundation. He has also presented many courses concerning the evolution of his appliance, technique, and treatment results in San Diego and throughout the world.

In many instances, worthwhile technical advances in our specialty have come from private practitioners working at the chair. Larry Andrews is no exception. His observation of a lack of consensus among orthodontists about treatment goals, and the robotic repetition of wire-bending procedures without concern for precious time prompted his effort to design an improved appliance through analysis, consolidation, and simplification. Insatiably inquisitive and goal oriented, he painstakingly collected, studied, and measured 120 naturally occurring optimal occlusions. The development of the straight-wire appliance was not the result of a single discovery, but rather the product of a long and tedious process. Many individual innovations were distilled and combined for Andrews's intricate design.

In September 1972 he published the "Six Keys to Normal Occlusion" and demonstrated the need for orthodontic goals to mimic the occlusions of naturally optimal dentitions. Indeed, the teeth and jaws are the foundations from which we may recontour the orofacial complex. His forward thinking created an appliance designed to eliminate repetitive, time-consuming, and difficult-to-reproduce archwire bends, so that the clinician can focus on diagnosis and attaining predictable results. His new concept makes it unnecessary to place bends in an archwire other than for the fine tuning of normal variety. The appliance is versatile, and a broad range of techniques can be applied.

It follows that this book should be studied diligently by all who must evaluate the myriad appliances presented by companies, together with their claims of efficacy. This text is the first of two volumes and presents the concept that it is feasible to build many treatment goals into an appliance. The achievement of optimum occlusion is difficult, but the clinician is propelled more efficiently toward this goal with an appliance that is fully programmed. Dr. Andrews has always been an innovative clinician and a master at documentation of progress and results. His imagination has indeed given us a powerful tool to pursue our treatment goals. He has created a force field that bridges the three planes of space in bracket design.

Authorship of a high-quality text is more than a labor of love. It is a commitment to accuracy and clarity, with discipline to persist until completion. Writing demands unwavering intellectual and physical vigor, a total immersion. This book is a concise and extremely well illustrated discourse on the evolution of the straight-wire appliance. The text is constructively critical of some of our inconsistencies in treatment goals. Its intention is not to present an exhaustive review and analysis of the research literature. It is not a compendium of statistical data. Rather, it is structured to present the straight-wire concept and appliance in a lucid, concise but complete manner. Accuracy and clarity are derived from explicit but simple language and supplemented with extensive illustrations rather than many pages of burdensome narrative. Larry Andrews presents efficiency in content, simplicity in syntax, and a logical sequence in the development of the text, with conclusions that are substantiated with clear illustrations.

Submission of a book for review by expert peers, some with opposing points of view, is a hallmark of high quality and the search for truth. Books often differ from scientific journals in that no review by peers is necessary prior to publication. Some texts are a series of anecdotal presentations and opinions with extended conclusions, often suggesting science in action, but they seldom stand the test of time or promote progress. This text has been reviewed by many consultants with differing points of view. The author has diligently revised the text many times over a period of seven years to ensure accuracy in presentation and a symphonic blend of text with illustrations. This book fills a vacuum in the clinical evaluation of a fully programmed appliance. The concepts and appliance description are based on thirty years of clinical practice and research.

Many books are written on how to construct appliances or perform a procedure. Few verify whether they reach the objective. Larry Andrews lives a life of creative involvement, evolution, and determination, all combined with common sense and a pursuit of high ideals. His ambition is to present a concept that encourages our specialty toward objective goals. Mechanics is recognized as a vital line in the therapeutic chain, and appliances have been a traditional battleground in orthodontics. This is predictable, since there has been a

disconcerting lack of continuity between goal and appliance. A straight-wire appliance is not a product of serendipity, but is poetry in design. It is an appliance fully programmed with a combination of simplicity and effectiveness for the road to successful treatment. Experience and research are synthesized in a logical pattern and permit technique choices to be made by the clinician. Lawrence F. Andrews leaves a heritage of creativeness and synergism for those who follow.

WAYNE G. WATSON, D.D.S.

Editor, *American Journal of Orthodontics,* 1978–1985

Acknowledgments

Coenraad F. Moorrees, professor of orthodontics at the Harvard School of Dental Medicine, spent a great deal of time on this book and provided thoughtful, discerning advice. His welcome help was generously given, but his involvement does not in any way imply endorsement of the book's contents. Time did not permit Dr. Moorrees to see all the chapters or the final version of those chapters he did review before printing, so he cannot be held accountable for any errors.

John Valleau, a talented writer and editor, has worked closely with me on everything I have published, and has collaborated on the defining of new terms. He helped construct the original Six Keys article, which is now on the required reading list in all but three orthodontic departments in North America. He edited my writings that appeared in German, English, and Japanese professional journals, as well as the six-part series about the Straight-Wire Appliance in the *Journal of Clinical Orthodontics* (JCO). Eugene L. Gottlieb, JCO editor, later said, "There have been more requests for reprints of those articles than for any other in the history of this publication." John helped

with my teaching syllabus (the prelude to this book), all four editions of which sold out. John is my chief editor, confidant, and friend.

For eighteen years, Jackie Nevelow has managed my office—a place that is as much involved in research, writing, and teaching as in providing clinical services. She has processed innumerable versions of the text, and has made a number of valuable contributions to the organization of the entire volume. Jackie is resourceful and durable, and the most upbeat and self-motivated person I know.

Julie Olfe is a freelance editor who has coordinated all aspects of preparing the text for printing.

Lisa Schirmer is a skilled medical illustrator. Approximately 80 percent of the illustrations in this book were done by her, requiring several years of her full-time work. Walter Stuart, Carol Frick, Darryl Millsap, John Molinar, and Kalan Brunik provided the other illustrations.

Those interested in functional occlusion appreciate Ron Roth for discovering that the Straight-Wire Appliance is useful for more than attaining the Six Key goals more easily.

Ron has spearheaded the move to include functional occlusion as a treatment goal for normal malocclusions.

Although the straight-wire concept and appliance are now being taught in most orthodontic departments in North America and in several foreign countries, there has been no textbook. In an attempt to fill that need, I sent an early draft of this volume to a number of orthodontic department chairmen, for counsel concerning its content in relation to the needs of their schools. The following chairpersons and staff members took the time to provide suggestions about editing and content:

Rolf G. Behrents, assisted by Joe L. Wasson, University of Tennessee

Dennis O. Bernard, West Virginia University

Gerald Borell, assisted by Daubert Telsey, New York University

Alan J. Borislow, Albert Einstein Medical Center

Douglas L. Buck, Oregon Health Sciences University

Zeev Davidovich, assisted by Dennis L. Johnson and James A. Tetz, Ohio State University

LaForrest D. Garner, Indiana University

Anthony A. Gianelly, Boston University

Kenneth E. Glover, assisted by William K. Lobb, University of Alberta

W. Stuart Hunter, University of Western Ontario

Alex Jacobson, University of Alabama in Birmingham

Lysle E. Johnston, St. Louis University Medical Center

Lewis Klapper, Loyola University of Chicago

Mladen M. Kuftinec, University of Louisville

Richard A. Litt, University of California, San Francisco

Coenraad F. Moorrees, Harvard School of Dental Medicine

Ram S. Nanda, University of Oklahoma

Harold T. Perry, Jr., Northwestern University

Donald R. Poulton, University of the Pacific

William R. Proffit, University of North Carolina

Michael L. Riolo, University of Detroit

Leo S. Shanley, Washington University

Everett Shapiro, Tufts University

Arthur T. Storey, University of Manitoba

J. Daniel Subtelny, assisted by Edward W. Sommers, Eastman Dental Center

Orhan C. Tuncay, University of Kentucky

Robert L. Vanarsdall, Jr., University of Pennsylvania

Roland D. Walters, Loma Linda University

Morris H. Wechsler, University of Montreal

Dan C. West, University of Texas

Thomas J. Zwemer, assisted by Jerry L. Boshell, Medical College of Georgia.

Other individuals have followed the development of the straight-wire appliance since its inception, and remained available to help in any way possible during the writing of this book. My thanks for counsel and editorial suggestions go to these friends and associates:

Eugene L. Gottlieb

Jack E. King

Arthur B. Lewis

Robert E. Matthews

Richard P. McLaughlin

Brainerd F. Swain

Wayne G. Watson.

My thanks also extend to the diplomates of the American Board of Orthodontics, whose treatment casts provide historical documentation of occlusal aspects of the state of the art of orthodontics from the mid-1960s through the mid-1980s.

Introduction

This book reports the results of fourteen research projects. One led to the six key elements in optimal occlusion. Five led to the concept of the straight-wire appliance.* Eight were designed to explain and justify the concept.

The Straight-Wire Appliance is used as an example because it is currently the only fully programmed appliance. When patents expire, there will probably be as many fully programmed appliances as there are manufacturers. The principles taught here are fundamental and should apply to all appliances that adhere to the concept.

A fully programmed appliance—or any other appliance, for that matter—is not a treatment philosophy. This book does not teach or require any treatment procedures or goals except for Six-Key occlusion and optimal arch lines. Additional goals and most treatment procedures used with any edgewise appliance can be used with a fully programmed appliance, but with less wire bending. (A second volume is planned to explain the Andrews treatment philosophy and its clinical application.)

Regardless of one's expertise in other aspects of orthodontics, fitting the teeth together as well as they can be is essential to being a good orthodontist. Brackets stand between the teeth and the orthodontist: which ones are prescribed play a large role in the quality of the results and in treatment efficiency. This book teaches the importance of using an appliance whose slots' planes indirectly represent the planes of the crowns. Without this symbiotic condition, the orthodontist is at a distinct tactical disadvantage.

Some new methods and terms are introduced because the straight-wire appliance concept is new and because traditional methods and terms are sometimes inadequate or incorrect. Essential for understanding this book is that tooth positions are referenced from the crown's facial axis, not from the tooth's or crown's long axis, as is more traditional. *Optimal* is used for *correct*; *normal* is used to mean *not abnormal*.

Also new in this book is the concept of three arch lines. The term *arch length* must

---

*Throughout the book *straight-wire* refers conceptually to any fully programmed appliance; *Straight-Wire* refers to the appliance designed by the author and trademarked and manufactured by "A"-Co., San Diego, CA, USA, a Johnson & Johnson company.

now be modified. The optimal length of each arch line may be known, but it is difficult to achieve orthodontically with an appliance that is not fully programmed, because of the unpredictable slot siting and the wire-bending and wire-forming side effects inherent in such appliances. A distinct advantage of a fully programmed appliance is that when sited as prescribed it targets the slots predictably and eliminates the need for wire bends. It does not, however, eliminate the need for wire forming.

A fully programmed appliance will not cause teeth to move faster than is biologically possible; it can only match that limit and achieve it as directly as possible. A part of the individualized straight-wire appliance concept is that it is effective for 90 percent of patients that have normal malocclusions. *Effective* means that it will be more efficient in moving teeth over the most direct route with fewer wire bends than will other appliances that are not fully programmed; *normal* means treatable to optimal standards without the need for surgery.

Not all is new in this book: the contents of some chapters have been separately published by the author in various journals and teaching syllabi. But nowhere is there more complete information about the fully programmed appliance.

Chapter 1

Posttreatment Occlusion

The concept that an edgewise appliance could be fully programmed evolved from a series of five studies. The first began in 1960. It involved examination of posttreatment dental casts to assess the state of the art of orthodontics in terms of static occlusion. The research was undertaken for a thesis then required for certification by the American Board of Orthodontics. There was no intent, at the time of the initial study, to develop a new appliance.

The American Board of Orthodontics, the Edward H. Angle Society, and the Tweed Foundation require submission of pretreatment and posttreatment records as a prerequisite for certification or membership. Each organization has its own standards for diagnosis, treatment planning, aesthetics, and occlusal results. The posttreatment casts displayed by members or prospective members at the meetings of these organizations provided an ideal opportunity for assessing the quality of American orthodontics in terms of static occlusion.

Analysis of hundreds of posttreatment casts in the early 1960s led to preliminary conclusions about the occlusal standards then considered to represent good treatment (Fig. 1.1).

Several conditions were consistently present, just as they would be in a satisfactory setup of denture teeth: the incisors were not rotated; the interarch relationship had no crossbite or overjet; and the molar interarch relationship was as prescribed by Edward H. Angle in 1899 [6],* except where teeth were extracted in only one arch.

Except for these few consistencies, the dominant feature of treatment results seemed to be variation. Such variation would not be found in denture setups. However, none of the differences in occlusal results triggered disqualification by either the submitting orthodontist or the examiners. The articulation of occlusal surfaces often did not match the classic textbook description. The long axes of teeth on either side of extraction sites were not always parallel. Though different for extraction than for nonextraction treatment, the range of crown inclination and angulation of any tooth type was moderate within the dental casts submitted by any one orthodontist,

---

*References are listed at the end of this book.

3

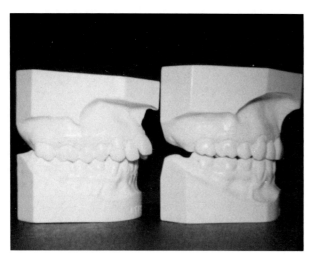

Fig. 1.1. Posttreatment casts (*right*) showing the tooth positions and the interarch relationships that were acceptable in the early 1960s. Pretreatment casts are on the left.

but varied considerably from one clinician to another. The permanent second molars were not routinely included in treatment. Interdental spaces (at extraction sites and other locations) occurred frequently and often seemed to result from incomplete treatment rather than from mesiodistal crown-size discrepancies. Rotations of teeth requiring translation were common. Dental casts were not mounted on articulators for assessing functional occlusion, nor were intraoral photographs used for this purpose. There was no standardization as to whether dental casts were registered in centric relation or centric occlusion.

Although orthodontists are experts on occlusion, their treatment results do not always satisfy the occlusal standards of other specialists or of generalists. One must ask, in matters of occlusion, whether the goals of orthodontists are different from those of others in dentistry, or whether there are clinical limitations that prevent orthodontists from reaching the goals considered exemplary by others.

For the prosthodontist, optimal occlusion is not difficult to achieve or to critically evaluate when artificial teeth are set in wax and mounted on an articulator. Under these conditions, the characteristics of occlusion can be viewed with ease from both the lingual and the facial aspect, and, if the occlusion is not correct, the crowns can be moved readily in warm wax until their occlusal surfaces articulate properly.

Similarly, dentists reconstructing a dentition on an articulator can change the occlusal surface of a waxed crown instantly with a hot spatula and immediately see the results. But the occlusion of natural teeth is not as readily improved as that of denture teeth set in wax or that of waxed crowns; weeks may pass before orthodontists can judge the effects of their adjustments. Additional problems for orthodontists include rebound, different rates of jaw growth, and degrees of patient cooperation. Also, when the teeth in an arch are connected with a wire, the positioning of one tooth often is accompanied by unwanted movement of adjacent teeth.

Other problems inherent in orthodontics concern judging the progress of treatment clinically. Examples include interarch relationship, which may appear more satisfactory than it actually is because the clinical perspective is from a 45° angle to the buccal segments rather than from 90° (Fig. 1.2); the lingual aspect of the occlusion, because it cannot be examined; and function, because centric closure and border movements made voluntarily by a patient may differ from ones carefully monitored, registered, and transferred to casts mounted on an articulator.

This initial attempt to assess the state of the art of orthodontics in terms of posttreatment static occlusion did not yield the consistent and adequate data required for firm conclusions. One implication, however, was clear: the paragon positions of natural teeth (perhaps the proper goal for orthodontists?) could be found only by studying dentitions with naturally optimal occlusion.

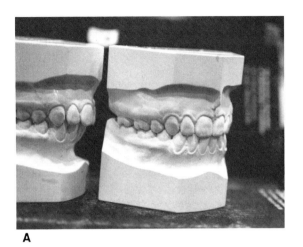
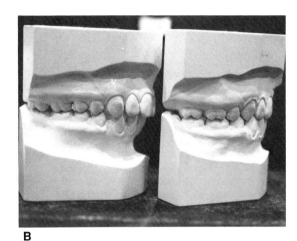

A

B

Fig. 1.2. An occlusion viewed from two perspectives. *A,* at 45° to the buccal segments, optical illusion may cause tooth positions and interarch relationships to appear better than they are. *B,* at 90°, the positions and relationships can be viewed as they actually are.

Chapter **2**

Naturally Occurring
Optimal Occlusion

On the hypothesis that naturally occurring optimal occlusion would be worthy of emulation, casts of such dentitions were collected over a four-year period. When notified of this project, some fifteen orthodontists and general dentists in the San Diego, California, area cooperated by referring candidates. Other subjects included personal friends and acquaintances. Dr. A. G. Brodie's help was especially valuable: he arranged to duplicate a collection of casts with naturally good-to-excellent occlusion at the University of Illinois orthodontic department. By 1964 the sample comprised 120 casts. The gathering of these casts constituted the second of the five steps that led to the development of the first fully programmed orthodontic appliance.

The collecting continues, with many of the casts supplemented by headfilms and extraoral photographs.* Casts collected since mid-1985 have been mounted; lateral headfilms have been taken with the patient's head in true vertical position; and, in addition to conventional extraoral photographs, a lateral extraor-

al photograph has been taken to show both a bared forehead and the patient smiling enough to fully expose the maxillary incisors. The casts are continually reexamined, and the less exemplary are screened out. The casts reported on here are the 120 best of the total sample, as of 1988. These dentitions (1) have never been subjected to orthodontic treatment, (2) are well aligned and pleasing in appearance, (3) appear to have excellent occlusion, and (4) would not benefit from orthodontic treatment.

Twenty of the 120 casts have been photographed to illustrate some of the consistencies found in the positions and interarch relationship of the crowns (Figs. 2.1–2.20). All of the following photographs were taken at a right angle to the center portion of the right buccal

*Contributors: University of Illinois orthodontic department, orthodontic graduate students at Loyola University of Chicago, San Diego dentists and orthodontists, and other orthodontists throughout the United States. The sample therefore represents the judgment of a broad panel of professionals in dentistry, with their selections later examined by numerous orthodontists—often with the aid of color slides.

segment. Facial axes on the posterior crowns (dominant groove for molars, and prominent facial ridge for all others) were marked before being photographed so that crown angulation can be easily assessed. The midpoint of the height of each clinical crown was also marked.

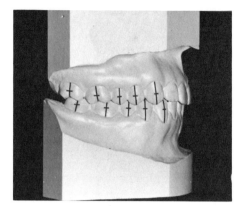

Fig. 2.3

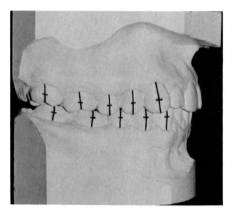

Fig. 2.1

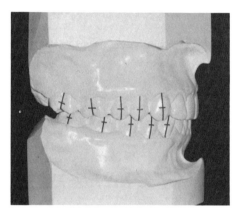

Fig. 2.4

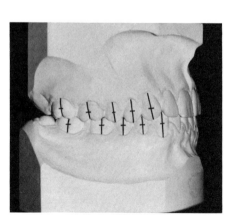

Fig. 2.2

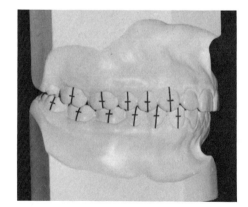

Fig. 2.5

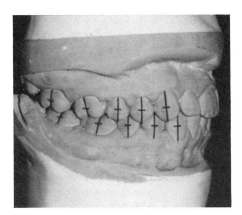

Fig. 2.6

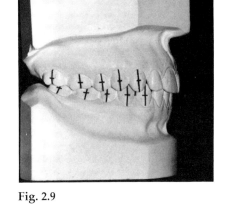

Fig. 2.9

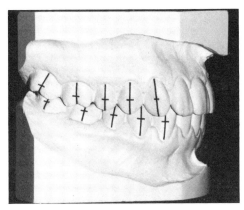

Fig. 2.7

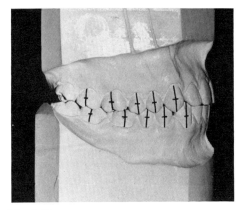

Fig. 2.10

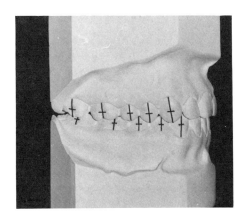

Fig. 2.8

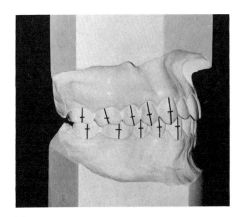

Fig. 2.11

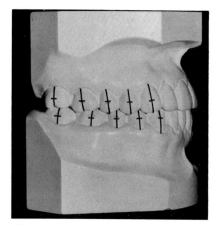

Fig. 2.12

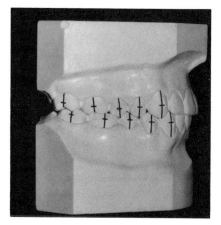

Fig. 2.15

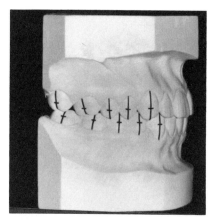

Fig. 2.13

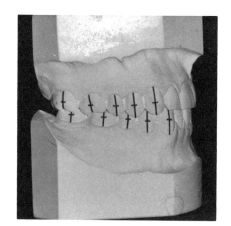

Fig. 2.16

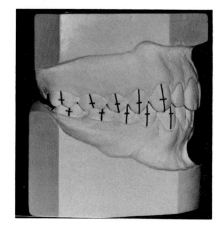

Fig. 2.14

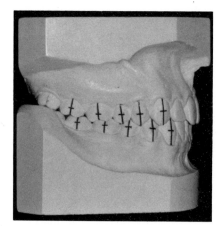

Fig. 2.17

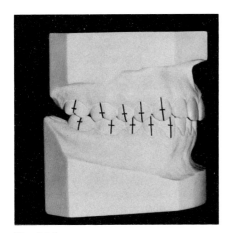

Fig. 2.18

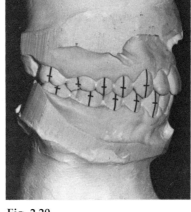

Fig. 2.20

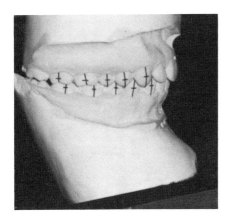

Fig. 2.19

11

Chapter 3

The Six Keys to Optimal Occlusion*

The third and—in retrospect—the most important step leading to the development of a fully programmed appliance was the discovery of six characteristics that were consistently present in the collection of 120 casts of naturally optimal occlusion [4]. These qualities will be referred to as the Six Keys to Optimal Occlusion. The individual keys are not entirely new, but together they have special value for the orthodontist, because (1) they are a complete set of indicators of optimal occlusion; (2) they can be judged from tangible landmarks; and (3) they can be judged from the facial and occlusal surfaces of the crowns, reducing the need for a lingual view or for articulating paper to confirm occlusal interfacing.

Many writers have described in detail how the occlusal surfaces of teeth should fit together, but that information has not been adequate for orthodontists, who must work chiefly with the facial surfaces of the teeth. The extent to which the facial surfaces of each

tooth type have dependable angular relationships to their occlusal surfaces at all times, and to the occlusal plane when the teeth are optimally positioned, has not been known. Some such correlations have been assumed, but verification and quantitative specifics have been absent. Treatment, therefore, has proceeded by trial and error in some respects. This factor may be partly responsible for disparate treatment results.

The traditional guidelines used by orthodontists to indirectly assess occlusion have been individually inadequate and collectively incomplete. One such guideline is the classic concept of the interarch relationship of the permanent first molars. In 1899 Angle postulated that, as a *sine qua non* of optimal occlusion, the mesiobuccal cusp of the maxillary first molar must occlude in the buccal groove between the mesial and middle buccal cusps of the mandibular first molar [6]. Angle did not contend that this factor alone would yield proper occlusion. Many occlusions, before or after treatment, are inadequate even though Angle's preferred molar relationship is present.

A more recent (1953) guideline for judging

*Called the Six Keys to Normal Occlusion in earlier writings, but *optimal* is more correct.

13

one aspect of occlusion uses roentgenographic cephalometry. The guideline sets forth recommended inclinations of the maxillary and mandibular central incisors for various interjaw relationships [23]. This guideline cannot be applied intraorally or with the cast itself, because it concerns the tooth's long axis, which cannot be seen clinically. For that matter, even when optimal incisor inclinations are attained along with Angle's preferred molar relationship, the total occlusion may still not be optimal.

So the question arose whether a complete set of guidelines for judging occlusal interfacing without articulating paper and without a lingual view could be found. Ideally, this would make it possible to assume an occlusion to be optimal or at least equilibratable if all guidelines were present.

The positions and interarch relationships of all the crowns in the collection of 120 dental casts with optimal occlusion were studied intensively to learn what characteristics, if any, occurred consistently. Angle's insight about the molar cusp-groove relationship was again validated. However, the articulation of the molars in these dental casts exhibited three cardinal elements rather than one, and the other two are just as important as the cusp-groove requirement (see Key I, p.18).

Other characteristic features of optimal occlusion became apparent. For instance, in a dentition with optimal occlusion, nearly every tooth type has its independent amount of crown angulation and inclination; but the amounts for each tooth type are similar for other dentitions that are optimal. The depth of the curve of Spee varied only moderately and was clearly an important attribute of optimal occlusion.

In all, the Six Keys make it possible to assess occlusion from facial and occlusal sites without using measuring devices. Later, for purposes of designing the new appliance, instruments were used to measure angulation, inclination, relative facial prominence of each crown, and other relevant factors.

The following terms (introduced alphabetically through p. 18) are necessary for discussing the Six Keys.

Andrews plane. The surface or plane on which the midtransverse plane of every crown in an arch will fall when the teeth are optimally positioned (Fig. 3.1). If the plane is concave or convex, technically it is a surface; but in all instances it will be referred to here as the Andrews plane.

Clinical crown. Normally, the amount of crown that can be seen intraorally or with a study cast.

In this book *clinical crown* means the amount visible in late mixed dentitions and adult dentitions with gingiva that is healthy and not recessed (Fig. 3.2). Orban has defined the clinical crown as the anatomical crown height minus 1.8 mm [21]. In young patients or those with hypertrophied or receding gingiva, the clinical-crown height can be found by measuring the distance from the incisal edge or cusp tip of the crown to the cemento-enamel junction, and then subtracting 1.8 mm.

Crown angulation. The angle formed by the facial axis of the clinical crown (FACC) and a line perpendicular to the occlusal plane (Fig. 3.3).

Crown angulation is considered positive

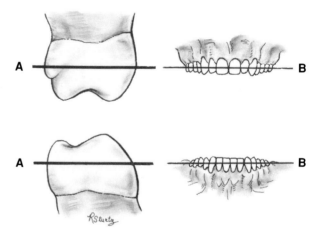

Fig. 3.1. When a crown is optimally positioned, its midtransverse plane (*A*) falls on the Andrews plane (*B*).

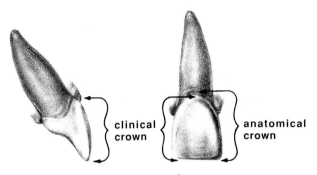

Fig. 3.2. Clinical and anatomical crown.

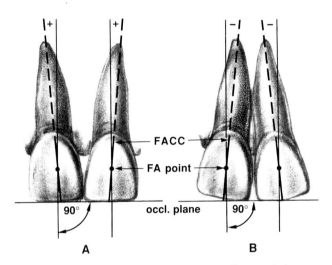

Fig. 3.3. Crown angulation: *A*, positive; *B*, negative.

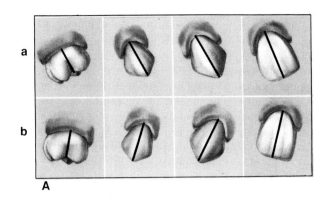

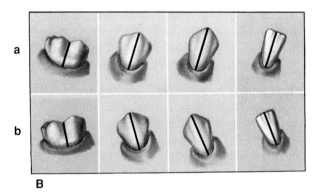

Fig. 3.4. Examples of crown angulation for each tooth class: *A*, maxillary positive *(a)* and negative *(b)*; *B*, mandibular positive *(a)*, and negative *(b)*.

when the occlusal portion of the FACC is mesial to the gingival portion (Fig. 3.3A), negative when distal (Fig. 3.3B).

The exact degree of crown angulation cannot be judged, but the nature of the angulation (positive or negative) and whether it is excessive can be (Fig. 3.4).

Crown inclination. The angle between a line perpendicular to the occlusal plane and a line that is parallel and tangent to the FACC at its midpoint (the FA point). Crown inclination is determined from the mesial or distal perspective. It is sometimes incorrectly called torque, which means a twisting force. "Tangent to" means that the line representing the

inclination of the FACC should be equidistant from each end of the clinical crown, while touching the FACC.

Crown inclination is considered positive if the occlusal portion of the crown, tangent line, or FACC is facial to its gingival portion, negative if lingual (Fig. 3.5). The exact degree of crown inclination cannot be judged, but the nature of the inclination (positive or negative) and whether it is excessive can be (Fig. 3.6).

Facial axis of the clinical crown (FACC)*. For all teeth except molars, the most prominent portion of the central lobe on each

---

*Called the long axis of the clinical crown (LACC) in earlier writings. Anatomically and geometrically, *facial axis* is the more correct term.

15

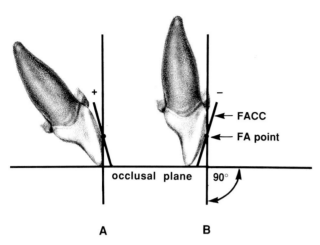

Fig. 3.5. Crown inclination: *A,* positive; *B,* negative.

crown's facial surface (Fig. 3.7); for molars, the buccal groove that separates the two large facial cusps (Fig. 3.8).

Crowns develop from the fusion of embryonic lobes. Upon maturation, these lobes retain their identity with areas of prominence (cusps and ridges) and boundary lines (fissures and grooves) (Fig. 3.9). Clinically, the FACC for all teeth except molars can be highlighted with the side of a pencil lead (Fig. 3.10); for molars, it can be highlighted with the point of a pencil (Fig. 3.11). From the facial perspective, the FACC is observed as a straight line (Figs. 3.7 and 3.8). From the mesial or distal perspective this landmark is used to judge inclination by visualizing a straight line that is parallel to the FACC and tangent to a point on the FACC that separates the gingival half of the crown from the occlusal half (Fig. 3.12).

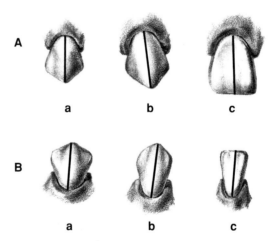

Fig. 3.7. Facial axes of premolars *(a),* canines *(b),* and incisors *(c)*: *A,* maxillary; *B,* mandibular.

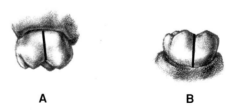

Fig. 3.8. Facial axes of molars: *A,* maxillary; *B,* mandibular.

Fig. 3.6. Examples of crown inclination for each tooth class: *A,* maxillary positive *(a)* and negative *(b)*; *B,* mandibular positive *(a)* and negative *(b)*.

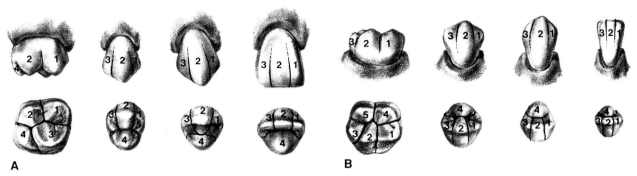

Fig. 3.9. Facial and occlusal views of each tooth class with their lobes numbered: *A,* maxillary teeth; *B,* mandibular teeth.

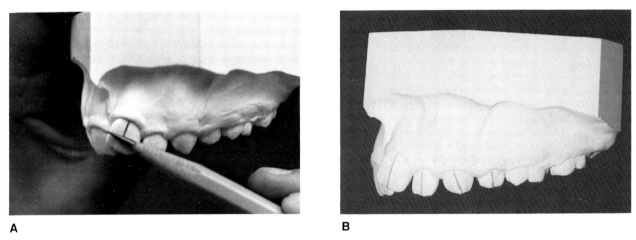

Fig. 3.10. *A,* Highlighting a central incisor's FACC (the prominent ridge of the crown's central lobe) with the side of a pencil. *B,* FACC marked on each maxillary crown except molars.

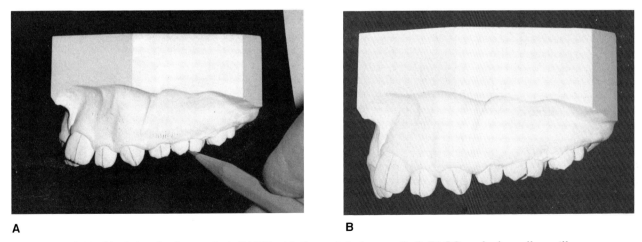

Fig. 3.11. *A,* Highlighting the first molar's FACC with the point of a pencil. *B,* FACC marked on all maxillary crowns.

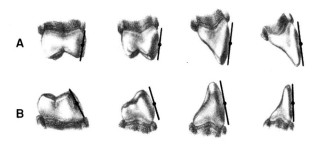

Fig. 3.12. From the mesial or distal perspective, the facial axis is an imaginary line tangent to the FA point. Examples are for each maxillary *(A)* and mandibular *(B)* tooth class.

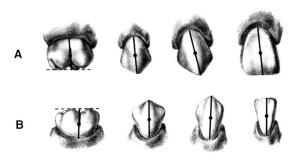

Fig. 3.13. The facial-axis point (FA point) is the point on the FACC that separates the gingival half of the clinical crown from the occlusal half. Examples are for each maxillary *(A)* and mandibular *(B)* tooth class.

It should be noted that the FACC differs from conventional referents (the long axis of the crown or tooth, contact points, marginal ridges, incisal edges) for judging angulation and inclination. These traditional referents are impractical for reasons that will be explained in detail in Chapter 7.

Facial-axis point (FA point)*. The point on the facial axis that separates the gingival half of the clinical crown from the occlusal half (Fig. 3.13).

The distances between the occlusal and gingival extremities of the facial surfaces are not equal for all crowns within an arch, but

---

*Called the long axis point (LA-point) in earlier writings. Anatomically and geometrically, *facial-axis point* is the more correct term.

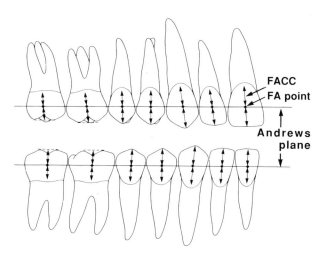

Fig. 3.14. The distance between the occlusal and gingival borders varies for each crown in an arch. However, the borders are equidistant from the crown's FA point at all times, and equidistant from the Andrews plane when the teeth are optimally positioned.

for each crown they are equidistant from the FA point (Fig. 3.14).

Tooth class. A group of teeth having similar shape and function. Classes are incisors, canines, premolars, and molars.

Tooth type. A subordinate category within a class of teeth. Premolars are a class of teeth and are similar; a mandibular first premolar is a type and is different from any other tooth type, such as a mandibular second premolar.

Key I: Interarch Relationships

Key I is the first of the six significant characteristics that were consistently present in the sample of 120 dental casts with optimal occlusion. Key I pertains to the occlusion and the interarch relationships of the teeth. This key consists of seven parts.

1. The mesiobuccal cusp of the permanent maxillary first molar occludes in the groove between the mesial and middle buccal cusps of the permanent mandibular first molar (Fig. 3.15Ab), as explained by Angle [6].

2. The distal marginal ridge of the maxillary first molar occludes with the mesial marginal ridge of the mandibular second molar (Fig. 3.15Aa).

3. The mesiolingual cusp of the maxillary first molar occludes in the central fossa of the mandibular first molar (Fig. 3.15Bd, Ce).

4. The buccal cusps of the maxillary premolars have a cusp-embrasure relationship with the mandibular premolars (Fig. 3.15Ac, D).

5. The lingual cusps of the maxillary premolars have a cusp-fossa relationship with the mandibular premolars (Fig. 3.15Cf).

6. The maxillary canine has a cusp-embrasure relationship with the mandibular canine and first premolar. The tip of its cusp is slightly mesial to the embrasure (Fig. 3.15D).

7. The maxillary incisors overlap the mandibular incisors (Fig. 3.15D), and the midlines of the arches match.

The cusp-groove and the marginal-ridge conditions of the molars, the cusp-embrasure relationship of the premolars and canines, and incisor overjet can be observed directly from the buccal perspective (Fig. 3.15). The FACC permits assessment of the lingual-cusp occlusion of the molars and premolars when these teeth are viewed from their mesiobuccal aspect, as explained below.

Interarch relationship of the posterior teeth of two dentitions can be the same, but the interfacing of the occlusal surfaces of the two dentitions may differ because of differing crown inclinations. Judging crown inclination (and therefore occlusal interfacing) is ineffective from the buccal perspective. It can be compared to attempting to learn whether the flanges of a hinge are together or apart by looking only at its joint (Fig. 3.16).

Correct occlusal interfacing depends on correct interarch relationship, angulation, and crown inclination. Interarch relationship and angulation are best judged from the buccal perspective (Fig. 3.16); crown inclination for

Fig. 3.15. Key I: Optimal interarch relationships and occlusal interfacing. *A,* Interarch relationships of molars and premolars: *a,* marginal-ridge occlusion; *b,* molar cusp-groove relationship; *c,* premolar cusp-embrasure relationship. *B,* Mesial perspective of occlusal interfacing of molar or premolar: *d,* cusp-fossa relationship. *C,* Lingual perspective of occlusal interfacing: *e,* cusp-fossa occlusion of molars; *f,* cusp-fossa occlusion of premolars. *D,* Interarch relationships of canines and incisors.

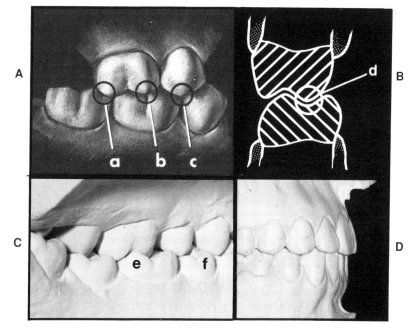

posterior teeth is best judged from the dentition's mesiobuccal perspective (Fig. 3.17). Judging posterior occlusion first from the buccal (for angulation and interarch relationship) then from the mesiobuccal aspect (for inclination) provides a perspective that can be systematically described and quantified. Such information, along with other nonocclusal guidelines, provides a set of standards against which occlusal deviations can be identified.

Key II: Crown Angulation

Essentially all crowns in the sample have a positive angulation* (Fig. 3.18). All crowns of each tooth type are similar in the amount of angulation (Chapter 2). (Wheeler [29] notes the similarity of contact-area position for each

---

*Maxillary second molars are positive in angulation only if they have completed their eruption. Third molars were not present often enough to be evaluated.

tooth type, which supports the optimal sample findings.)

Key III: Crown Inclination

As they do in angulation, consistent patterns also prevail in crown inclination, with the following characteristics for individual teeth.

1. Most maxillary incisors (81.5%) have a positive inclination (Fig. 3.19A,B); mandibular incisors have a slightly negative inclination (Fig. 3.19A,C). In most of the optimal sample, the interincisal crown angle is less than 180°. The crowns of maxillary incisors are more positively inclined, relative to a line 90° to the occlusal plane, than the mandibular incisors are negatively inclined to the same line (Fig. 3.20).

2. The inclinations of the maxillary incisor crowns are generally positive—the centrals more positive than the laterals. Canines and

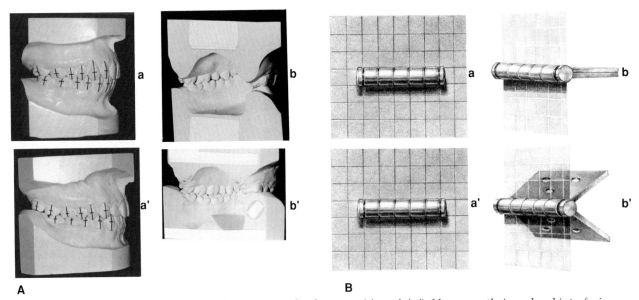

A
B

Fig. 3.16. Interarch relationship of two dentitions can be the same (*Aa and Aa'*). However, their occlusal interfacing can differ (*Ab and Ab'*). Similarly, the joint portions of two hinges (*Ba and Ba'*) look the same whether the flanges are together (*Bb*) or apart (*Bb'*). Vertical lines on crowns indicate facial axes; junctions of horizontal and vertical lines indicate FA points.

20

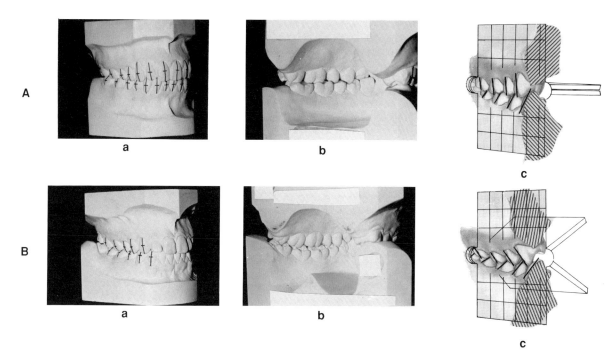

Fig. 3.17. From the mesiobuccal perspective the inclination of the crowns permits indirect judging of occlusal interfacing. *A,* Correct inclination and correct occlusal interfacing: *a,* mesiobuccal perspective; *b,* lingual perspective; *c,* inclination correlated with occlusal interfacing. *B,* Incorrect inclination and incorrect occlusal interfacing: *a,* mesiobuccal perspective; *b,* lingual perspective; *c,* inclination correlated with occlusal interfacing. Vertical lines on crowns indicate facial axes; junctions of vertical and horizontal lines indicate FA points.

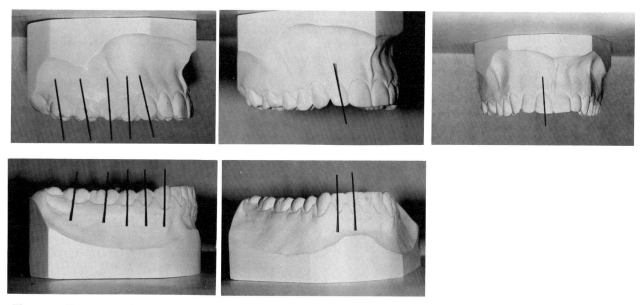

Fig. 3.18. Positive FACC angulation for each tooth type in the optimal sample. Wires are glued at the FA points, parallel to each crown's FACC.

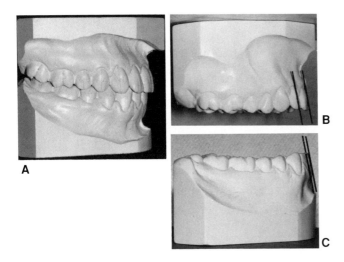
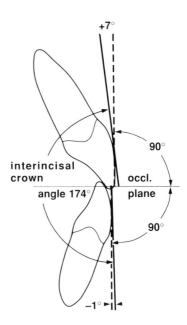

Fig. 3.19. Incisor inclination. Maxillary incisor inclination is consistently positive *(A, B)*; mandibular incisor inclination is consistently negative *(A, C)*.

Fig. 3.20. Interincisal crown angle for the majority of the optimal sample was less than 180°.

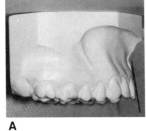
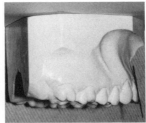
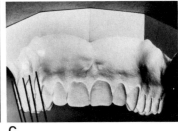

Fig. 3.21. Maxillary crown inclinations. Central incisors *(A)* are more positive than lateral incisors *(B)*; posterior teeth are negative *(C)*. Wires are glued at the FA points, parallel to each crown's FACC.

premolars are negative and quite similar. The inclinations of the maxillary first and second molars are also similar and negative, but slightly more negative than those of the canines and premolars (Fig. 3.21). The molars are more negative because they are measured from the groove instead of from the prominent facial ridge, from which the canines and premolars are measured.

3. The inclinations of the mandibular crowns are progressively more negative from the incisors through the second molars (Fig. 3.22).

Key IV: Rotations

The fourth key to optimal occlusion is an absence of tooth rotations (Fig. 3.23).

Key V: Tight Contacts

Contact points should abut unless a discrepancy exists in mesiodistal crown diameter (Fig. 3.23).

22

Fig. 3.22. Mandibular crown inclinations. Central and lateral incisors *(A)* have the same inclination (generally slightly negative). The posterior teeth are increasingly negative from the canines through the molars *(B)*. Wires are glued at the FA points, parallel to each crown's FACC.

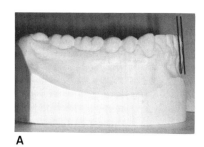

A

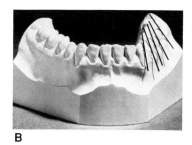

B

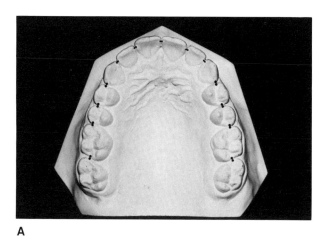

A

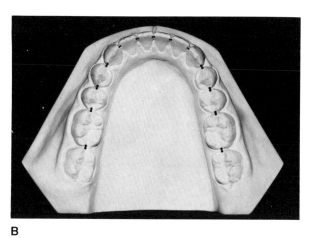

B

Fig. 3.23. Maxillary arch *(A)* and mandibular arch *(B)* showing no rotations and no interdental spacing. Dots indicate contact points.

Key VI: Curve of Spee

The depth of the curve of Spee ranges from a flat plane to a slightly concave surface (Fig. 3.24).

Discussion

Although the 120 dentitions with naturally occurring optimal occlusion show individual differences in arch form and size of teeth, they generally possess the Six Key characteristics described above. Absence of any of the six qualities results in an occlusion that is proportionally inferior to the naturally optimal sample.

The Six Keys are interdependent ele-

ments of the structural system of optimal occlusion. As such, they serve as a base for evaluating occlusion. More important, the Six Keys can be used as treatment objectives for most patients. In 1974 at the seventeenth annual meeting of the Saint Louis University Orthodontic Education and Research Foundation, Ronald H. Roth reported his experience with the Six Key guidelines: ". . . if I were to define very simply the requirements of an ideal occlusion, both anatomically and functionally, for the natural dentition, I would have to say: 'It would incorporate the Six Keys . . . with mandible in gnathologic centric relation.' " To achieve these goals may not be feasible in all instances, but to stop short when they are attainable may be unacceptable.

The optimal sample revealed similarities in the patterns of angulation, inclination, shape, and relative size (facial prominence) of tooth types. It appeared that these characteristics could be incorporated into an orthodontic appliance to enhance precision and consistency in treatment results. But this was not enough for appliance design. The next steps were to explore and quantify the extent to which position, shape, and relative size were, within each tooth type, shared. This information was vital for determining the extent to which an appliance could be programmed and yet be suitable for most patients.

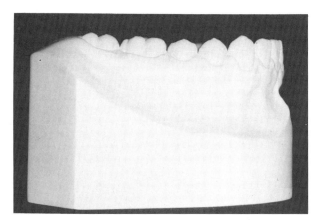

Fig. 3.24. Mandibular arch with a curve of Spee within the 0–2.5-mm depth range.

Chapter 4

Measurements

Design of the Experiment

The fourth study leading to the development of the first fully programmed appliance involved thousands of measurements of the crowns in the 120-cast sample. The purpose was to learn the extent to which position and, in certain ways, shape were constant within each tooth type, and how relative size was consistent within an arch. The findings would later supply data for the design of the new appliance. Figure 4.1 illustrates the measurements made: (a) the bracket area of each tooth type, (b) vertical crown contour, (c) crown angulation, (d) crown inclination, (e) maxillary molar offset, (f) horizontal crown contour, (g) facial prominence of each crown, and (h) depth of the curve of Spee.

The facial axis of the clinical crown (FACC) and its midpoint, the facial-axis point (FA point), were marked on each crown of the dental casts (Fig. 4.2). The FACC is the reference line from which crown angulation and inclination are measured (Fig. 4.1c,d).

Duplicates were made of the 120 casts.

On the duplicate casts the occlusal half of each crown was ground away (Fig. 4.3).

A line was drawn on the trimmed surfaces of the casts, connecting the most facial aspects of the contact areas. This is called the embrasure line (Fig. 4.4).

The maxillary molar offset and the most facially prominent portion of each crown were measured from the embrasure line (Fig. 4.1e,g). Ultimately these data were used in bracket design to eliminate the need for first-order archwire bends.

The following equipment was used to obtain the measurements:

1. Two arch-shaped templates constructed of 2-mm-thick, rigid, flat plastic. The template for the maxillary arch was larger than the one for the mandibular arch (Fig. 4.5). Each template was used to represent the occlusal plane of its respective arch. The canine areas of each template were recessed.

2. A protractor with an adjustable readout arm (Fig. 4.6) for measuring angulation, inclination, and molar offset (Fig. 4.1c,d,e).

25

3. A Boley gauge with sharpened points (Fig. 4.7) for measuring bracket area, crown prominence, and depth of the curve of Spee (Fig. 4.1a,g,h).

4. A template with a series of circles ranging from 1/4" to 2" in diameter (Fig. 4.8) for measuring vertical and horizontal facial crown contour (Fig. 4.1b,f).

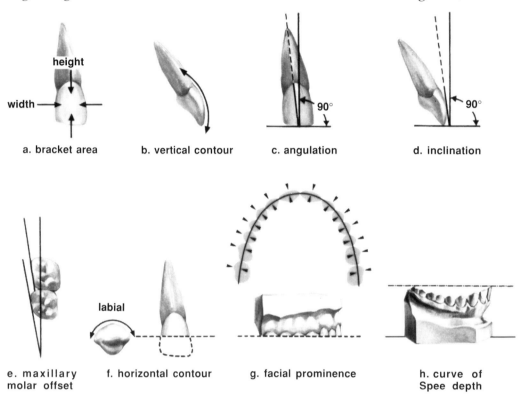

Fig. 4.1. Measurements made on sample casts.

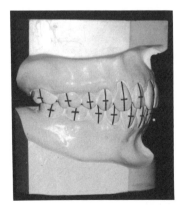

Fig. 4.2. The FACC (*vertical line*) and the FA point (*junction of vertical and horizontal lines*) marked on each crown.

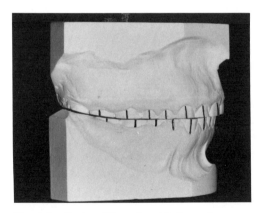

Fig. 4.3. Casts with occlusal halves of crowns trimmed away. Lines represent FACC.

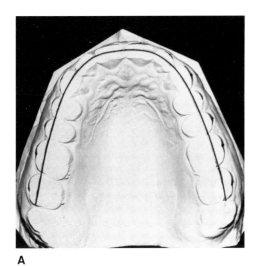

A

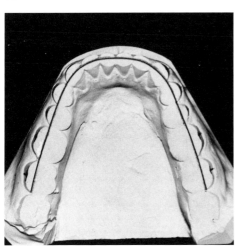

B

Fig. 4.4. The embrasure line: *A*, maxillary arch; *B*, mandibular arch.

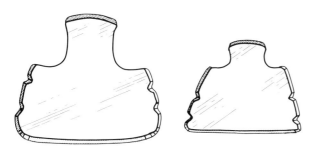

Fig. 4.5. Templates with recessed areas for canines: *left*, maxillary; *right*, mandibular.

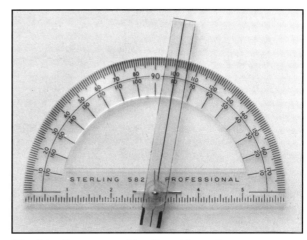

Fig. 4.6. Protractor with adjustable readout arm.

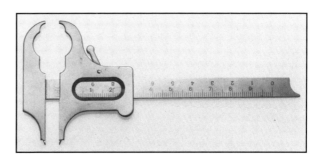

Fig. 4.7. Boley gauge with sharpened points.

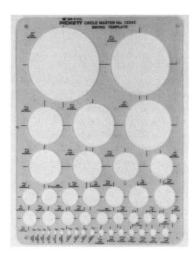

Fig. 4.8. Template of circles.

27

Methods of Measurement

Bracket Area

On the facial aspect of each crown, the height and width of the potential bracket area were measured with a Boley gauge (Figs. 4.1a, 4.9). The smallest crowns of each normal tooth type ultimately determined the occlusogingival height and mesiodistal width limits for each bracket base, since a base must not be too large to fit its designated tooth.

Vertical Crown Contour

The vertical contour of the facial surface of each crown in the bracket area was ascertained by superimposing a series of arcs from the template of circles until a match was found (Figs. 4.1b, 4.10). These measurements revealed the extent of constancy of each tooth type's vertical anatomy. This information was later used to design the vertical anatomy of each bracket base.

Crown Angulation

Crown angulation is the angle between the FACC of each crown and a line perpendicular to the occlusal plane (Fig. 4.1c). The procedure for measuring was as follows:

1. The arch-shaped plastic template was positioned over the occlusal surfaces to represent the occlusal plane of the arch (Fig. 4.11).

2. The base of the protractor was placed on the plastic template parallel to a line that would connect the contact points of the crown being measured (Fig. 4.12).

3. The protractor's readout arm was adjusted to parallel the crown's FACC (Fig. 4.13).

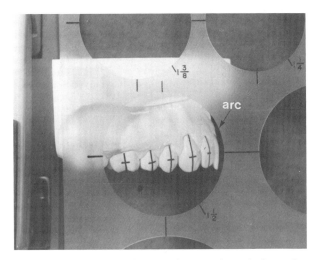

Fig. 4.10. Matching the arc of a template circle to the vertical contour of a maxillary central incisor.

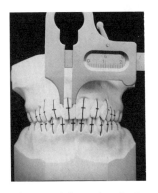 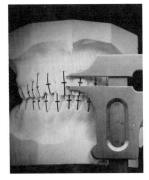

Fig. 4.9. Measuring for bracket size.

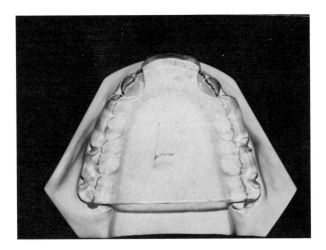

Fig. 4.11. Plastic template set on the teeth.

28

4. The angulation of the crown was read from where the center line of the readout arm fell on the protractor's scale (Fig. 4.14).

These measurements established the range of crown angulation for each tooth type. Later the measurements were used to determine how much the slots needed to be angled within each bracket.

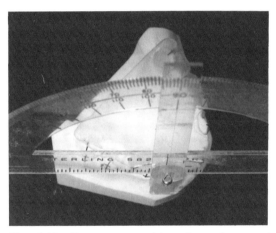

Fig. 4.12. Protractor positioned on the template to measure crown angulation.

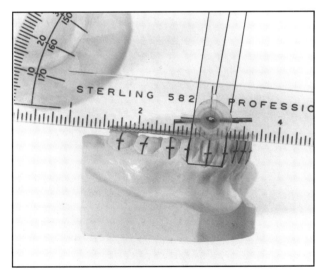

Fig. 4.13. Protractor readout arm adjusted to parallel the mandibular canine's facial axis.

Crown Inclination

Crown inclination is the angle between a line perpendicular to the occlusal plane and a line parallel and tangent to the FACC (Fig. 4.1d). The plastic templates were again used to represent each arch's occlusal plane. The protractor was positioned at right angles to a line that would connect the contact points of the crown being measured (Fig. 4.15).

The protractor's readout arm was adjusted to be parallel and tangent to the FACC at the FA point (Fig. 4.16), and the inclination of the crown was read on the protractor's scale.

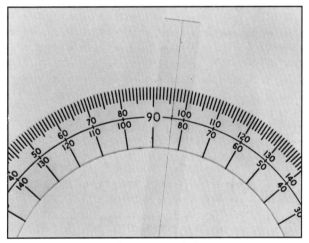

Fig. 4.14. Degrees of crown angulation.

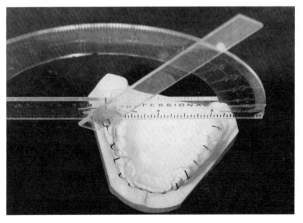

Fig. 4.15. Protractor positioned on the occlusal template to measure crown inclination.

These measurements established the range of crown inclination for each tooth type. Ultimately this information, when incorporated into each bracket for each tooth type, would reduce or eliminate the need for third-order archwire bends for attaining the correct inclination of the teeth.

Offset of Maxillary Molars

The facial cusps of maxillary molars are not equally prominent. For each molar, a straight section of wire was placed level with the trimmed occlusal surface, connecting the facial cusps (Fig. 4.17). The angle between that wire and the embrasure line is the offset angle (Fig. 4.18). These offset measurements were later used as design data to reduce or eliminate the maxillary molar offset bends that are needed with less-sophisticated edgewise brackets.

Horizontal Crown Contour

The horizontal radius of each cusp was measured at the junction of the crown's facial surface and the trimmed "occlusal" surface on the duplicate casts (Fig. 4.1f). Circle segments in the template were superimposed on each cusp until a match was obtained (Fig. 4.19). These measurements revealed the constancy of the horizontal contour of each tooth type's facial surface. Eventually these data were used to establish the horizontal contour for each bracket base.

Crown Facial Prominence

On the occlusally trimmed casts, the distance from the embrasure line to each crown's most prominent facial point was measured with a Boley gauge (Figs. 4.1g, 4.20). These measurements established the relative constancy of crown prominence within an arch. Later this information was applied inversely for designing bracket prominence.

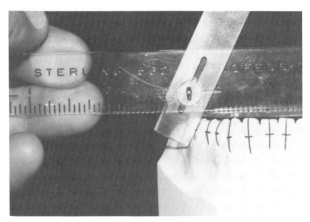

Fig. 4.16. Protractor readout arm adjusted to be parallel and tangent to the FACC at the FA point.

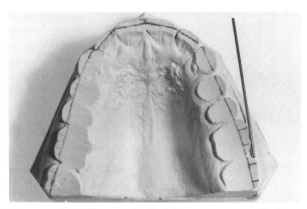

Fig. 4.17. Maxillary molar facial cusps connected with a straight wire at the level of the crown's midtransverse plane. The occlusal halves of the crowns have been trimmed away. Lines at right angles to the embrasure line show the unequal prominence of the buccal cusps.

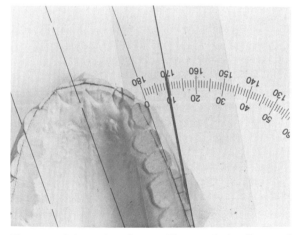

Fig. 4.18. Measuring the maxillary molar's offset angle.

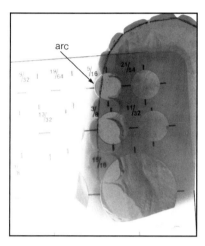

Fig. 4.19. Arc of a template circle matched to the buccal cusp of a maxillary first premolar.

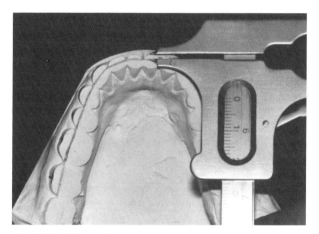

Fig. 4.20. Measuring crown prominence.

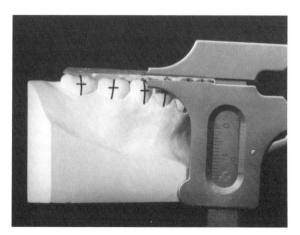

Fig. 4.21. Measuring the depth of the curve of Spee.

Depth of the Curve of Spee

To measure the curve of Spee (Fig. 4.1h), the plastic template was placed over the occlusal surfaces of the mandibular arch . Usually the template touched only the incisal edges of the mandibular incisors and the distal cusps of the permanent second molars. The template was recessed in the canine areas to prevent its rocking over the tips of the cusps (Fig. 4.5). On each side, the depth of the curve of Spee was determined by measuring, in millimeters, the distance from the side of the template facing the teeth to the buccal cusp tip farthest from it (Fig. 4.21).

An optimal curve of Spee is an essential key to optimal occlusion. The depth of the curve is important to bracket design because the slots of a fully programmed appliance must collectively be on a surface that is nearly parallel to the occlusal surface of an arch when the occlusion is correct.

Findings

The measurements in six of the eight categories (all except bracket size and curve of Spee) were averaged for each tooth type, and the results served as norms for the design of the new appliance. The averages of the angulation, inclination, prominence, offset, and Spee measurements are as follows.

Maxillary Teeth

Angulation of the maxillary crowns averaged 5° for the central incisors, 9° for the lateral incisors, 11° for the canines, 2° for the first and second premolars, and 5° for the molars (Fig. 4.22).

Crown inclination averaged 7° for the central incisors, 3° for the lateral incisors, –7° for the canines and the first and second premolars, and –9° for the molars (Fig. 4.23).

Crown prominence, relative to the embrasure line, is greatest for the first and second molars (2.9 mm). The premolars and canines (2.4 mm and 2.5 mm) are next in prominence. The lateral incisor (1.65 mm) has the smallest crown prominence; the central incisor (2.1 mm) has the second smallest (Fig. 4.24).

Maxillary molar offset averaged 10° relative to the embrasure line (Fig. 4.25).

Mandibular Teeth

Angulation for the mandibular crowns averaged 2° for the central and lateral incisors, 5° for the canines, and 2° for the premolars and molars (Fig. 4.26).

Inclination averaged –1° for central and lateral incisors, –11° for the canines, –17° for first premolars, –22° for second premolars, –30° for permanent first molars, and –35° for permanent second molars (Fig. 4.27).

Crown prominence, relative to the embrasure line, is greatest for the molars (2.5 mm) and is progressively less for other tooth

categories: premolars (2.35 mm), canines (1.9 mm), and incisors (1.2 mm) (Fig. 4.28).

No offset is needed for mandibular molars because the middle and mesiobuccal cusps are equally prominent (Fig. 4.29).

The curve of Spee ranged from flat to 2.5 mm deep.

Measurement data for angulation, inclination, and prominence are listed in the Appendix.

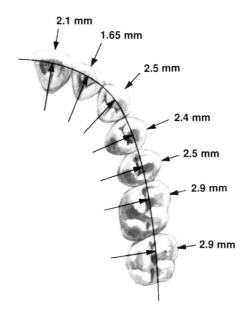

Fig. 4.24. Average maxillary crown prominence.

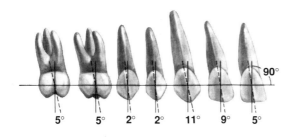

Fig. 4.22. Average maxillary crown angulation.

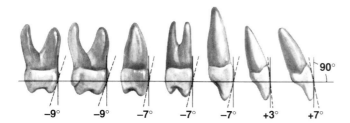

Fig. 4.23. Average maxillary crown inclination.

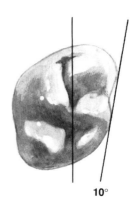

Fig. 4.25. A line connecting the buccal cusps of maxillary molars falls at 10° to the embrasure line.

32

Conclusions

This study revealed consistencies of position (except for incisor inclination), morphology, and relative facial prominence for the crowns of each tooth type within an arch. The differences in incisor inclination were attributable to interjaw disharmony. Thus, special consideration must be given in bracket design to correlating the inclination of incisors with the interjaw relationship.

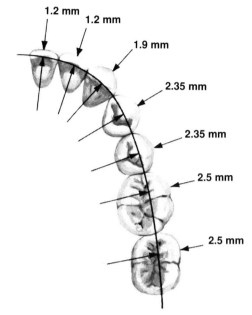

Fig. 4.28. Average mandibular crown prominence.

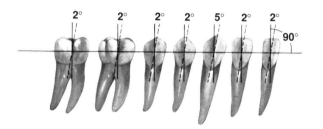

Fig. 4.26. Average mandibular crown angulation.

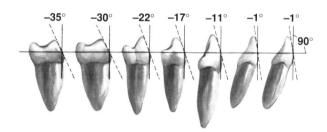

Fig. 4.27. Average mandibular crown inclination.

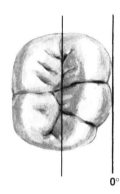

Fig. 4.29. A line connecting the mesial and middle buccal cusps of a mandibular molar parallels the embrasure line.

Chapter 5

Naturally Optimal
versus Treated Occlusion

The first two studies (Chapters 1 and 2) led to, and studies 3 and 4 (Chapters 3 and 4) established the conceptual feasibility of a fully programmed appliance; the fifth study, reported in this chapter, established the need. In this fifth project the occlusal characteristics of the posttreatment dental casts displayed at meetings of the American Association of Orthodontics, the Tweed Foundation, and the Angle Society were compared with those in the untreated optimal sample. The comparison yielded perspective on the state of the art of posttreatment static occlusion by revealing the extent to which the Six Keys were present in honors-quality treatment results.*

For this study 1150 of the exhibited post-

treatment dental casts were evaluated. The project began in the mid-1960s and continued for 10 years. A supplemental study involving posttreatment casts was made in the mid-1980s.

Why report 10- and 20-year-old treatment results? Because orthodontics is, justifiably, slow to change. It takes years of testing before new ideas are adopted by clinicians or taught at the university level. For this reason, most universities still teach some of the methods, objectives, and appliances that were used in the 1960s and 1970s. But adoption of the six occlusal guidelines introduced in 1972 began in the late 1970s and by 1988 was widespread. This was evidenced by the Six Keys' being present more often among treatment results in

---

*An important acknowledgment must be made here: The standards for orthodontic treatment in America are among the finest in the world. Most of our leaders in this field spent many years in successful practice before submitting their records at the national meetings, and there can be no disparagement of their competence. The fact that some range of excellence was found among the 1150 models implies no adverse criticism; instead, the findings simply reflected the state of the art. Few

would claim that orthodontics, even on the high level seen at these meetings, had (or has) reached its ultimate development. Last to make such a claim would be those whose work was displayed for close scrutiny by other experienced professionals, recent graduates, and students. Some of the posttreatment results, though lacking in occlusal attributes, may reflect treatment limitations, and were in fact the best that could be done.

the mid-1980s sample; also, the article "The Six Keys to Normal Occlusion"[4] had become mandatory reading in all but three orthodontic departments at American and Canadian universities and colleges.

Each posttreatment cast (not postretention) in the 1150-cast sample was examined for the presence or lack of each of the Six Keys.

Methods and Results

The subjectiveness of the process for judging some of the Six Keys is reduced when the objective information about optimal occlusion presented in Chapters 2, 3, 4, and 5 is employed. When one has an ideal in mind, deviations from it are readily determined.

Key I: Interarch Relationships

The traditional method for measuring only the cusp-groove relationship of the first molars may misrepresent the true nature of the interarch relationship. Figure 5.1 demonstrates premolars and canines that are 3 mm Class II even though the first molars are Class I as determined solely from the traditional cusp-groove relationship. Another example of the fallacy of the cusp-groove standard occurs when second deciduous molars cause a temporary end-to-end relationship of the permanent molars (Fig. 5.2). Pseudo-Class II molar relationships found in the mixed dentition must be correctly interpreted.

Another condition that misrepresents the interarch relationship is incorrect angulation (Fig. 5.5C). In this case the actual cusp-groove or cusp-embrasure condition must be adjusted to reflect what that condition would be if the teeth were correctly angulated without the help of nonreciprocal force. Figure 5.3 demonstrates Class I relationships.

The interarch relationship of a side can be correctly interpreted and conveyed only when the effects of deciduous molars and incorrect angulation are compensated for; when the interarch relationship for each molar, premolar, and canine is measured; and when these measurements are totaled and averaged.

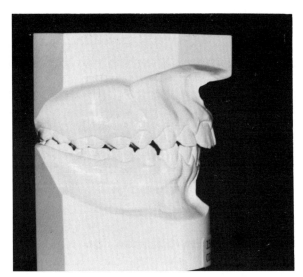

Fig. 5.1. A Class I molar cusp-groove condition. All other interarch relationships are 3 mm Class II.

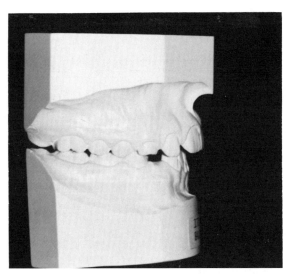

Fig. 5.2. A Class II tendency of molars caused by the presence of a mandibular deciduous molar. Premolars are Class I.

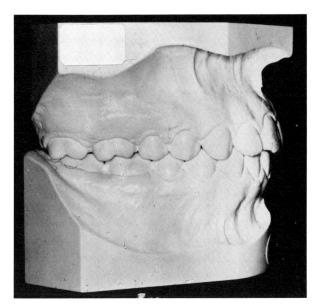

Fig. 5.3. Class I molars, premolars, canines, and incisors.

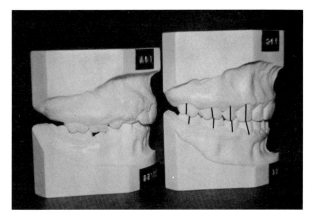

Fig. 5.4. A posttreatment example *(right)* lacking most aspects of Key I. Lines on teeth represent estimated FACC. (Pretreatment casts are on left.)

For the dentition, the interarch relationship is determined by adding and averaging the interarch relationship for each side, to get one number.

Although most of the 1150 posttreatment casts satisfied Angle's criterion for the molar relationship, 932 (80%) differed from the Key I condition found in the optimal sample. In most instances, the distal marginal ridge of the maxillary first molar did not occlude with the mesial marginal ridge of the mandibular second molar, and the premolars and canines did not have a cusp-embrasure relationship (Fig. 5.4).

Key II: Angulation

If the angulation of the FACC varies more than plus or minus 2° from the optimal for that tooth type, it is considered incorrect (Fig. 5.5).

In 91% of the posttreatment casts the crowns had one or more teeth whose angulation obviously differed from those of the optimal sample. The maxillary lateral incisor (Fig. 5.5A) and canine angulations (Fig. 5.5B) fre-

quently were negative, in contrast to positive in the optimal sample. Maxillary molar angulation often was negative or insufficiently positive in nonextraction treatment (Fig. 5.5C), and excessively positive in extraction treatment (Fig. 5.5D).

Key III: Inclination

If the inclination of the FACC varies more than plus or minus 2° from the optimal for that tooth type, it is considered incorrect (Fig. 5.6).

The interincisor FACC angle was more than 180° in 78% of the posttreatment casts (Fig. 5.6A), whereas this angle was less than 180° in 81.5% of the optimal sample. Also, maxillary posterior crown inclination was not always negative in the posttreatment casts (Fig. 5.6B); it was, however, in the optimal sample.

Key IV: Rotations

If a line connecting the contact points of a crown varies more than 2° from parallel to a line representing the arch form, the tooth is rotated. A rotated tooth can sometimes be detected from the facial perspective of the casts

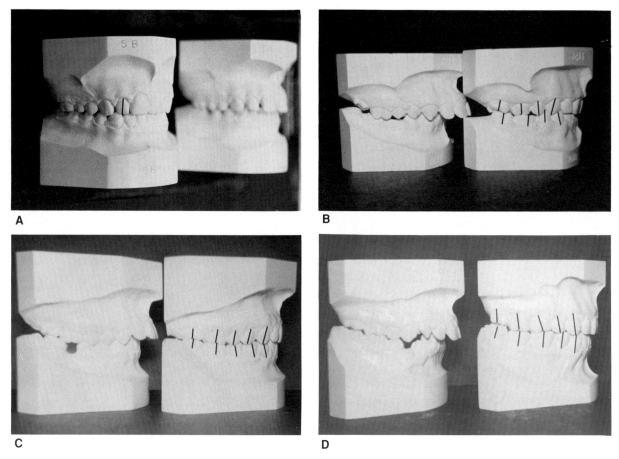

Fig. 5.5. Examples of incorrect posttreatment angulation (on right in each pair). *A*, Negative maxillary incisor angulation; *B*, negative canine angulation; *C*, negative maxillary molar, premolar, and canine angulation; *D*, excessively positive angulation of the maxillary first molar. Lines on teeth represent estimated FACC.

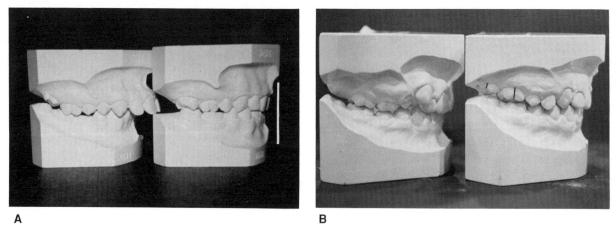

Fig. 5.6. Examples of incorrect posttreatment inclination (on right in each pair): *A*, negative maxillary incisor inclination and interincisor FACC angle larger than 180°; *B*, insufficient negative maxillary molar inclination. Lines on teeth represent estimated FACC. (Pretreatment casts are on left.)

(Fig. 5.6B), but the condition can be best observed from the occlusal perspective (Fig. 5.7).

In 67% of the posttreatment casts, rotations were evident. Most of the rotated teeth were those that had required translation during treatment.

Key V: Tight Contacts

Barring missing teeth or tooth size discrepancy, interdental space indicates incorrect maxillary incisor angulation (Fig. 5.8A), incorrect incisor inclination (Fig. 5.8B), or incorrect mesiodistal or faciolingual position of a tooth or teeth (Fig. 5.8C).

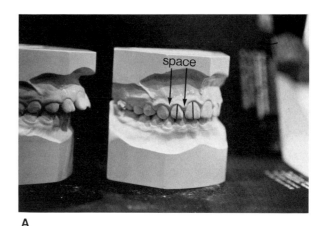

A

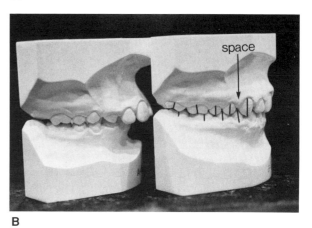

B

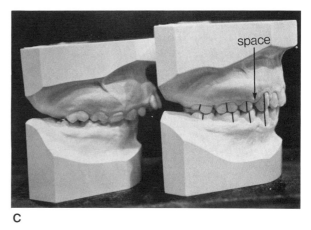

C

Fig. 5.8. Examples of posttreatment interdental space: *A*, space resulting from insufficient maxillary lateral incisor angulation; *B*, space resulting from insufficient maxillary incisor inclination; *C*, extraction site space resulting from incorrect mesiodistal tooth position. Lines on teeth represent estimated FACC. (Pretreatment casts are on left.)

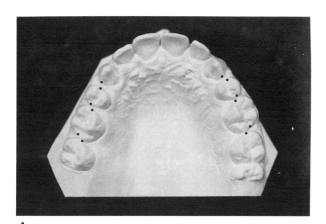

A

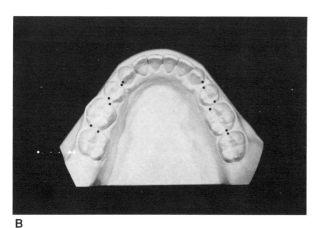

B

Fig. 5.7. Posttreatment examples of rotated teeth: *A*, maxillary arch; *B*, mandibular arch. Black dots represent estimated contact points.

One or more spaces ascribed to incomplete treatment rather than to tooth size discrepancy were evident in 43% of the posttreatment casts.

Key VI: Curve of Spee

The curve of Spee is incorrect if it is less than 0 or more than 2.5 mm (Fig. 5.9).

A curve of Spee estimated to be greater than 2.5 mm was noted in 56% of the posttreatment casts.

Photographic Evidence

Several hundred pretreatment and posttreatment casts of the 1150-cast sample were photographed to support the reported data. In the mid-1960s, 128 pairs were photographed (Figs. 5.12–5.144); in the mid-1970s, 186 were photographed (Figs. 5.146–5.297). All of these casts were displayed at national meetings of the American Association of Orthodontists, and represent the efforts of some of the diplo-mates certified at those times. Most of the treatment had been with an edgewise appliance with no built-in features; some of the brackets may have been angulated; some slots may have been inclined.

The pretreatment and posttreatment casts photographed in the mid-1960s were limited to *every* Class II malocclusion.* Each tooth or condition that does not meet the Six Key standards is recorded below each photograph, and each key is graded. Following each group of casts is a summary of the work of each orthodontist.

Dental casts photographed from the buccal perspective best illustrate the presence or absence of Key I. Also evident, however, are the angulation of the posterior teeth, the inclination of the incisors (and sometimes the posterior teeth), the interincisor FACC angle, and—to some extent—spaces, rotations, and

---

*To preserve the anonymity of patients and orthodontists, the precise years these photographs were taken are not given.

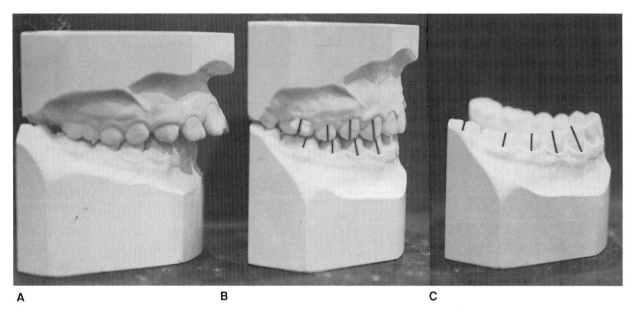

A	B	C

Fig. 5.9. A deep curve of Spee: *A,* pretreatment casts; *B,* posttreatment casts; *C,* mandibular posttreatment cast. Lines on teeth represent estimated FACC.

depth of the curve of Spee. The FACC of each crown in the posttreatment casts was estimated and marked on the photographs.

The 1970s sample was not limited to Class II malocclusions, as the 1960s sample had been. Some of the mid-1970s sample were also photographed from the labial and occlusal perspectives to better illustrate keys not easily discernible from the buccal view.

Again in the mid-1980s, 210 American Board casts were photographed, but this sample was not a part of the formal study. It represents the results of 14 orthodontists who became diplomates in the mid-1980s and agreed to anonymously display their work in this book. Most of the mid-1980s sample were treated with the edgewise appliance, some with built-in features; by then some orthodontists had adopted the Six Key guidelines. The mid-1980s sample is shown at the end of Chapter 14.

Altogether, the photographs provide (1) visual evidence of the reported findings, (2) an opportunity to compare the ranges of positions and interarch relationships found in the posttreatment casts with those in the optimal sample, (3) examples of how orthodontists differ in their treatment priorities and results, and (4) an opportunity to compare the quality of the occlusal results of three decades.

Posttreatment Grading

The 1960s samples show posttreatment casts from only the right sides. The quality of the Six Keys from that perspective is recorded and graded. Figure 5.10 shows a pretreatment and a posttreatment example and a form with the pertinent data recorded. At the top of the form are the orthodontist's and patient's assigned numbers (in lieu of names), and whether the treatment was nonextraction (NE) or included extractions (E). Below that information are six Roman numerals indicating the keys; to the immediate right of each numeral is either a space for recording errant conditions or a Palmer bar for recording errant teeth. To the far right of each numeral is a space for recording the grade for each key.

How to judge each key is explained earlier in this chapter. The information to be recorded is: Key I, interarch relationship of the buccal segment in millimeters; Key II, the teeth that are incorrectly angulated; Key III, the teeth that are incorrectly inclined; Key IV, the teeth that are rotated; Key V, the location of spaces not related to tooth size discrepancy; and Key VI, the depth of the curve of Spee when it is greater than 2.5 mm.

The grade of A is assigned when all aspects of a key are within the specified range.

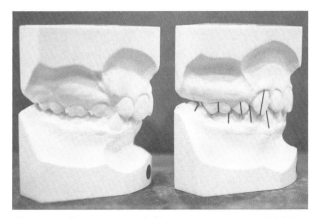

Fig. 5.10. Pretreatment *(left)* and posttreatment *(right)* casts and grading form.

Grades of B through E are based on: for Key I, the number of millimeters by which the interarch relationship is incorrect; for Keys II, III, and IV, the number of errant teeth; for Key V, the number of spaces; for Key VI, the depth of the curve of Spee. The criteria for each grade are shown in Table 1.

Following the work of each orthodontist is a summary form. Figure 5.11 illustrates an example of a completed form. It serves to summarize the strengths and weaknesses of a single orthodontist. At the top of the form is the orthodontist's assigned number, the number of patients analyzed, and how many were treated with and without extractions. Below are Roman numerals I–VI for the Six Keys. The first space to the right of each key is for recording the deviant teeth or conditions present in 50% or more of the orthodontist's casts. The second space is for recording the errant teeth or conditions present in fewer than 50% of the casts but showing a trend significant enough to be noted. The third space is for recording the average grade for that key for all the casts for that orthodontist.

The information to be recorded for each key in the column labeled "50% or more" on the summary form is: Key I, the number of casts not Class I; Key II, the teeth that are incorrectly angulated; Key III, the teeth that are incorrectly inclined; Key IV, the teeth that are rotated; Key V, the number of casts with spaces that are not related to tooth size discrepancy; and Key VI, the number of casts with deep curves of Spee. The second column is for documenting treatment flaws that occur frequently but in fewer than 50% of the casts. The criteria for the information are the same as for column one, except for frequency of occurrence.

The grade is arrived at by converting the letter grade assigned to each key for each treatment result to a numerical equivalent (A = 4.0, B = 3.0, C = 2.0, D = 1.0, E = 0.0); averaging these numbers; and then converting back to a letter equivalent (Table 2).

Summary for Orthodontist 15

Patients 8 NE 4 E 4

Keys	50% or more	Less than 50%, but significant	Grade
I	8 casts		D–
II	76 3 / 3	/ 65	D–
III	21 / 21	7 /	C
IV		765 /	B
V			A
VI	6 casts		C

Fig. 5.11. Summary form.

Table 1
Criteria for Grading Casts

	Each grade's variation from optimal conditions				
	A	B	C	D	E
Key I	—	0.5–1.5 mm	1.6–2.0 mm	2.1–2.5 mm	2.6 mm or more
Key II	—	1–2 incorrect teeth	3–4 incorrect teeth	5–6 incorrect teeth	7 or more incorrect teeth
Key III	—	1–2 incorrect teeth	3–4 incorrect teeth	5–6 incorrect teeth	7 or more incorrect teeth
Key IV	—	1–2 rotated teeth	3–4 rotated teeth	5–6 rotated teeth	7 or more rotated teeth
Key V	—	1 space	2 spaces	3 spaces	4 or more spaces
Key VI	—	3 mm	4 mm	5 mm	6 mm or more

Conclusions

When dentitions with naturally optimal occlusions are compared with dentitions treated by orthodontists, the following conclusions are apparent:

- Few of the posttreatment results meet the Six Key standards.

- Treatment priorities and results of a given orthodontist share characteristic features not always observed in the results of other orthodontists.

- During the 10-year span of the formal study no discernible improvement occurred in the presence of the Six Keys.

Table 2
Grading Equivalents

A	4.0–3.7
A–	3.6–3.5
B+	3.4–3.3
B	3.2–2.7
B–	2.6–2.5
C+	2.4–2.3
C	2.2–1.7
C–	1.6–1.5
D+	1.4–1.3
D	1.2–0.7
D–	0.6–0.5
E+	0.4–0.3
E	0.2–0.0

43

Photographs from 1960s Samples

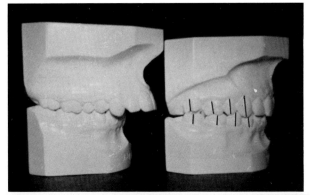

ORTHODONTIST # 1

Ortho 1	Patient 1	NE___	E _x_
Key	Grade	Key	Grade
I 2mm Cl II	C	IV 76	B
II ___ 3	B	V	A
III 7 21	C	VI 3mm	B

Fig. 5.12

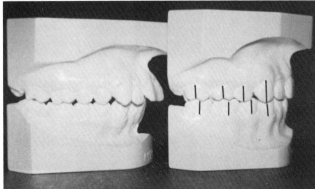

Ortho 1	Patient 2	NE___	E _x_
Key	Grade	Key	Grade
I 2.5mm Cl II	D	IV 76	B
II 76 3 3	C	V	A
III 76 21	C	VI	A

Fig. 5.13

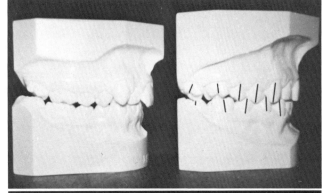

Ortho 1	Patient 3	NE _x_	E___
Key	Grade	Key	Grade
I 2mm Cl II	C	IV 6	B
II 7 543 6543	E	V	A
III 76 21	C	VI	A

Fig. 5.14

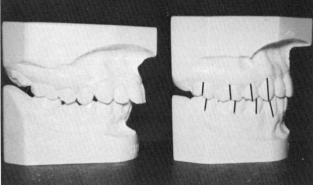

Ortho 1	Patient 4	NE___	E _x_
Key	Grade	Key	Grade
I 2.5mm Cl II	D	IV 65	B
II 7 3 3	C	V	A
III	A	VI	A

Fig. 5.15

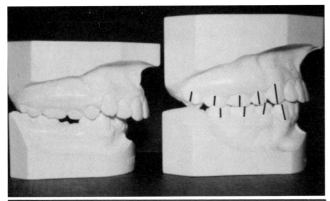

Ortho	1	Patient	5		NE		E	x
Key				Grade	Key			Grade
I	2mm Cl II			C	IV			A
II	876 / 7 5 3			D	V			A
III				A	VI			A

Fig. 5.16

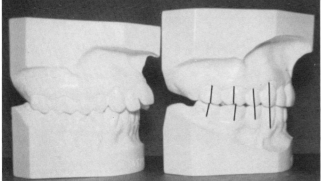
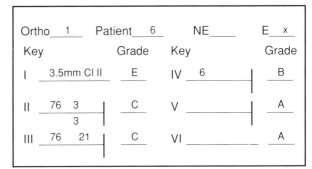

Ortho	1	Patient	6		NE		E	x
Key				Grade	Key			Grade
I	3.5mm Cl II			E	IV	6		B
II	76 3 / 3			C	V			A
III	76 21			C	VI			A

Fig. 5.17

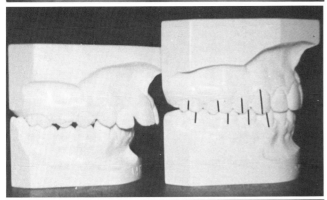
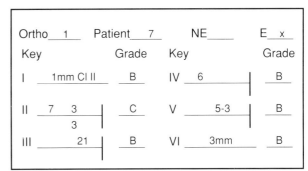

Ortho	1	Patient	7		NE		E	x
Key				Grade	Key			Grade
I	1mm Cl II			B	IV	6		B
II	7 3 / 3			C	V	5-3		B
III	21			B	VI	3mm		B

Fig. 5.18

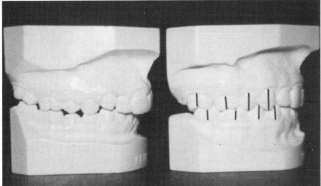

Ortho	1	Patient	8		NE		E	x
Key				Grade	Key			Grade
I	Cl I			A	IV			A
II	3 / 7 3			C	V			A
III	21 / 21			C	VI	3mm		B

Fig. 5.19

45

Summary for Orthodontist 1			
Patients 8	NE 1	E 7	
Keys	50% or more	Less than 50%, but significant	Grade
I	7 casts		C
II	7 3 3	6 7 5	C
III	7 21	6	B–
IV	6	7	B
V			A
VI		3 casts	A–

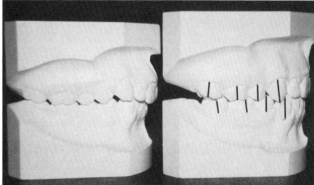
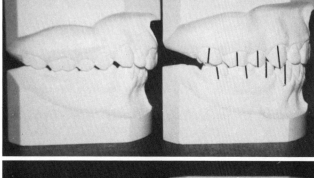
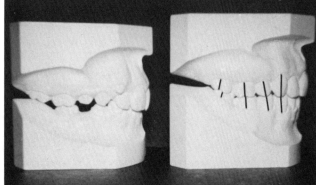
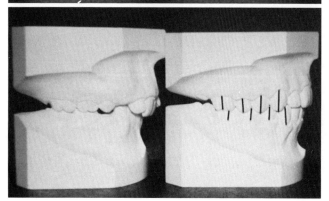

ORTHODONTIST # 2

Ortho 2	Patient 1		NE	E x
Key		Grade	Key	Grade
I	1mm Cl II	B	IV 6	B
II	76 76 3	D	V 5-3	B
III	7 21	C	VI	A

Fig. 5.20

Ortho 2	Patient 2		NE	E x
Key		Grade	Key	Grade
I	3.5mm Cl II	E	IV 6	B
II	765 3 65 3	E	V	A
III	21	B	VI 4mm	C

Fig. 5.21

Ortho 2	Patient 3		NE x	E
Key		Grade	Key	Grade
I	0.5mm Cl II	B	IV	A
II	43 3	C	V	A
III	21	B	VI	A

Fig.5.22

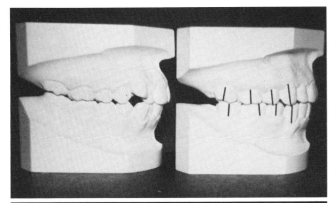

Ortho __2__	Patient __4__	NE ____	E __x__
Key	Grade	Key	Grade
I 2.5mm Cl II D		IV _____|	A
II 76 / 6 |	C	V _____|	A
III 21 |	B	VI _____	A

Fig. 5.23

Ortho __2__	Patient __5__	NE __x__	E ____
Key	Grade	Key	Grade
I 3mm Cl II E		IV 6 ____|	B
II 76 / 3 |	C	V _____|	A
III 21 / 21 |	C	VI _____	A

Fig. 5.24

Ortho __2__	Patient __6__	NE __x__	E ____
Key	Grade	Key	Grade
I 3mm Cl II E		IV 6 ____|	B
II 543 / 3 |	C	V _____|	A
III 21 |	B	VI _____	A

Fig. 5.25

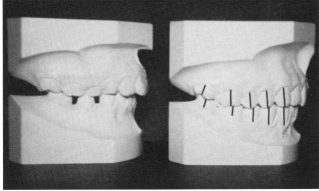
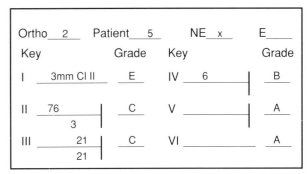
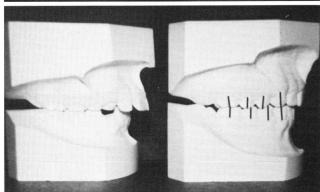

Summary for Orthodontist __2__			
Patients __6__ NE __3__ E __3__			
Keys	50% or more	Less than 50%, but significant	Grade
I	6 casts	_____	D
II	76 3 / 6 3 |	54 |	C–
III!	21 / 21 |	_____|	B
IV	6 |	_____|	B+
V	_____	_____	A
VI	_____	_____	A

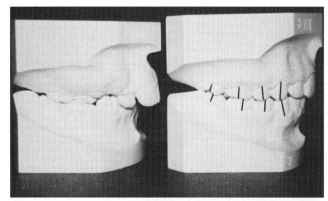

ORTHODONTIST #3

Ortho ___3___ Patient ___1___ NE _____ E __x__

Key			Grade	Key			Grade
I	3mm Cl II		E	IV	6	|	B
II	76 3		C	V		|	A
	3	|					
III	21	|	C	VI	4mm		C
	21	|					

Fig. 5.26

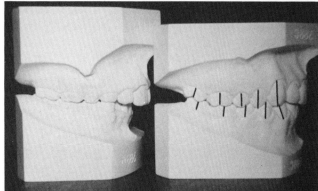

Ortho ___3___ Patient ___2___ NE __x__ E _____

Key			Grade	Key			Grade
I	1.5mm Cl II		B	IV	5	|	B
II	76 3		C	V		|	A
	3	|					
III	21	|	B	VI	4mm		C

Fig. 5.27

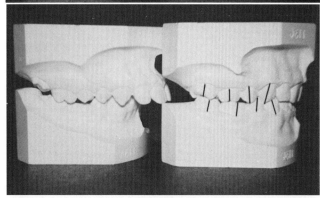

Ortho ___3___ Patient ___3___ NE _____ E __x__

Key			Grade	Key			Grade
I	2.5mm Cl II		D	IV	76	|	B
II	76 3		E	V		|	A
	765 3	|					
III	7 21	|	D	VI	4mm		C
	21	|					

Fig. 5.28

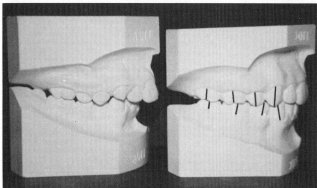

Ortho ___3___ Patient ___4___ NE _____ E __x__

Key			Grade	Key			Grade
I	2mm Cl II		C	IV	76	|	B
II	7 3		D	V		|	A
	65 3	|					
III	21	|	B	VI			A

Fig. 5.29

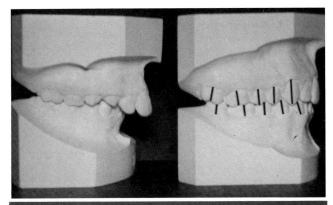

Ortho 3	Patient 5	NE x	E ___
Key	Grade	Key	Grade
I 0.5mm Cl II	B	IV 5	B
II 7 3 / 6 43	D	V	A
III 21 / 21	C	VI 3mm	B

Fig. 5.30

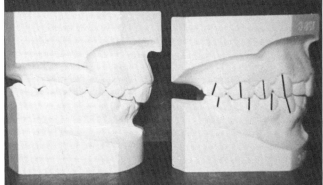

Ortho 3	Patient 6	NE ___	E x
Key	Grade	Key	Grade
I 1mm Cl II	B	IV	A
II 7 / 3	B	V 5-3	B
III 21	B	VI 3mm	B

Fig. 5.31

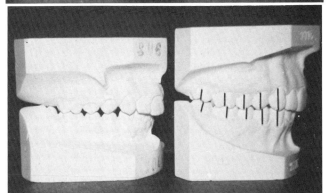

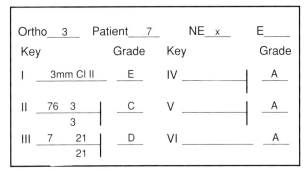

Ortho 3	Patient 7	NE x	E ___
Key	Grade	Key	Grade
I 3mm Cl II	E	IV	A
II 76 3 / 3	C	V	A
III 7 21 / 21	D	VI	A

Fig. 5.32

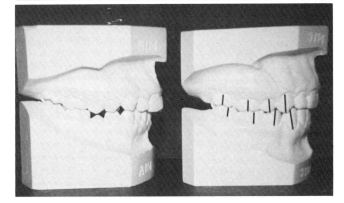

Ortho 3	Patient 8	NE ___	E x
Key	Grade	Key	Grade
I 2.5mm Cl II	D	IV 5	B
II 76 3 / 5 3	D	V	A
III 21	B	VI 3mm	B

Fig. 5.33

49

Summary for Orthodontist __3__

Patients __8__   NE __3__   E __5__

Keys	50% or more	Less than 50%, but significant	Grade
I	8 casts		C−
II	76 3		C−
	3	65	
III	21		C+
	21		
IV		65	B+
V			A
VI	6 casts		B

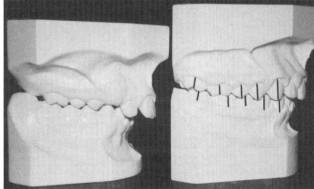

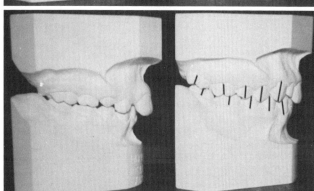

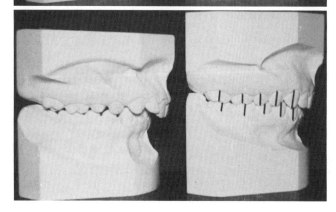

ORTHODONTIST #4

Ortho __4__   Patient __1__   NE __x__   E ____

Key		Grade	Key		Grade
I	2mm Cl II	C	IV	5	B
II	7 3	C	V		A
	6 3				
III		A	VI	3mm	B

Fig. 5.34

Ortho __4__   Patient __2__   NE __x__   E ____

Key		Grade	Key		Grade
I	1mm Cl II	B	IV		A
II	7 543	D	V		A
	3				
III	21	B	VI	4mm	C

Fig. 5.35

Ortho __4__   Patient __3__   NE __x__   E ____

Key		Grade	Key		Grade
I	2mm Cl II	C	IV		A
II	76 3	C	V		A
	3				
III	21	C	VI	3mm	B
	21				

Fig. 5.36

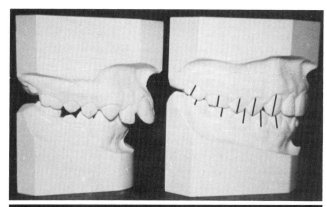

Ortho 4		Patient 4		NE x		E ___	
Key		Grade		Key		Grade	
I	1.5mm Cl II	B		IV	_____|	A	
II	76543 / 43	E		V	_____|	A	
III	21 / 21 |	C		VI	5mm	D	

Fig. 5.37

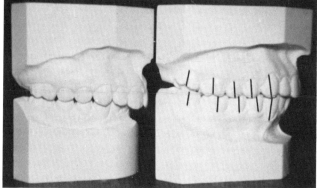

Ortho 4		Patient 5		NE x		E ___	
Key		Grade		Key		Grade	
I	2.5mm Cl II	D		IV	6 |	B	
II	7 / 54 |	C		V	_____|	A	
III	7 / 21 |	C		VI	_____	A	

Fig. 5.38

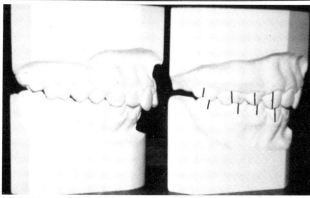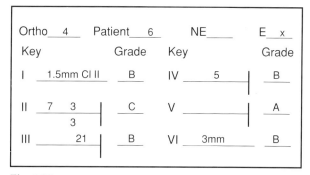

Ortho 4		Patient 6		NE ___		E x	
Key		Grade		Key		Grade	
I	1.5mm Cl II	B		IV	5 |	B	
II	7 3 / 3 |	C		V	_____|	A	
III	21 |	B		VI	3mm	B	

Fig. 5.39

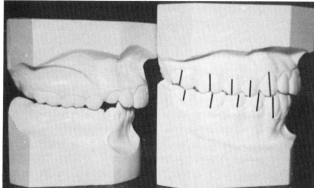

Ortho 4		Patient 7		NE x		E ___	
Key		Grade		Key		Grade	
I	2mm Cl II	C		IV	65 |	B	
II	7 / 3 |	B		V	_____|	A	
III	21 / 21 |	C		VI	4mm	C	

Fig. 5.40

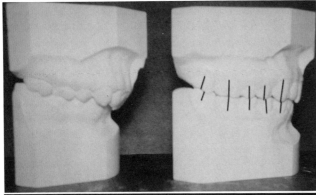

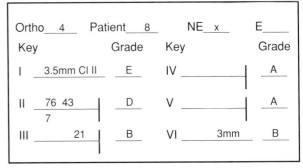

Ortho 4	Patient 8	NE x	E ___
Key	Grade	Key	Grade
I 3.5mm Cl II	E	IV _____|	A
II 76 43 / 7	D	V _____|	A
III 21	B	VI _____ 3mm	B

Fig. 5.41

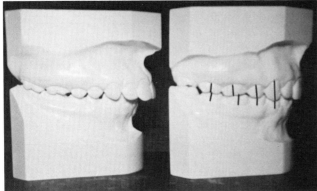

Ortho 4	Patient 9	NE ___	E x
Key	Grade	Key	Grade
I 3.5mm Cl II	E	IV _____|	A
II 7 3 / 3	C	V _____|	A
III 21 / 21	C	VI ____ 4mm	C

Fig. 5.42

Summary for Orthodontist 4			
Patients 9	NE 7	E 2	
Keys	50% or more	Less than 50%, but significant	Grade
I	9 casts	_____	C
II	7 3 / 3 |	6 4 |	C
III	21 / 21 |	_____	B–
IV	_____|	5 |	A–
V	_____		A
VI	8 casts	_____	B–

ORTHODONTIST #5

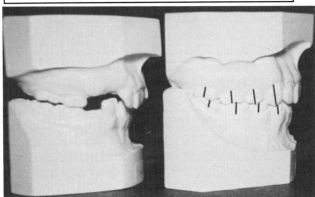

Ortho 5	Patient 1	NE ___	E x
Key	Grade	Key	Grade
I 2mm Cl II	C	IV _____|	A
II 7 / 3	B	V _____|	A
III 21 |	B	VI ____ 4mm	C

Fig. 5.43

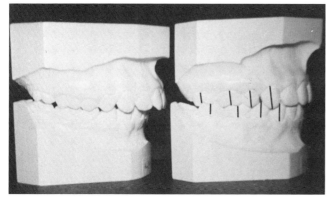

Ortho 5	Patient 2	NE	E x
Key	Grade	Key	Grade
I Cl I	A	IV	A
II	A	V 5-3	B
III 21	B	VI	A

Fig. 5.44

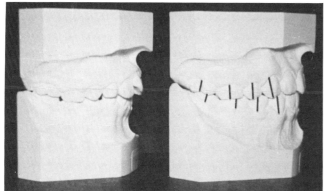

Ortho 5	Patient 3	NE	E x
Key	Grade	Key	Grade
I 1mm Cl II	B	IV	A
II	A	V	A
III	A	VI 3mm	B

Fig. 5.45

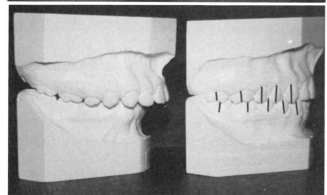

Ortho 5	Patient 4	NE x	E
Key	Grade	Key	Grade
I 1mm Cl II	B	IV	A
II 543 43	D	V	A
III 21	B	VI	A

Fig. 5.46

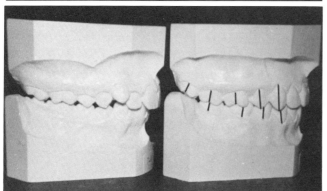

Ortho 5	Patient 5	NE	E x
Key	Grade	Key	Grade
I 2.5mm Cl II	D	IV	A
II 876 3	C	V	A
III	A	VI 3mm	B

Fig. 5.47

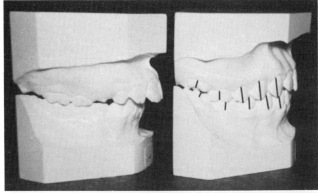

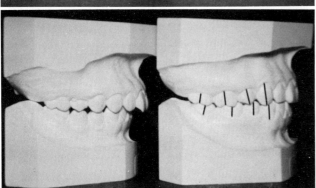

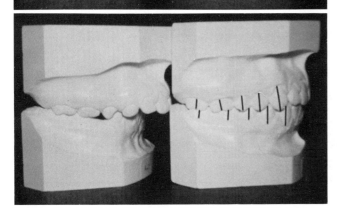

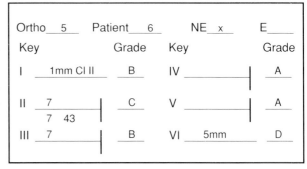

Ortho 5	Patient 6	NE x	E
Key	Grade	Key	Grade
I 1mm Cl II	B	IV	A
II 7 / 7 43	C	V	A
III 7	B	VI 5mm	D

Fig. 5.48

Ortho 5	Patient 7	NE	E x
Key	Grade	Key	Grade
I 2.5mm Cl II	D	IV 5	B
II 7 5 / 7 3	C	V	A
III	A	VI 3mm	B

Fig. 5.49

Ortho 5	Patient 8	NE x	E
Key	Grade	Key	Grade
I Cl I	A	IV 5	B
II 7	B	V	A
III	A	VI	A

Fig. 5.50

Summary for Orthodontist 5			
Patients 8	NE 3	E 5	
Keys	50% or more	Less than 50%, but significant	Grade
I	6 casts		B–
II	7 / 3	5 / 4	B–
III		21	A–
IV		5	A
V			A
VI	5 casts		B

54

ORTHODONTIST #6

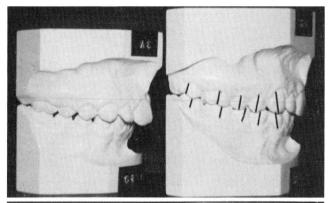

Ortho 6	Patient 1	NE x	E
Key	Grade	Key	Grade
I 2mm Cl II	C	IV 6 |	B
II 7654 / 543 |	E	V |	A
III 21 |	B	VI 3mm	B

Fig. 5.51

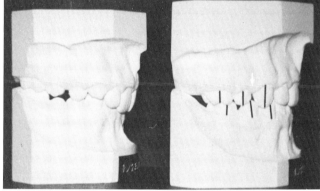

Ortho 6	Patient 2	NE	E x
Key	Grade	Key	Grade
I 2mm Cl II	C	IV 6 |	B
II 6 3 / 5 3 |	C	V 5-3 |	B
III 21 / 21 |	C	VI 3mm	B

Fig. 5.52

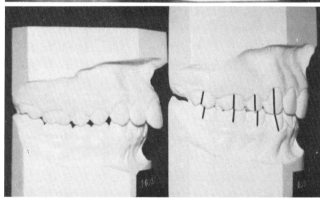

Ortho 6	Patient 3	NE	E x
Key	Grade	Key	Grade
I 3.5mm Cl II	E	IV 6 |	B
II 76 3 / 3 |	C	V |	A
III 21 / 21 |	C	VI 3mm	B

Fig. 5.53

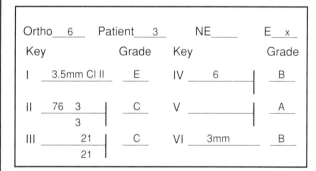
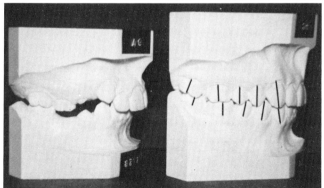

Ortho 6	Patient 4	NE x	E
Key	Grade	Key	Grade
I 2mm Cl II	C	IV 65 |	B
II 7 / 6543 |	D	V |	A
III 21 / 21 |	C	VI 3mm	B

Fig. 5.54

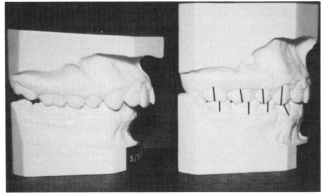

Ortho 6	Patient 5	NE	E x
Key	Grade	Key	Grade
I 1.5mm Cl II	B	IV	A
II 3 / 3	B	V	A
III 21 / 21	C	VI 3mm	B

Fig. 5.55

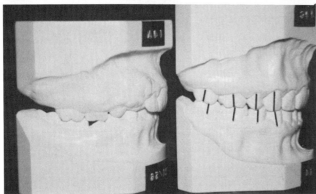

Ortho 6	Patient 6	NE	E x
Key	Grade	Key	Grade
I 3mm Cl II	E	IV 65	B
II 7 3 / 3	C	V	A
III 21 / 21	C	VI 3mm	B

Fig. 5.56

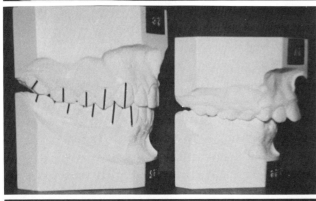

Ortho 6	Patient 7	NE x	E
Key	Grade	Key	Grade
I 1mm Cl II	B	IV	A
II 7 43 / 3	C	V	A
III 21 / 21	B	VI	A

Fig. 5.57

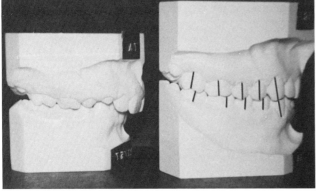

Ortho 6	Patient 8	NE x	E
Key	Grade	Key	Grade
I 2mm C II	C	IV 5	B
II 7 / 3	B	V	A
III 21 / 21	C	VI 4mm	C

Fig. 5.58

56

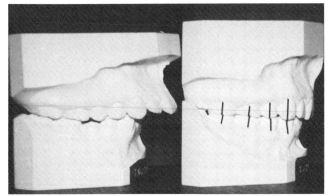

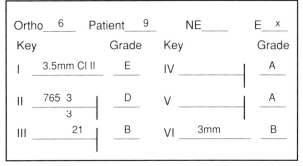

Ortho 6	Patient 9	NE	E x
Key	Grade	Key	Grade
I 3.5mm Cl II	E	IV	A
II 765 3 / 3	D	V	A
III 21	B	VI 3mm	B

Fig. 5.59

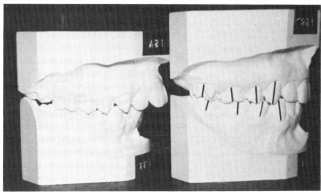

Ortho 6	Patient 10	NE	E x
Key	Grade	Key	Grade
I 2mm Cl II	C	IV 65	B
II 7 3 / 5 3	C	V	A
III 21 / 21	C	VI	A

Fig. 5.60

Summary for Orthodontist 6			
Patients 10	NE 4	E 6	
Keys	50% or more	Less than 50%, but significant	Grade
I	10 casts		C–
II	7 3 / 3	6 / 5	C
III	21 / 21		C+
IV	6	5	B+
V			A
VI	8 casts		B

ORTHODONTIST #7

Ortho 7	Patient 1	NE x	E
Key	Grade	Key	Grade
I 3mm Cl II	E	IV 6	B
II 87	B	V	A
III 21 / 21	C	VI 3mm	B

Fig. 5.61

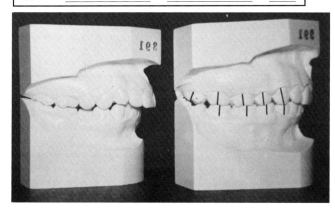

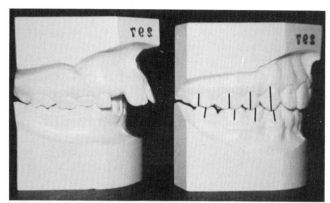

Ortho 7	Patient 2		NE		E x
Key	**Grade**		**Key**		**Grade**
I	2.5mm Cl II	D	IV		A
II	76 3 / 3	C	V	5-3	B
III	21 / 21	C	VI	3mm	B

Fig. 5.62

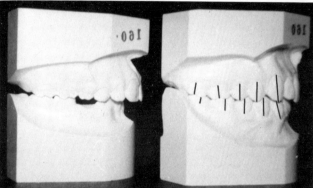

Ortho 7	Patient 3		NE x		E
Key	**Grade**		**Key**		**Grade**
I	1.5mm Cl II	B	IV		A
II	7 3 / 3	C	V		A
III	21 / 21	C	VI	4mm	C

Fig. 5.63

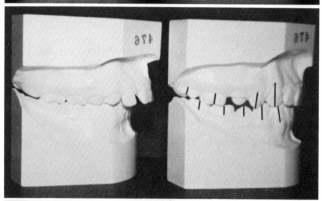

Ortho 7	Patient 4		NE x		E
Key	**Grade**		**Key**		**Grade**
I	1mm Cl II	B	IV		A
II	76 43 / 3	D	V		A
III	21	B	VI		A

Fig. 5.64

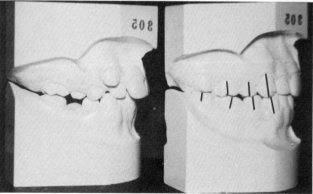

Ortho 7	Patient 5		NE		E x
Key	**Grade**		**Key**		**Grade**
I	2.5mm Cl II	D	IV	6	B
II	65 3	C	V		A
III	21 / 21	C	VI	4mm	C

Fig. 5.65

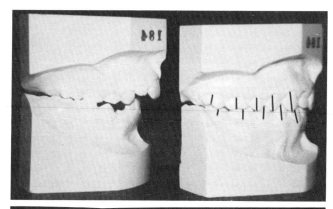

Ortho 7	Patient 6	NE x	E
Key	Grade	Key	Grade
I 1mm Cl II	B	IV	A
II 7 / 43	C	V	A
III 7 21 / 21	D	VI 4mm	C

Fig. 5.66

Ortho 7	Patient 7	NE x	E
Key	Grade	Key	Grade
I 1mm Cl II	B	IV	A
II 6543 / 7 3	D	V	A
III 21 / 21	C	VI 5mm	D

Fig. 5.67

Summary for Orthodontist 7			
Patients 7	NE 5	E 2	
Keys	50% or more	Less than 50%, but significant	Grade
I	7 casts		C
II	7 3 / 3	6 4	C
III	21 / 21		C
IV		6	A
V			A
VI	6 casts		C+

ORTHODONTIST #8

Ortho 8	Patient 1	NE x	E
Key	Grade	Key	Grade
I 3.5mm Cl II	E	IV	A
II 7 43 / 7 3	D	V	A
III 21	B	VI 3mm	B

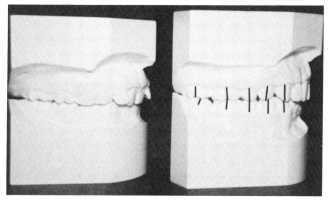

Fig. 5.68

59

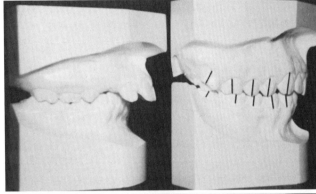

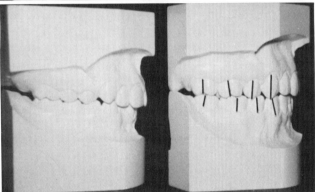

Ortho __8__	Patient __2__	NE __x__	E ____
Key	**Grade**	**Key**	**Grade**
I ___3mm Cl II___	E	IV ___6___	B
II ___7 543___ / ___43___	D	V _____	A
III ___7 21___	C	VI ___3mm___	B

Fig. 5.69

Ortho __8__	Patient __3__	NE ____	E __x__
Key	**Grade**	**Key**	**Grade**
I ___2.5mm Cl II___	D	IV ___6___	B
II ___7 5 3___ / ___3___	C	V _____	A
III ___21___	B	VI _____	A

Fig. 5.70

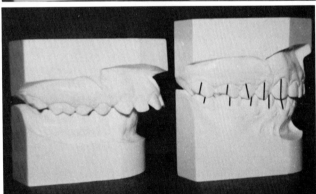

Ortho __8__	Patient __4__	NE __x__	E ____
Key	**Grade**	**Key**	**Grade**
I ___2mm Cl II___	C	IV _____	A
II ___765 3___ / ___5 3___	D	V _____	A
III ___21___	B	VI ___3mm___	B

Fig. 5.71

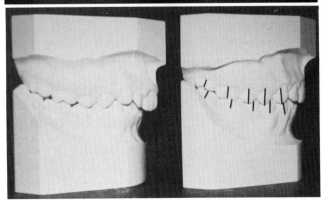

Ortho __8__	Patient __5__	NE __x__	E ____
Key	**Grade**	**Key**	**Grade**
I ___1mm Cl II___	B	IV _____	A
II ___7___ / ___7 3___	C	V _____	A
III ___7 21___ / ___21___	D	VI ___5mm___	D

Fig. 5.72

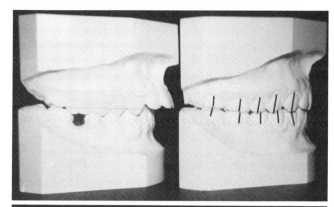

Ortho	8		Patient	6		NE	x		E	
Key			Grade		Key				Grade	
I	3.5mm Cl II		D		IV	6			B	
II	76543		E		V				A	
	43									
III	21		B		VI	4mm			C	

Fig. 5.73

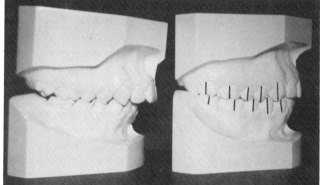

Ortho	8		Patient	7		NE	x		E	
Key			Grade		Key				Grade	
I	1mm Cl II		B		IV	6			B	
II	76543		D		V				A	
	3									
III	21		C		VI	3mm			B	
	21									

Fig. 5.74

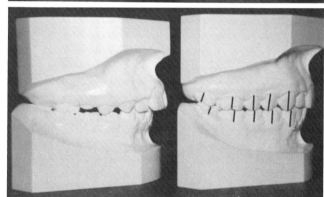

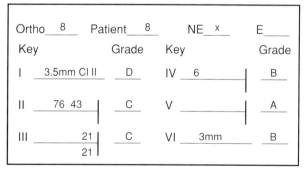

Ortho	8		Patient	8		NE	x		E	
Key			Grade		Key				Grade	
I	3.5mm Cl II		D		IV	6			B	
II	76 43		C		V				A	
III	21		C		VI	3mm			B	
	21									

Fig. 5.75

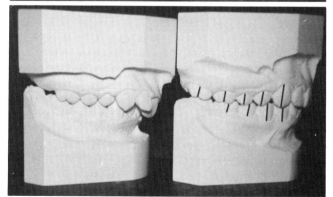

Ortho	8		Patient	9		NE	x		E	
Key			Grade		Key				Grade	
I	2mm Cl II		C		IV				A	
II	76543		E		V				A	
	65 3									
III	21		C		VI	3mm			B	
	21									

Fig. 5.76

61

Summary for Orthodontist ___8___

Patients ___9___   NE ___8___   E ___1___

Keys	50% or more	Less than 50%, but significant	Grade
I	9 casts		D
II	76543 3		D
III	21	21	C+
IV	6		B
V			A
VI	8 casts		B

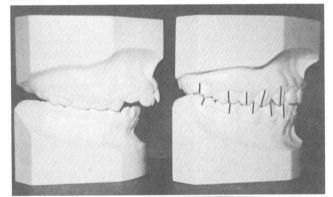

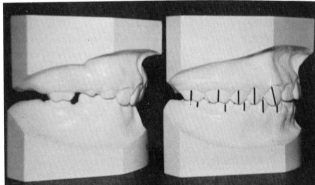

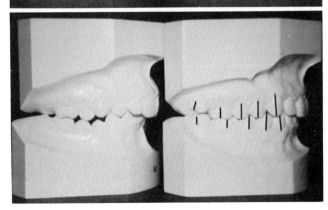

ORTHODONTIST #9

Ortho ___9___   Patient ___1___   NE __x__   E ____

Key		Grade	Key		Grade
I	2mm Cl II	C	IV	6	B
II	43 43	C	V		A
III	21 21	C	VI	4mm	C

Fig. 5.77

Ortho ___9___   Patient ___2___   NE __x__   E ____

Key		Grade	Key		Grade
I	1mm Cl II	B	IV	6	B
II	76 3	C	V		A
III		A	VI	3mm	B

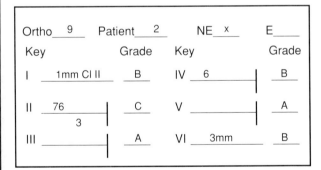

Fig. 5.78

Ortho ___9___   Patient ___3___   NE __x__   E ____

Key		Grade	Key		Grade
I	1mm Cl II	B	IV		A
II	76 7 3	C	V		A
III		A	VI	3mm	B

Fig. 5.79

62

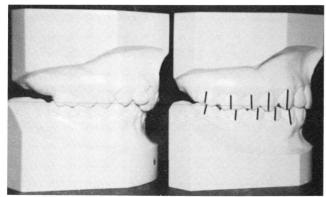

Ortho 9	Patient 4	NE x	E
Key	Grade	Key	Grade
I 2.5mm Cl II	D	IV 65	B
II 76 3	C	V	A
3			
III 21	B	VI	A

Fig. 5.80

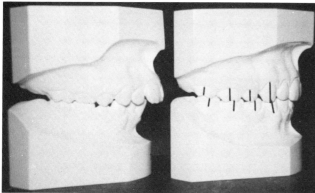

Ortho 9	Patient 5	NE	E x
Key	Grade	Key	Grade
I 2.5mm Cl II	D	IV	A
II 76 3	C	V 5-3	B
3			
III 21	B	VI 3mm	B

Fig. 5.81

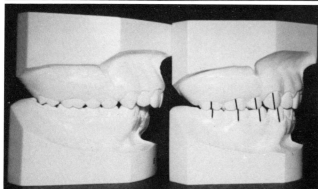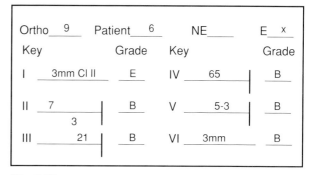

Ortho 9	Patient 6	NE	E x
Key	Grade	Key	Grade
I 3mm Cl II	E	IV 65	B
II 7	B	V 5-3	B
3			
III 21	B	VI 3mm	B

Fig. 5.82

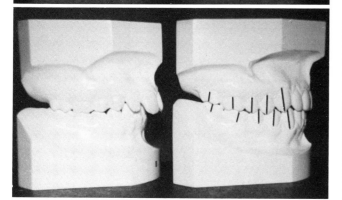

Ortho 9	Patient 7	NE x	E
Key	Grade	Key	Grade
I 2mm Cl II	C	IV 6	B
II 4	C	V	A
65 3			
III	A	VI 3mm	B

Fig. 5.83

63

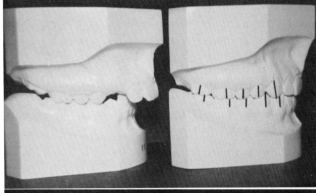

Ortho 9	Patient 8	NE x	E
Key	Grade	Key	Grade
I 2.5mm Cl II	C	IV 6	B
II 7 3	B	V	A
III 21	B	VI 3mm	B

Fig. 5.84

Ortho 9	Patient 9	NE x	E
Key	Grade	Key	Grade
I 3.5mm Cl II	D	IV	A
II 7 3 / 7 5 3	D	V	A
III 21	B	VI 4mm	C

Fig. 5.85

Summary for Orthodontist 9			
Patients 9	NE 6	E 3	
Keys	50% or more	Less than 50%, but significant	Grade
I	9 casts		C
II	7	6 3	C
III	21		B
IV	6		B+
V			A
VI	8 casts		B

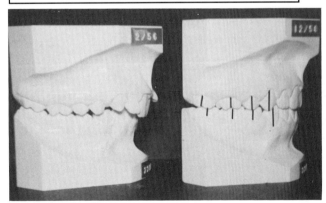

ORTHODONTIST #10

Ortho 10	Patient 1	NE	E x
Key	Grade	Key	Grade
I 3mm Cl II	E	IV 6	B
II 76 3 / 3	C	V	A
III 21	B	VI	A

Fig. 5.86

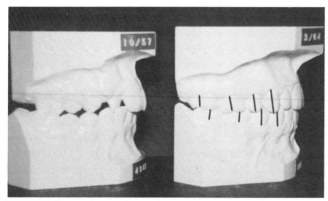

Ortho 10	Patient 2	NE	E x
Key	Grade	Key	Grade
I Cl I	A	IV	A
II	A	V	A
III	A	VI	A

Fig. 5.87

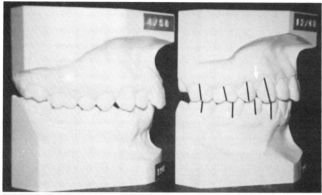

Ortho 10	Patient 3	NE	E x
Key	Grade	Key	Grade
I Cl I	A	IV	A
II	A	V 5-3	B
III 21	B	VI	A

Fig. 5.88

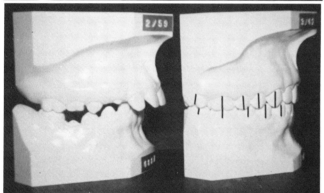

Ortho 10	Patient 4	NE x	E
Key	Grade	Key	Grade
I 2mm Cl II	C	IV 6	B
II 76 3	C	V	A
III 21	B	VI	A

Fig. 5.89

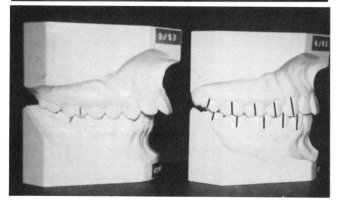

Ortho 10	Patient 5	NE	E x
Key	Grade	Key	Grade
I Cl I	A	IV	A
II	A	V	A
III	A	VI	A

Fig. 5.90

65

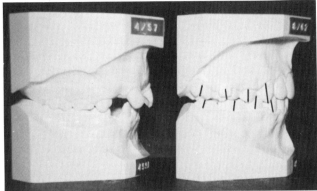

Ortho	10	Patient	6	NE		E	x
Key		Grade	Key			Grade	
I	1mm Cl II	B	IV	7	|	B	
II	7 / 765 3	D	V		|	A	
III	7	B	VI	3mm		B	

Fig. 5.91

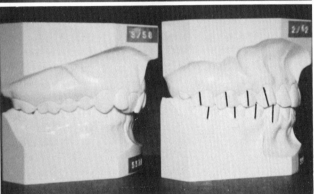
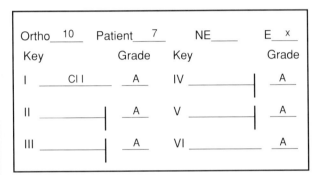

Ortho	10	Patient	7	NE		E	x
Key		Grade	Key			Grade	
I	Cl I	A	IV		|	A	
II		A	V		|	A	
III		A	VI			A	

Fig. 5.92

Ortho	10	Patient	8	NE	x	E	
Key		Grade	Key			Grade	
I	1mm Cl II	B	IV		|	A	
II	7 3 / 3	C	V		|	A	
III		A	VI			A	

Fig. 5.93

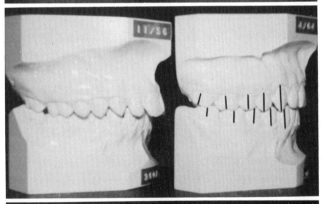
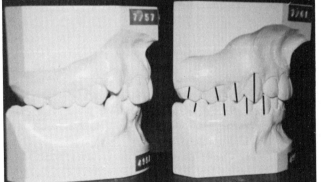

Ortho	10	Patient	9	NE		E	x
Key		Grade	Key			Grade	
I	Cl I	A	IV		|	A	
II	7 3 / 6	C	V		|	A	
III		A	VI			A	

Fig. 5.94

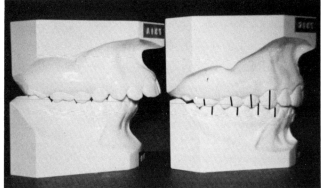

Ortho __10__	Patient __10__	NE ____	E __x__
Key	Grade	Key	Grade
I ___Cl I___	A	IV _____ |	A
II ___3___ |	B	V ___5-3___ |	B
III ___21___ | ___21___ |	C	VI ___3mm___	B

Fig. 5.95

Ortho __10__	Patient __11__	NE ____	E __x__
Key	Grade	Key	Grade
I ___Cl I___	A	IV _____ |	A
II __76 3__ | __5__	C	V _____ |	A
III _____ | __21__ |	B	VI _____	A

Fig. 5.96

Summary for Orthodontist __10__			
Patients __11__ NE __2__ E __9__			
Keys	50% or more	Less than 50%, but significant	Grade
I	___7 casts___	_____	B+
II	__7 3__ |	_____ |	B
		__3__ |	
III	_____ |	__21__ |	B+
		__21__ |	
IV	_____ |	_____ |	A
V	_____	_____	A
VI	_____	___3 casts___	A

ORTHODONTIST #11

Ortho __11__	Patient __1__	NE __x__	E ____
Key	Grade	Key	Grade
I __1mm Cl II__	B	IV __5__ |	B
II __76__ | __5 3__ |	C	V _____ |	A
III __21__ |	B	VI _____	A

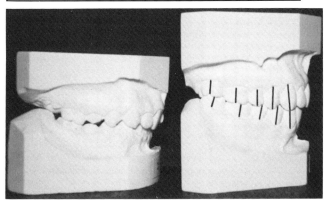

Fig. 5.97

67

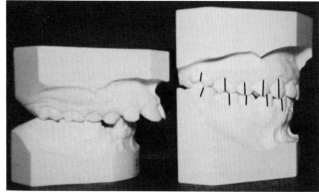

Ortho 11		Patient 2		NE x		E
Key		Grade	Key			Grade
I	3mm Cl II	E	IV			A
II	76 43 / 76 43	E	V			A
III	7 21 / 21	D	VI	3mm		B

Fig. 5.98

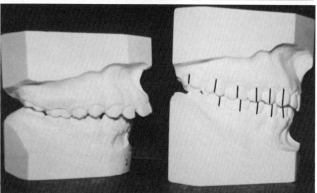

Ortho 11		Patient 3		NE x		E
Key		Grade	Key			Grade
I	2.5mm Cl II	D	IV	7		B
II	876 3 / 3	D	V			A
III	87 21	C	VI	3mm		B

Fig. 5.99

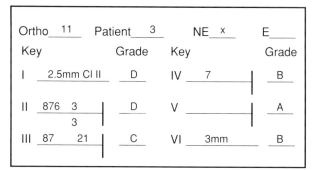

Ortho 11		Patient 4		NE x		E
Key		Grade	Key			Grade
I	2mm Cl II	C	IV			A
II	7 3 / 3	C	V			A
III	21	B	VI			A

Fig. 5.100

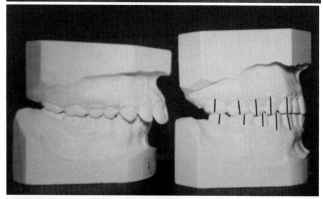

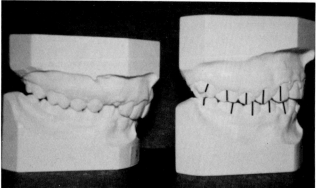

Ortho 11		Patient 5		NE x		E
Key		Grade	Key			Grade
I	2mm Cl II	C	IV	7		B
II	7 43 / 76 3	D	V			A
III	7 21	C	VI	4mm		C

Fig. 5.101

68

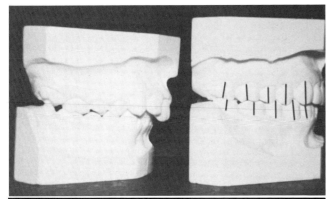

Ortho 11		Patient 6		NE x		E ___	
Key		Grade	Key		Grade		
I	1.5mm Cl II	B	IV		A		
II	76 3 / 43	D	V		A		
III	21	B	VI	3mm	B		

Fig. 5.102

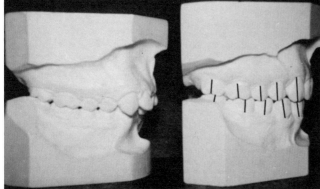

Ortho 11		Patient 7		NE x		E ___	
Key		Grade	Key		Grade		
I	2.5mm Cl II	D	IV		A		
II	7 3 / 43	C	V		A		
III	21	B	VI		A		

Fig. 5.103

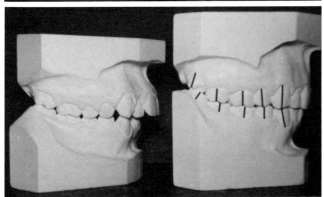
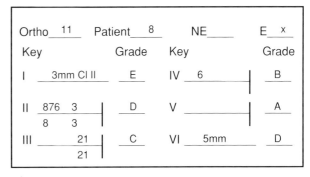
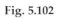

Ortho 11		Patient 8		NE ___		E x	
Key		Grade	Key		Grade		
I	3mm Cl II	E	IV	6	B		
II	876 3 / 8 3	D	V		A		
III	21 / 21	C	VI	5mm	D		

Fig. 5.104

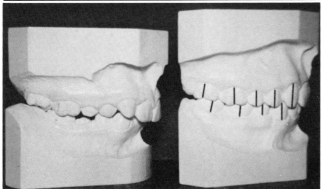

Ortho 11		Patient 9		NE ___		E x	
Key		Grade	Key		Grade		
I	Cl I	A	IV		A		
II	76 3 / 3	C	V		A		
III	3 1 / 21	C	VI		A		

Fig. 5.105

69

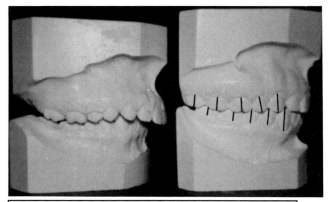

<table>
</table>

Ortho 11	Patient 10	NE	E x
Key	Grade	Key	Grade
I _Cl I_	A	IV _____|	A
II _5_	B	V _____|	A
III _____21|	B	VI _____	A

Fig. 5.106

Summary for Orthodontist __11__
Patients __10__   NE _7_   E _3_

Keys	50% or more	Less than 50%, but significant	Grade
I	8 casts		C
II	76 3 / 3		C–
		4	
III	21 / 21	7	C+
IV			A–
V			A
VI	5 casts		B

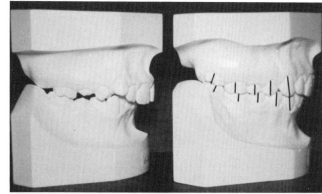

ORTHODONTIST #12

Ortho 12	Patient 1	NE x	E
Key	Grade	Key	Grade
I _2mm Cl II_	C	IV _____|	A
II _7_ / _7 3_	C	V _____|	A
III _7 21_ / _21_	D	VI _4mm_	C

Fig. 5.107

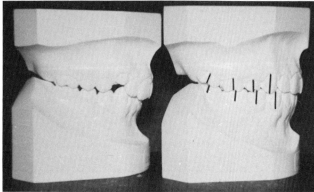

Ortho 12	Patient 2	NE	E x
Key	Grade	Key	Grade
I _2mm Cl II_	C	IV _6_|	B
II _7 3_ / _3_	C	V _____|	A
III _7 21_|	C	VI _____	A

Fig. 5.108

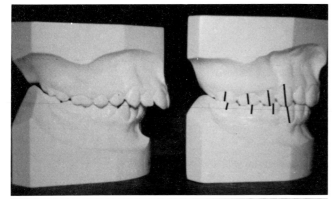

Ortho 12	Patient 3	NE	E x
Key	Grade	Key	Grade
I 2mm Cl II	C	IV	A
II 7 / 3	B	V 5-3	B
III 21 / 21	C	VI	A

Fig. 5.109

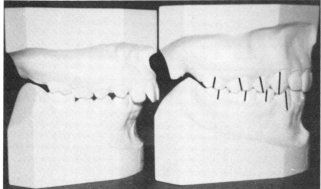

Ortho 12	Patient 4	NE	E x
Key	Grade	Key	Grade
I 1.5mm Cl II	B	IV	A
II 7 5 3 / 5 3	D	V	A
III 21	B	VI	A

Fig. 5.110

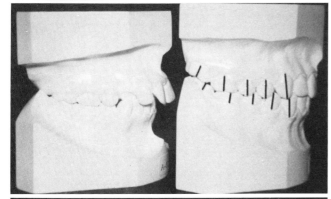

Ortho 12	Patient 5	NE x	E
Key	Grade	Key	Grade
I 1mm Cl II	B	IV	A
II 7 / 7 3	C	V	A
III / 21	B	VI 4mm	C

Fig. 5.111

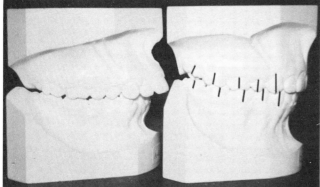

Ortho 12	Patient 6	NE	E x
Key	Grade	Key	Grade
I Cl I	A	IV	A
II 87 5 3	C	V	A
III	A	VI 4mm	C

Fig. 5.112

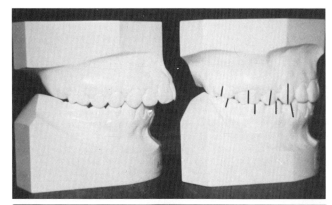

Ortho 12	Patient 7	NE	E x
Key	Grade	Key	Grade
I 2mm Cl II	C	IV 6	B
II 765 3 / 3	D	V	A
III	A	VI 3mm	B

Fig. 5.113

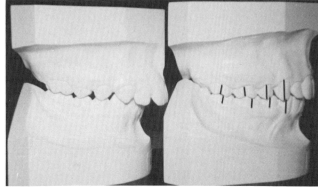

Ortho 12	Patient 8	NE	E x
Key	Grade	Key	Grade
I 2mm Cl II	C	IV	A
II 7 3	B	V 5-3	B
III 21 / 21	C	VI	A

Fig. 5.114

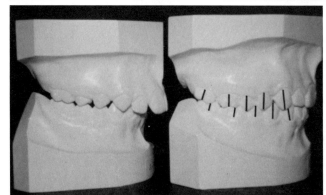

Ortho 12	Patient 9	NE x	E
Key	Grade	Key	Grade
I Cl I	A	IV	A
II 7 / 3	B	V 4-3	B
III 21	B	VI 3mm	B

Fig. 5.115

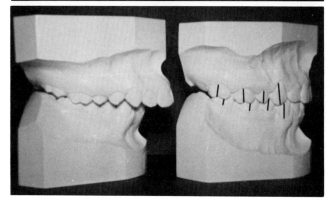

Ortho 12	Patient 10	NE	E x
Key	Grade	Key	Grade
I Cl I	A	IV	A
II 7 / 3	B	V	A
III	A	VI	A

Fig. 5.116

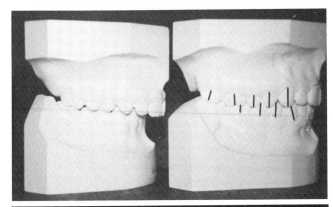

Ortho 12	Patient 11		NE x	E
Key		Grade	Key	Grade
I	Cl I	A	IV	A
II	7 3 / 3	C	V	A
III	21	B	VI 4mm	C

Fig. 5.117

Ortho 12	Patient 12		NE x	E
Key		Grade	Key	Grade
I	1.5mm Cl II	B	IV	A
II	76 3	C	V	A
III	21	B	VI 4mm	C

Fig. 5.118

Summary for Orthodontist 12			
Patients 12	NE 5	E 7	
Keys	50% or more	Less than 50%, but significant	Grade
I	8 casts		B
II	7 3 / 3	5	C
III	21	21	B
IV			A
V			A
VI	7 casts		B

ORTHODONTIST #13

Ortho 13	Patient 1		NE	E x
Key		Grade	Key	Grade
I	1mm Cl II	B	IV	A
II	76 3 / 3	C	V	A
III	21 / 21	C	VI 3mm	B

Fig. 5.119

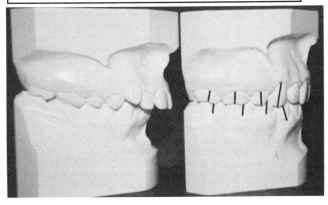

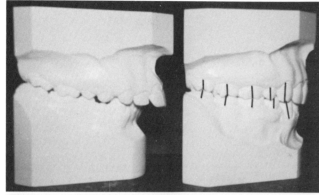

Ortho 13	Patient 2	NE	E x
Key	Grade	Key	Grade
I 3mm Cl II	E	IV 7	B
II 3 / 3	B	V	A
III 8 21 / 21	D	VI	A

Fig. 5.120

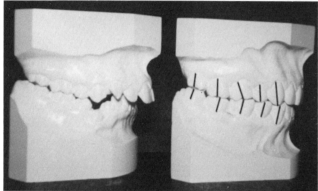

Ortho 13	Patient 3	NE	E x
Key	Grade	Key	Grade
I 2.5mm Cl II	D	IV	A
II 6 / 765	C	V	A
III 21	B	VI	A

Fig. 5.121

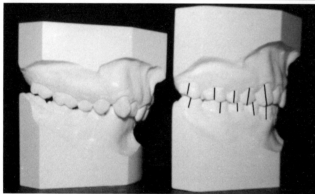

Ortho 13	Patient 4	NE x	E
Key	Grade	Key	Grade
I 2mm Cl II	C	IV 65	B
II 76 4 / 543	D	V	A
III 21	B	VI 3mm	B

Fig. 5.122

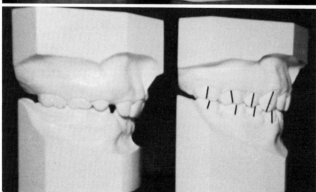

Ortho 13	Patient 5	NE	E x
Key	Grade	Key	Grade
I 2.5mm Cl II	C	IV	A
II 7 5 3 / 3	C	V	A
III 21 / 21	C	VI 3mm	B

Fig. 5.123

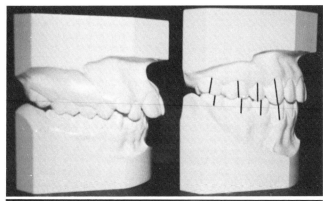

Ortho 13	Patient 6	NE ___	E x
Key	Grade	Key	Grade
I 2mm Cl II	C	IV 765	C
II 7 / 3	B	V	A
III	A	VI 3mm	B

Fig. 5.124

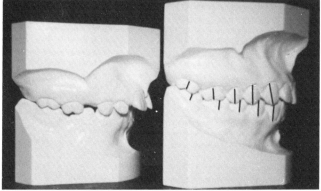

Ortho 13	Patient 7	NE x	E ___
Key	Grade	Key	Grade
I 1mm Cl II	B	IV	A
II 7 / 7	B	V	A
III	A	VI 5mm	D

Fig. 5.125

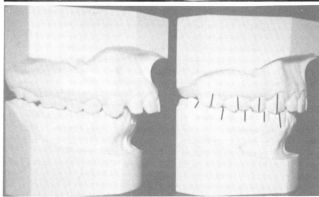

Ortho 13	Patient 8	NE ___	E x
Key	Grade	Key	Grade
I 2mm Cl II	C	IV 6	B
II 7 3 / 7 3	C	V	A
III 21	B	VI 4mm	C

Fig. 5.126

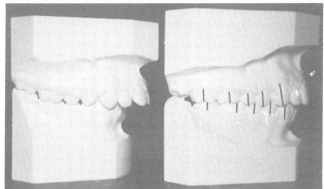

Ortho 13	Patient 9	NE x	E ___
Key	Grade	Key	Grade
I 0.5mm Cl II	B	IV	A
II 3	B	V	A
III 21 / 21	C	VI	A

Fig. 5.127

75

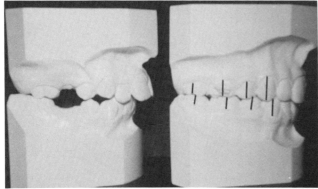

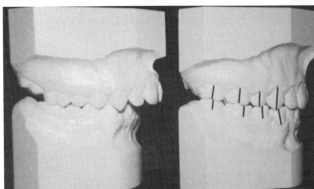

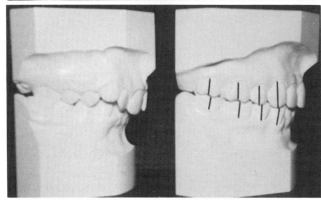

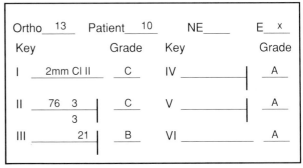

Ortho 13	Patient 10	NE	E x
Key	Grade	Key	Grade
I 2mm Cl II	C	IV _____|	A
II 76 3 / 3	C	V _____|	A
III 21|	B	VI _____	A

Fig. 5.128

Ortho 13	Patient 11	NE	E x
Key	Grade	Key	Grade
I 3mm Cl II	E	IV 6 __|	B
II 76 3 / 5 3	D	V _____|	A
III 21|	B	VI _____	A

Fig. 5.129

Ortho 13	Patient 12	NE	E x
Key	Grade	Key	Grade
I 3mm Cl II	E	IV 6 __|	B
II 76 3|	C	V _____|	A
III 21| / 21|	C	VI 3mm	B

Fig. 5.130

Summary for Orthodontist 13			
Patients 12	NE 3	E 9	
Keys	50% or more	Less than 50%, but significant	Grade
I	12 casts	_____	C–
II	76 3 / 3 |	_____ 5 ____|	C
III	21 |	_____ 21 |	B
IV	_____|	_____ 6 ____|	B+
V	_____	_____	A
VI	7 casts	_____	B

76

ORTHODONTIST #14

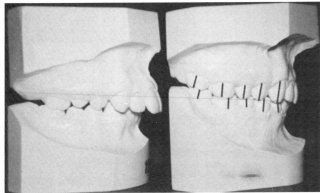

Ortho 14	Patient 1		NE x	E ___
Key		Grade	Key	Grade
I	3mm Cl II	E	IV	A
II	76543 / 6 3	E	V	A
III	21 / 21	C	VI 4mm	C

Fig. 5.131

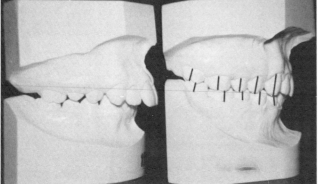

Ortho 14	Patient 2		NE x	E ___
Key		Grade	Key	Grade
I	3.5mm Cl II	E	IV 6	B
II	76543 / 3	D	V	A
III	1	B	VI 4mm	C

Fig. 5.132

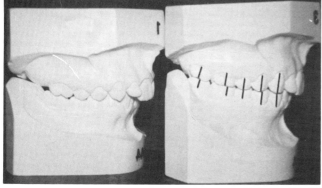
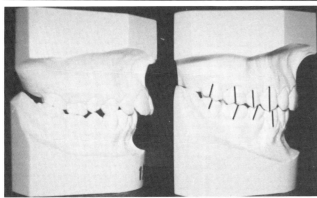
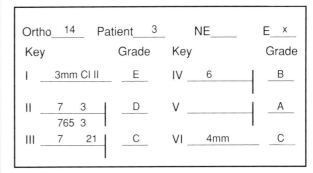

Ortho 14	Patient 3		NE ___	E x
Key		Grade	Key	Grade
I	3mm Cl II	E	IV 6	B
II	7 3 / 765 3	D	V	A
III	7 21	C	VI 4mm	C

Fig. 5.133

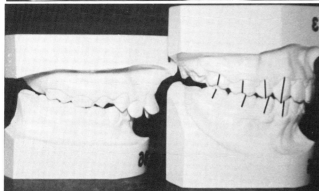

Ortho 14	Patient 4		NE ___	E x
Key		Grade	Key	Grade
I	3.5mm Cl II	E	IV	A
II	765 3 / 765	E	V	A
III	7 21 / 21	D	VI 3mm	B

Fig. 5.134

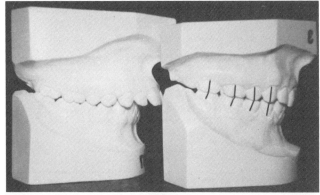

Ortho 14	Patient 5	NE	E x
Key	Grade	Key	Grade
I 3.5mm Cl II	E	IV 6	B
II 76 3 / 765	D	V	A
III 21 / 21	C	VI	A

Fig. 5.135

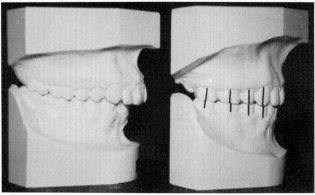

Ortho 14	Patient 6	NE	E x
Key	Grade	Key	Grade
I 3.5mm Cl II	E	IV 6	B
II 76 3	C	V	A
III 21 / 21	C	VI	A

Fig. 5.136

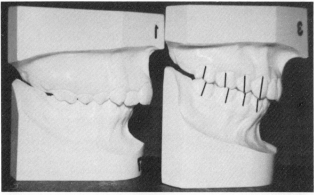

Ortho 14	Patient 7	NE	E x
Key	Grade	Key	Grade
I 3.5mm Cl II	E	IV	A
II 7 3 / 765 3	D	V	A
III 21 / 21	C	VI	A

Fig. 5.137

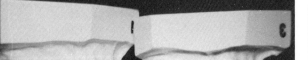

Ortho 14	Patient 8	NE	E x
Key	Grade	Key	Grade
I 2.5mm Cl II	D	IV	A
II 76 3 / 7 3	D	V 5-3	B
III 21 / 21	C	VI 3mm	B

Fig. 5.138

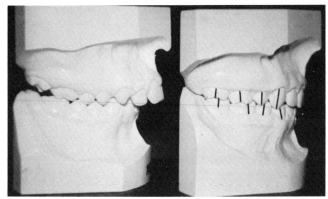

Ortho __14__	Patient __9__	NE____	E __x__
Key	Grade	Key	Grade
I ___2mm Cl II___	C	IV _____⌐	A
II ___7___3___ 65 3	D	V _____⌐	A
III _____21⌐	B	VI _____	A

Fig. 5.139

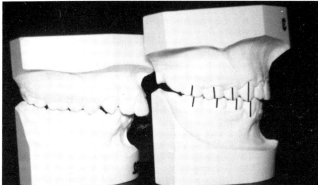

Ortho __14__	Patient __10__	NE____	E __x__
Key	Grade	Key	Grade
I ___2.5mm Cl II___	D	IV _____⌐	A
II ___7___3___ 3	C	V _____⌐	A
III _____⌐	A	VI _____	A

Fig. 5.140

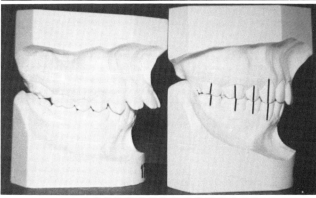

Ortho __14__	Patient __11__	NE____	E __x__
Key	Grade	Key	Grade
I ___3.5mm Cl II___	D	IV ___6___⌐	B
II ___76___3___ 3	C	V _____⌐	A
III _____2⌐ 21	C	VI _____	A

Fig. 5.141

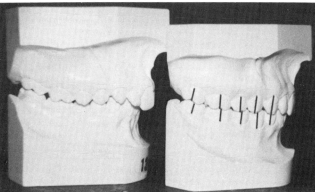

Ortho __14__	Patient __12__	NE __x__	E____
Key	Grade	Key	Grade
I ___3.5mm Cl II___	E	IV ___6___⌐	B
II ___76___43⌐	C	V _____⌐	A
III _____21⌐	B	VI ___3mm___	B

Fig. 5.142

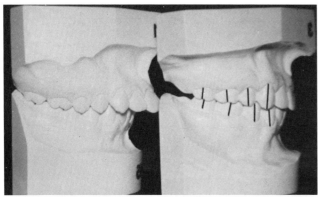

Ortho 14	Patient 13	NE	E x
Key	Grade	Key	Grade
I 2mm Cl II	C	IV	A
II 7 3 / 5 3	C	V	A
III 21	B	VI	A

Fig. 5.143

Ortho 14	Patient 14	NE	E x
Key	Grade	Key	Grade
I 3.5mm Cl II	E	IV 6	B
II 7 5 / 765 3	D	V	A
III 21 / 21	C	VI 3mm	B

Fig. 5.144

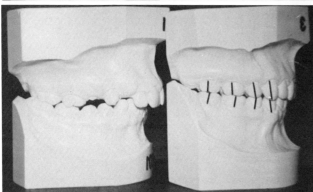

Summary for Orthodontist 14			
Patients 14	NE 3	E 11	
Keys	50% or more	Less than 50%, but significant	Grade
I	14 casts		E+
II	76 3 / 65 3	5 / 7	D
III	21 / 21		C+
IV	6		A–
V			A
VI	7 casts		B+

Photographs from 1970s Samples

Some of the 1970s casts were photographed from more perspectives than were the 1960s casts. This was to show errant conditions not visible in the right-side-only 1960s photographs. To accommodate the expanded perspectives, the Palmer box for the 1970s grading form is full-size. This permits a more thorough recording of errant teeth and conditions. However, just as was done for the 1960s

sample, only the teeth and conditions that can be seen from the sides of the casts facing right were graded and summarized. This establishes a common basis for comparing the 1960s and 1970s samples. Figure 5.145 shows pretreatment casts, examples of posttreatment casts from several perspectives, and the expanded grading form. The methods for summarizing the treatment results for each orthodontist are the same as for the 1960s results.

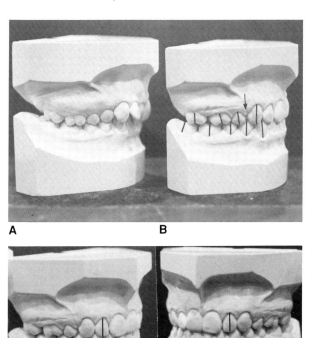

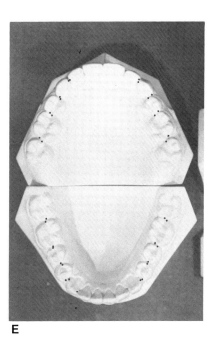

Ortho 1		Patient 2		NE____		E x
Key		Grade	Key			Grade
I	1mm Cl II	B	IV	65 3 | 654	6	D
II	6 32 | 2	C	V	5-3, 2-1| 1-2		C
III	21|	B	VI	|		A

Fig. 5.145. Pretreatment (*A*) and posttreatment (*B–E*) casts and grading form.

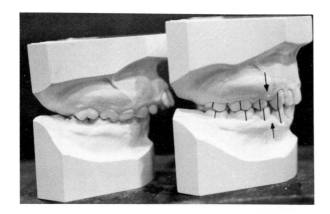

ORTHODONTIST #1

Ortho 1		Patient 1		NE		E x	
Key			Grade	Key			Grade
I	3mm Cl II		E	IV	⎮		A
II	76 3	⎮	D	V	5-3 ⎮		C
	65 3				5-3		
III		21⎮	B	VI			A

Fig. 5.146

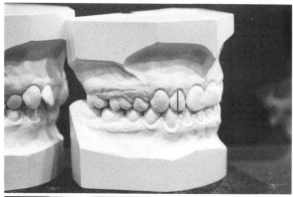

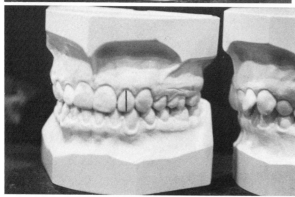

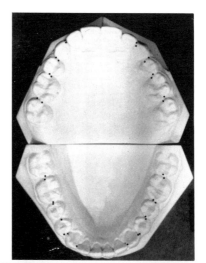

Ortho 1		Patient 2		NE		E x	
Key			Grade	Key			Grade
I	1mm Cl II		B	IV	65 3 ⎮ 3 56		D
					6 4 3 ⎮ 4 6		
II	6 32 ⎮ 2		C	V	5-3,2-1⎮1-2		C
	3						
III	21⎮		B	VI			A

Fig. 5.147

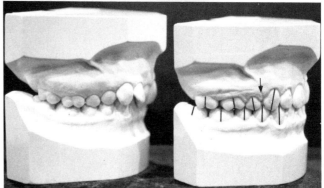

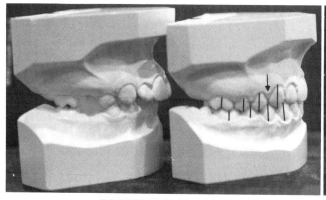

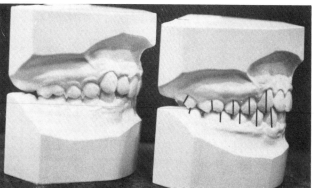

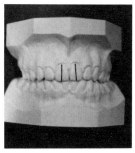

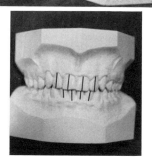

Ortho___1___   Patient___3___   NE_x___   E____

Key	Grade	Key	Grade
I 1mm Cl II	B	IV 65 |	B
II 6543 1|1 3 |	D	V 4-3, 1+1 |	C
III 6 21|	C	VI _____	A

Fig. 5.148

Ortho___1___   Patient___4___   NE_x___   E____

Key	Grade	Key	Grade
I 1mm Cl II	B	IV |	A
II 7 321|12 321|12	E	V |	A
III |	A	VI _____	A

Fig. 5.149

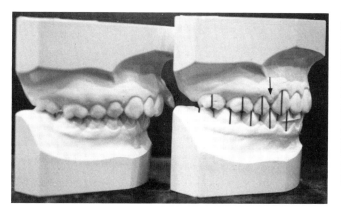

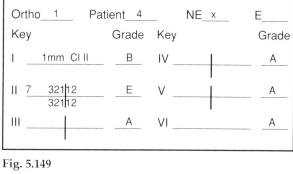

Ortho___1___   Patient___5___   NE____   E_x___

Key	Grade	Key	Grade
I 1mm Cl II	B	IV |	A
II 3 |	B	V 5-3 |	B
III | 21|	B	VI _____	A

Fig. 5.150

83

Summary for Orthodontist __1__

Patients __5__	NE __2__	E __3__	
Keys	50% or more	Less than 50%, but significant	Grade
I	5 casts		C+
II	6 3 / 3	7 21	D+
III		21 / 21	B
IV		65	B
V	4 casts		B−
VI			A

ORTHODONTIST #2

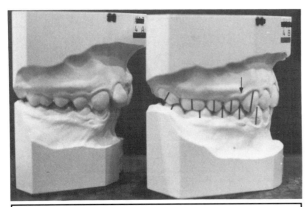

Ortho __2__	Patient __1__	NE __x__	E____	
Key		Grade	Key	Grade
I	1mm Cl II	B	IV	A
II	76 3 / 7	C	V 4-3	B
III	21 / 21	C	VI 3mm	B

Fig. 5.151

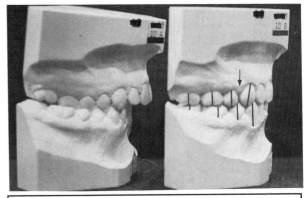

Ortho __2__	Patient __2__	NE____	E __x__	
Key		Grade	Key	Grade
I	2mm Cl II	C	IV	A
II	76 3 / 3	C	V 5-3	B
III	21	B	VI	A

Fig. 5.152

Summary for Orthodontist __2__

Patients __2__	NE __1__	E __1__	
Keys	50% or more	Less than 50%, but significant	Grade
I	2 casts		B−
II	76 3 / 7 3		C
III	21 / 21		B−
IV			A
V	2 casts		B
VI	1 cast		A−

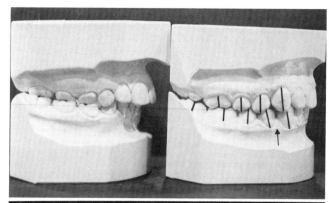

ORTHODONTIST #3

Ortho 3	Patient 1	NE x	E

Key		Grade	Key		Grade
I	1.5mm Cl II	B	IV		A
II	43	B	V	4-3	B
III		A	VI	3mm	B

Fig. 5.153

Ortho 3	Patient 2	NE	E x

Key		Grade	Key		Grade
I	2mm Cl II	C	IV	6	B
II	76 3 / 7 3	D	V	5-3	B
III	21	B	VI	3mm	B

Fig. 5.154

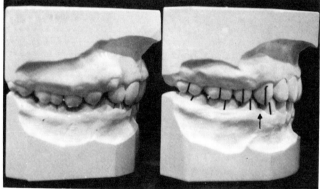

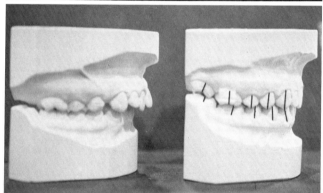

Ortho 3	Patient 3	NE x	E

Key		Grade	Key		Grade
I	2.5mm Cl II	D	IV		A
II	76543 / 76 43	E	V		A
III	21	B	VI	4mm	C

Fig. 5.155

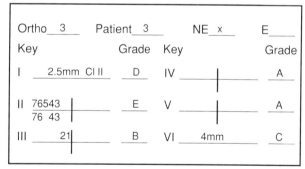

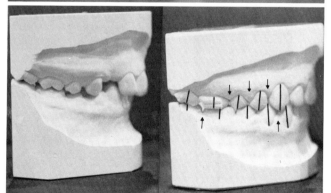

Ortho 3	Patient 4	NE x	E

Key		Grade	Key		Grade
I	1.5mm Cl II	B	IV		A
II	76543 / 43	E	V	6-5-4-3 / 7-6, 4-3	E
III	21	B	VI	3mm	B

Fig. 5.156

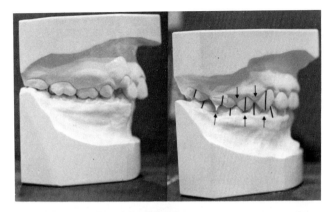

Ortho 3		Patient 5		NE		E x
Key		Grade	Key			Grade
I	1mm Cl II	B	IV			A
II	765 3 / 3	D	V	6-5-3 / 7-6-5-3		E
III	21	B	VI	4mm		C

Fig. 5.157

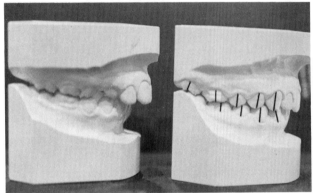

Ortho 3		Patient 6		NE x		E
Key		Grade	Key			Grade
I	2mm Cl II	C	IV			A
II	7 43 / 3	C	V			A
III	21	B	VI	4mm		C

Fig. 5.158

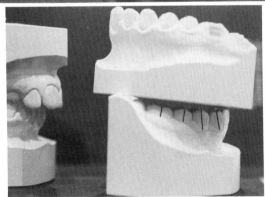

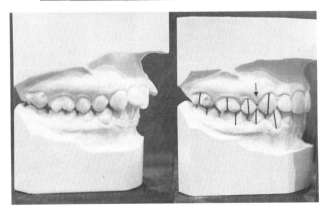

Ortho 3		Patient 7		NE		E x
Key		Grade	Key			Grade
I	1mm Cl II	B	IV	6		B
II	7 3 / 3	C	V	5-3		B
III	76 21	C	VI	3mm		B

Fig. 5.159

86

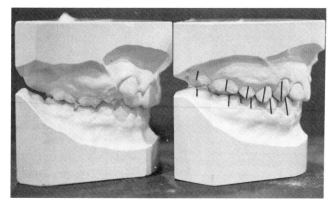

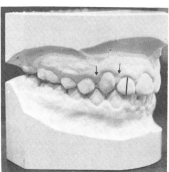

Ortho 3		Patient 8		NE x	E
Key		Grade	Key		Grade
I	2mm Cl II	C	IV 76 3		C
II	765432 / 76543	E	V 4-3-2		C
III	765	C	VI 3mm		B

Fig. 5.160

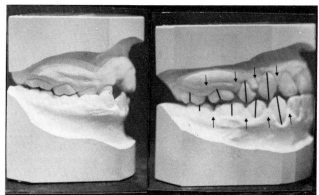

Ortho 3		Patient 9		NE	E x
Key		Grade	Key		Grade
I	Cl I	A	IV		A
II	6 3 / 7 3	C	V 7-6-5-3-2 / 7-6-5-3-2		E
III		A	VI		A

Fig. 5.161

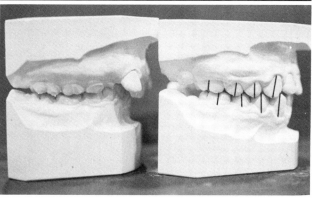

Ortho 3		Patient 10		NE x	E
Key		Grade	Key		Grade
I	1.5mm Cl II	B	IV		A
II	65 3 / 54	D	V		A
III	6	B	VI		A

Fig. 5.162

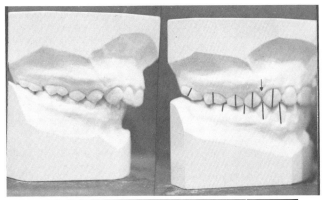

Ortho 3	Patient 11	NE x	E ___
Key	Grade	Key	Grade
I Cl I	A	IV |	A
II 7 3 |	C	V 4-3 |	B
43			
III 21 |	B	VI _____	A

Fig. 5.163

Summary for Orthodontist 3		
Patients 11 NE 7 E 4		
Keys	50% or more	Less than 50%, but significant	Grade
I	9 casts		B
II	76 3 |	54	D
	43	7	
III	21 |	6 |	B
IV	|	6 |	A–
V	8 casts		C+
VI	8 casts		B

ORTHODONTIST #4

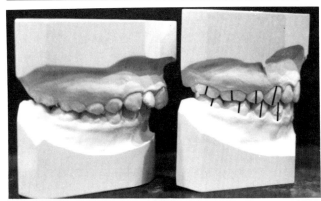

Ortho 4	Patient 1	NE ___	E x
Key	Grade	Key	Grade
I 2mm Cl II	C	IV 5 |	B
II 7 3 |	C	V |	A
3			
III 21 |	B	VI 3mm	B

Fig. 5.164

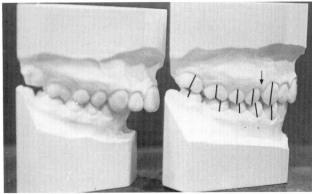

Ortho 4	Patient 2	NE x	E ___
Key	Grade	Key	Grade
I 3mm Cl II	E	IV 6 |	B
II 76 43 |	E	V 4-3 |	B
543			
III 21 |	B	VI 3mm	B

Fig. 5.165

ORTHODONTIST #2

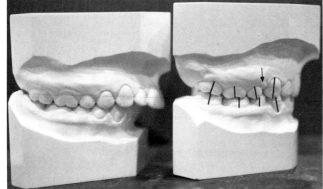

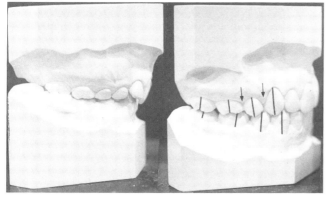

Ortho 4		Patient 3		NE		E x	
Key		Grade		Key			Grade
I	3mm Cl II	E		IV			A
II	7 5 3 / 3	C		V	5-3		B
III	7 21 /	C		VI	3mm		B

Fig. 5.166

Ortho 4		Patient 4		NE		E x	
Key		Grade		Key			Grade
I	2mm Cl II	C		IV			A
II	/	A		V	5-3 /		B
III	/	A		VI	3mm		B

Fig. 5.167

Ortho 4		Patient 5		NE		E x	
Key		Grade		Key			Grade
I	2mm Cl II	C		IV	6 /		B
II	7 5 3 /	C		V	6-5-3 /		C
III	21 /	B		VI			A

Fig. 5.168

Summary for Orthodontist 4			
Patients 5	NE 1	E 4	
Keys	50% or more	Less than 50%, but significant	Grade
I	5 casts		D
II	76 3 / 3	5 /	C
III	21 /	/	B
IV	/	6 /	B+
V	4 casts		B
VI	4 casts		B

89

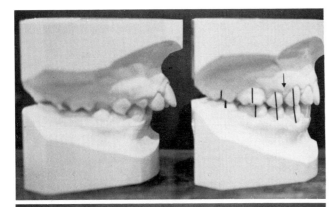

ORTHODONTIST #5

Ortho 5	Patient 1		NE		E x
Key		Grade	Key		Grade
I	3.5mm Cl II	E	IV		A
II	76 3 / 3	C	V	5-3	B
III		A	VI		A

Fig. 5.169

Ortho 5	Patient 2		NE x		E
Key		Grade	Key		Grade
I	1.5mm Cl II	B	IV		A
II	76 43	C	V	7-6-5-4-3	E
III	21 / 21	C	VI	3mm	B

Fig. 5.170

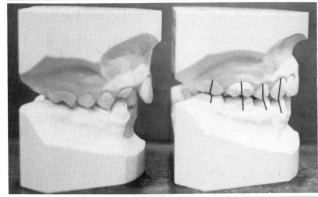

Ortho 5	Patient 3		NE		E x
Key		Grade	Key		Grade
I	3.5mm Cl II	E	IV		A
II	76 3 / 5 3	D	V		A
III	6 21	C	VI		A

Fig. 5.171

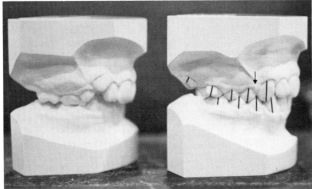

Ortho 5	Patient 4		NE x		E
Key		Grade	Key		Grade
I	1.5mm Cl II	B	IV		A
II	76543	D	V	5-3	B
III	21	B	VI		A

Fig. 5.172

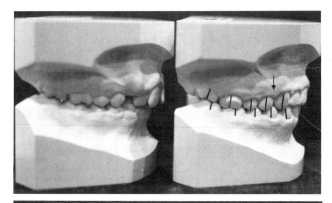

Ortho __5__	Patient __5__	NE __x__	E ____	
Key	Grade	Key		Grade
I __1.5mm Cl II__	B	IV __3__		B
II __76 43__ / __43__	D	V __4-3__		B
III __1__	B	VI __3mm__		B

Fig. 5.173

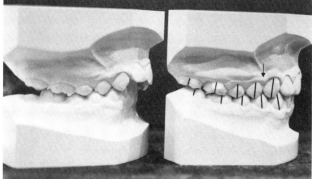

Ortho __5__	Patient __6__	NE __x__	E ____	
Key	Grade	Key		Grade
I __1.5mm Cl II__	B	IV ____		A
II __76 43__ / __43__	D	V __4-3__		B
III __1__	B	VI __3mm__		B

Fig. 5.174

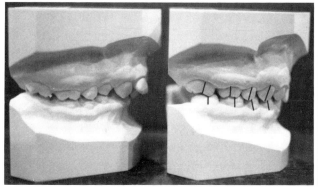

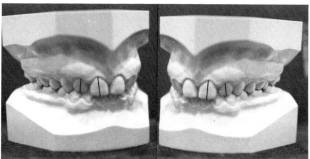

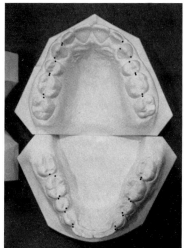

Ortho __5__	Patient __7__	NE ____	E __x__	
Key	Grade	Key		Grade
I __3mm Cl II__	E	IV __65__ / __65__	__3 5__ / __56__	E
II __765 3__ / __5 3__	D	V __5-3, 2-1__ / __1__	__1-2, 3-5__ / __1__	E
III __2__	__2__ B	VI __3mm__		B

Fig. 5.175

91

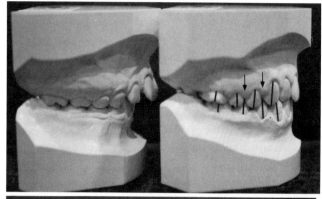

Ortho 5	Patient 8	NE x	E
Key	Grade	Key	Grade
I _2mm Cl II_	C	IV _5 3 |_	B
II _6 43 |_ / _43_	D	V _5-4-3 |_	C
III _2 |_	B	VI _4mm_	C

Fig. 5.176

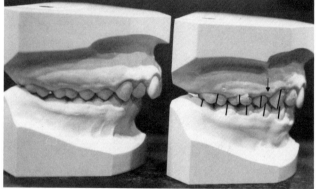

Ortho 5	Patient 9	NE	E x
Key	Grade	Key	Grade
I _2.5mm Cl II_	D	IV ___	A
II _7 3 |_ / _4_	C	V _5-3 |_	B
III _21|_	B	VI _3mm_	B

Fig. 5.177

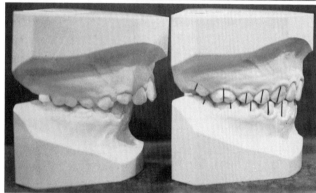

Ortho 5	Patient 10	NE x	E
Key	Grade	Key	Grade
I _3mm Cl II_	E	IV _5 |_	B
II _76543 |_ / _76_	E	V ___	A
III _21|_	B	VI ___	A

Fig. 5.178

Summary for Orthodontist 5			
Patients 10	NE 6	E 4	
Keys	50% or more	Less than 50%, but significant	Grade
I	_10 casts_		C–
II	_76 43 |_ / _3_	_5 |_ / _4_	D
III	_21|_	_|_	B
IV	_|_	_|_	A–
V	_8 casts_		B–
VI	_6 casts_		B+

ORTHODONTIST #6

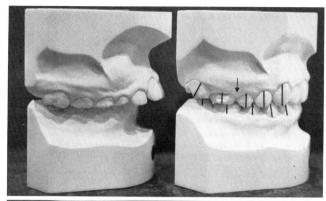

Ortho 6	Patient 1		NE x		E
Key		Grade	Key		Grade
I	1.5mm Cl II	B	IV	3	B
II	76 3 / 43	D	V	6-5	B
III	7 21	C	VI	3mm	B

Fig. 5.179

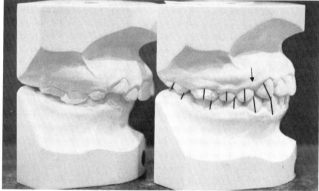

Ortho 6	Patient 2		NE x		E
Key		Grade	Key		Grade
I	Cl I	A	IV	3	B
II	76 3 / 43	D	V	4-3	B
III		A	VI	3mm	B

Fig. 5.180

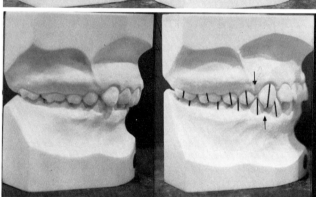

Ortho 6	Patient 3		NE x		E
Key		Grade	Key		Grade
I	Cl I	A	IV	3	B
II	7 3 / 3	C	V	4-3 / 4-3	C
III	3	B	VI		A

Fig. 5.181

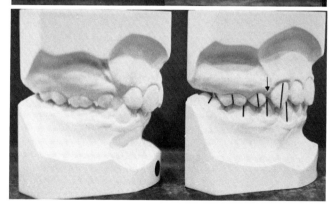

Ortho 6	Patient 4		NE		E x
Key		Grade	Key		Grade
I	1.5mm Cl II	B	IV	3	B
II	5 3 / 7 3	C	V	5-3	B
III	321	C	VI	3mm	B

Fig. 5.182

93

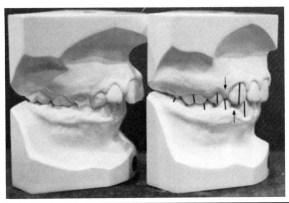

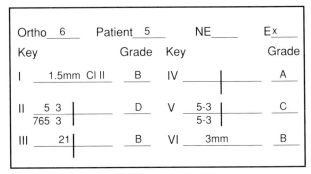

Ortho 6	Patient 5		NE___	Ex___
Key		Grade	Key	Grade
I 1.5mm Cl II		B	IV	A
II 5 3 / 765 3		D	V 5-3 / 5-3	C
III 21		B	VI 3mm	B

Fig. 5.183

Summary for Orthodontist 6			
Patients 5	NE 3	E 2	
Keys	50% or more	Less than 50%, but significant	Grade
I	3 casts		B+
II	7 3 / 3	6 / 7 4	D+
III	21	3	B
IV	3		B
V	5 casts		B–
VI	4 casts		B

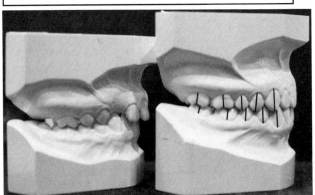

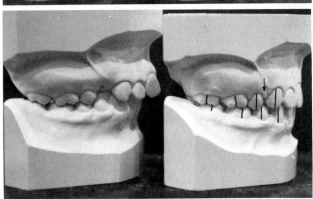

ORTHODONTIST #7

Ortho 7	Patient 1		NE x	E___
Key		Grade	Key	Grade
I 2mm Cl II		C	IV 6	B
II 7 43 / 3		C	V	A
III 21		B	VI	A

Fig. 5.184

Ortho 7	Patient 2		NE___	Ex___
Key		Grade	Key	Grade
I 2mm Cl II		C	IV 6	B
II 7 3 / 6		C	V 5-3	B
III		A	VI	A

Fig. 5.185

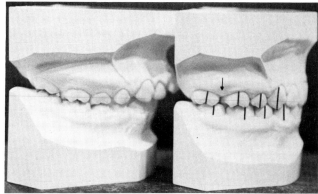

Ortho 7	Patient 3	NE	E x
Key	Grade	Key	Grade
I 2mm Cl II	C	IV 6 3 |	B
II 765 3 3 |	D	V 7-6 |	B
III 21 |	B	VI	A

Fig. 5.186

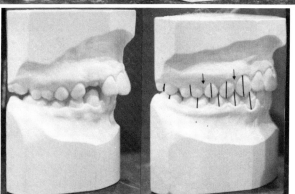

Ortho 7	Patient 4	NE x	E
Key	Grade	Key	Grade
I 1mm Cl II	B	IV |	A
II 7 43 | 43 |	D	V 6-5,4-3 |	C
III |	A	VI 3mm	B

Fig. 5.187

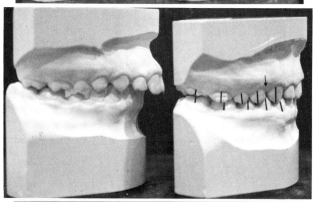

Ortho 7	Patient 5	NE x	E
Key	Grade	Key	Grade
I 2mm Cl II	C	IV |	B
II 76 3 | 4 3 |	D	V 4-3 |	B
III 21 |	B	VI 3mm	B

Fig. 5.188

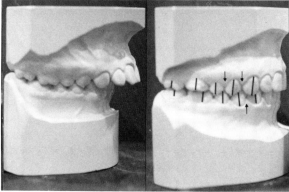

Ortho 7	Patient 6	NE x	E
Key	Grade	Key	Grade
I 2.5mm Cl II	D	IV |	A

II   76543 |
        43 |
	E	V 5-4-3 |
		        4-3 |
			D

III 21 |	B	VI	A

Fig. 5.189

95

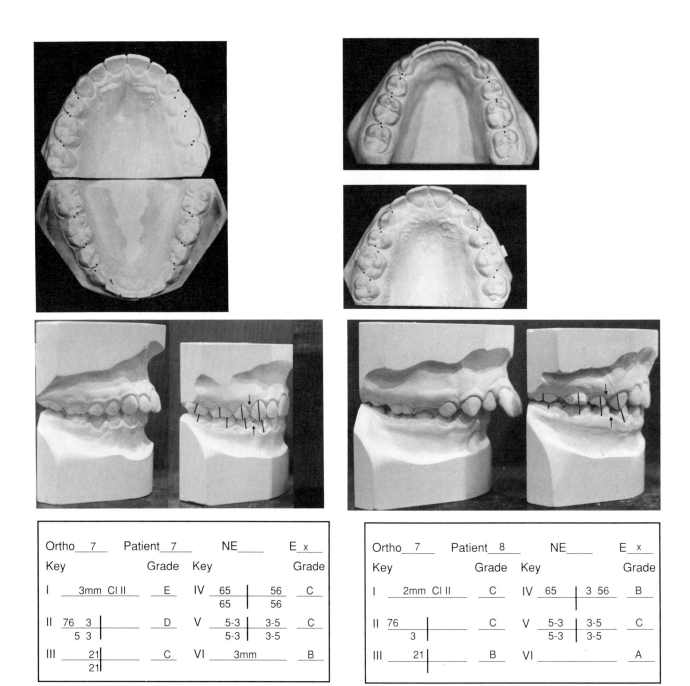

Ortho 7	Patient 7		NE___		E x	
Key		Grade	Key			Grade
I	3mm Cl II	E	IV	65 | 56		C
				65 | 56		
II	76 3 |	D	V	5-3 | 3-5		C
	5 3 |			5-3 | 3-5		
III	21|	C	VI	3mm		B
	21|					

Fig. 5.190

Ortho 7	Patient 8		NE___		E x	
Key		Grade	Key			Grade
I	2mm Cl II	C	IV	65 | 3 56		B
II	76	C	V	5-3 | 3-5		C
	3 |			5-3 | 3-5		
III	21|	B	VI			A

Fig. 5.191

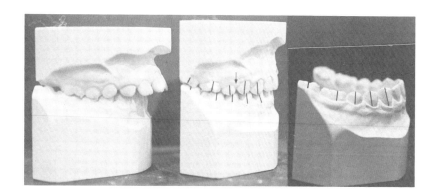

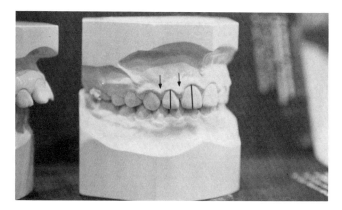

Ortho 7		Patient 9	NE x		E
Key		Grade	Key		Grade
I	2.5mm Cl II	D	IV		A
II	76 4 21 / 43	E	V	5-4,3-2-1	D
III		A	VI	4mm	C

Fig. 5.192

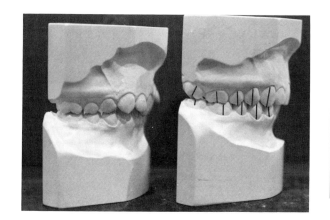

Ortho 7		Patient 10	NE x		E
Key		Grade	Key		Grade
I	2mm Cl II	C	IV		A
II	7 43 / 3	C	V		A
III	21 / 21	C	VI		A

Fig. 5.193

97

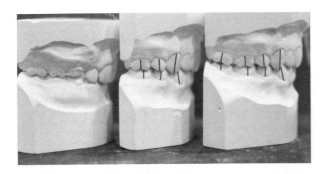

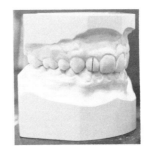

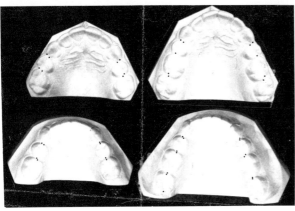

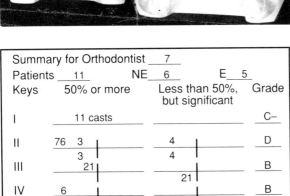

Ortho	7	Patient	11	NE		E	x
Key			Grade	Key			Grade
I	3.5mm Cl II		E	IV	65 | 56		C
					5 | 5 7		
II	76 32 |		D	V	|		A
	5 3 |						
III	21 |		C	VI			A
	21 |						

Fig. 5.194

Summary for Orthodontist	7			
Patients 11	NE 6		E 5	
Keys	50% or more	Less than 50%, but significant		Grade
I	11 casts			C–
II	76 3 |	4 |		D
	3 |	4 |		
III	21 |			B
		21 |		
IV	6 |			B
V	8 casts			B–
VI		4 casts		A–

ORTHODONTIST #8

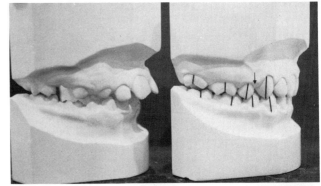

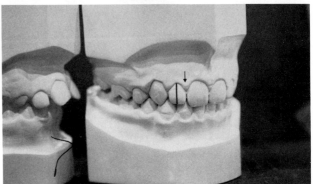

Ortho	8	Patient	1	NE		E	x
Key			Grade	Key			Grade
I	2mm Cl II		C	IV	|		A
II	765 32 |		E	V	5-3,2-1 |		C
	76 3 |						
III	76 21 |		C	VI	3mm		B
	|						

Fig. 5.195

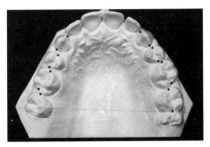

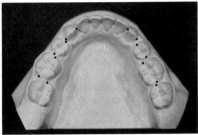

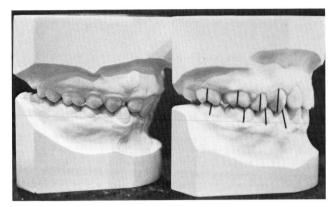

Ortho __8__   Patient __2__   NE____   E _x_

Key		Grade	Key		Grade
I	2mm Cl II	C	IV	65 3 | 56 / 65 3 | 3 56	D
II	765 3 | / 5 3 |	D	V	5-3 | 1-2,3-5 / 5-3 |	C
III	76 |	B	VI		A

Fig. 5.196

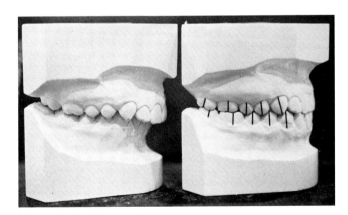

Ortho __8__   Patient __3__   NE _x_   E____

Key		Grade	Key		Grade
I	Cl I	A	IV	3 |	B
II	76 |	B	V	|	A
III	6 | / 6 |	B	VI		A

Fig. 5.197

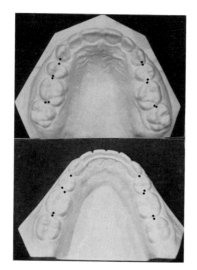

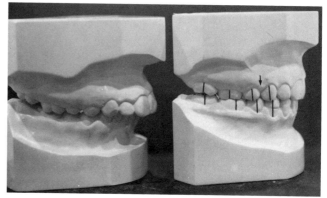

Ortho 8		Patient 4		NE		E x
Key	Grade			Key		Grade
I 2.5mm Cl II	D		IV	6 / 6 | 3 6 / 56		B
II 76 / 7 |	C		V	5-3 |		B
III 76 21 / 6 |	D		VI			A

Fig. 5.198

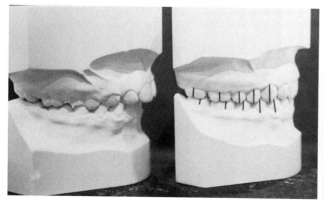

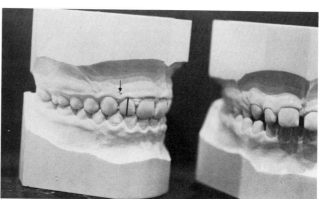

Ortho 8		Patient 5		NE x		E
Key	Grade			Key		Grade
I 2mm Cl II	C		IV |			A
II 76 32 / 3 |	D		V 3-2 |			B
III 21 |	B		VI			A

Fig. 5.199

Summary for Orthodontist 8			
Patients 5		NE 2	E 3
Keys	50% or more	Less than 50%, but significant	Grade
I	4 casts		C
II	76 3 / 3 |	5 |	D+
III	6 21 |	7 / 7 |	C+
IV	|	6 3 / 6 |	B
V	4 casts		B
VI			A

100

ORTHODONTIST #9

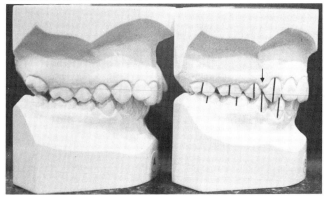

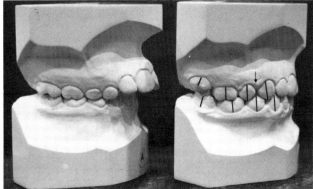

Ortho __9__ Patient __1__ NE ____ E _x_

Key	Grade	Key	Grade
I __2mm Cl II__	C	IV _____	A
II __76 3 |__	C	V __5-3 |__	B
III __21 |__	C	VI _____	A
__21 |__			

Fig. 5.200

Ortho __9__ Patient __2__ NE ____ E _x_

Key	Grade	Key	Grade
I __Cl I__	A	IV ____ | ____	A
II __76 |__	D	V __5-3 |__	B
__76 3__			
III __7 21 |__	C	VI _____	A

Fig. 5.201

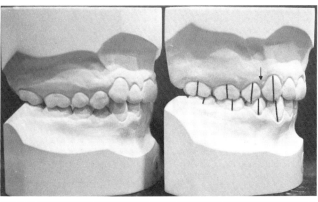

Ortho __9__ Patient __3__ NE ____ E _x_

Key	Grade	Key	Grade
I __2mm Cl II__	C	IV ____ | ____	A
II __7 5 32 |__	D	V __5-3-2 |__	C
__3__			
III __21 |__	B	VI _____	A

Fig. 5.202

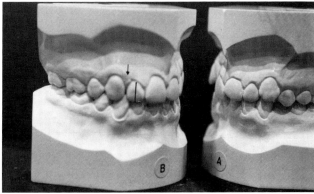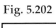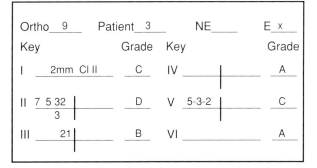

Summary for Orthodontist __9__

Patients __3__ NE ____ E __3__

Keys	50% or more	Less than 50%, but significant	Grade
I	2 casts		B
II	76 3 |	2 |	D+
	3 |	6	
III	21 |		C+
		21 |	
IV	____ | ____	____ | ____	A
V	3 casts		B
VI			A

101

ORTHODONTIST #10

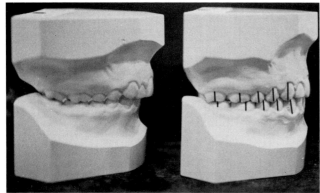

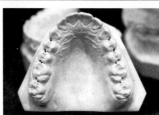

Ortho 10	Patient 1	NE x	E
Key	Grade	Key	Grade
I 2mm Cl II	C	IV 654 | 456	C
II 76 3 | 3	C	V |	A
III 21|	B	VI	A

Fig. 5.203

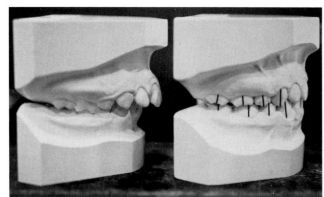

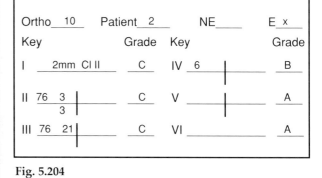

Ortho 10	Patient 2	NE	E x
Key	Grade	Key	Grade
I 2mm Cl II	C	IV 6 |	B
II 76 3 | 3	C	V |	A
III 76 21|	C	VI	A

Fig. 5.204

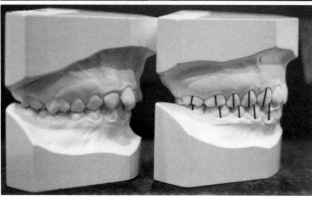

Ortho 10	Patient 3	NE x	E
Key	Grade	Key	Grade
I 1.5mm Cl II	B	IV 6 |	B
II 7 43 | 6	C	V |	A
III 76 21|	C	VI	A

Fig. 5.205

102

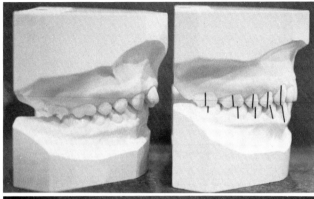

Ortho 10	Patient 4	NE x	E
Key	Grade	Key	Grade
I 2mm Cl II	C	IV 6	B
II 543 / 6 43	D	V	A
III	A	VI	A

Fig. 5.206

Ortho 10	Patient 5	NE	E x
Key	Grade	Key	Grade
I 1.5mm Cl II	B	IV	A
II 7 / 3	B	V 5-3	B
III	A	VI	A

Fig. 5.207

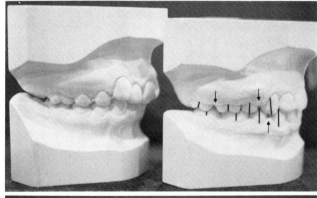

Ortho 10	Patient 6	NE	E x
Key	Grade	Key	Grade
I Cl I	A	IV	A
II 76	B	V 7-6,5-3 / 5-3	D
III	A	VI	A

Fig. 5.208

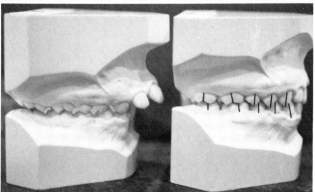

Ortho 10	Patient 7	NE x	E
Key	Grade	Key	Grade
I 2mm Cl II	C	IV 6	B
II 7 543 / 6 3	D	V	A
III 21	B	VI	A

Fig. 5.209

103

Summary for Orthodontist 10			
Patients 7	NE 4	E 3	
Keys	50% or more	Less than 50%, but significant	Grade
I	6 casts		B–
II	7 3 / 3	654 / 6	C
III	21	76	B
IV	6		B
V		2 casts	B+
VI			A

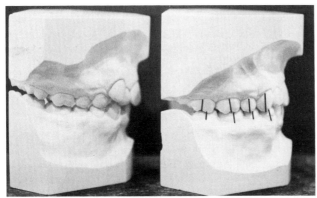

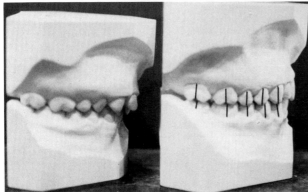

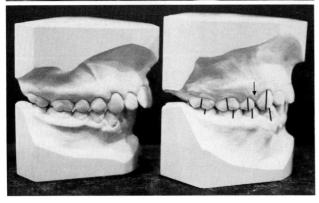

ORTHODONTIST #11

Ortho 11	Patient 1		NE		E x
Key		Grade	Key		Grade
I	2mm Cl II	C	IV		A
II	7 3 / 65 3	D	V		A
III		A	VI		A

Fig. 5.210

Ortho 11	Patient 2		NE x		E
Key		Grade	Key		Grade
I	3.5mm Cl II	E	IV	6	B
II	76543 / 43	E	V		A
III	21 / 21	C	VI	3mm	B

Fig. 5.211

Ortho 11	Patient 3		NE		E x
Key		Grade	Key		Grade
I	2mm Cl II	C	IV		A
II	7 3 / 3	C	V	5-3	B
III		A	VI	3mm	B

Fig. 5.212

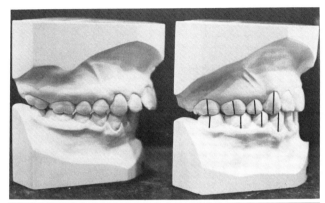

Ortho 11	Patient 4	NE	E x
Key	Grade	Key	Grade
I 1.5mm Cl II	B	IV 6 3	B
II 3	B	V	A
III 21	B	VI	A

Fig. 5.213

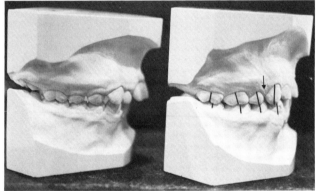

Ortho 11	Patient 5	NE	E x
Key	Grade	Key	Grade
I 3mm Cl II	E	IV	A
II 765 3 / 65 3	E	V 5-3	B
III	A	VI 3mm	B

Fig. 5.214

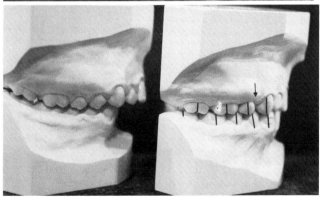

Ortho 11	Patient 6	NE	E x
Key	Grade	Key	Grade
I 2.5mm Cl II	D	IV	A
II 3 / 43	C	V 5-3	B
III	A	VI	A

Fig. 5.215

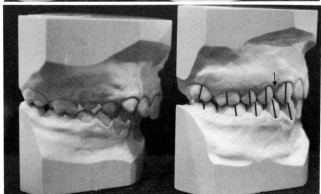

Ortho 11	Patient 7	NE x	E
Key	Grade	Key	Grade
I 1.5mm Cl II	B	IV 65	B
II 7 3 / 76 43	D	V 4-3	B
III 21	B	VI	A

Fig. 5.216

105

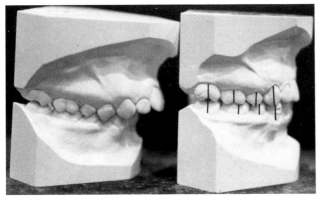

Ortho 11	Patient 8	NE	E x
Key	Grade	Key	Grade
I 2mm Cl II	C	IV |	A
II 76 3 | 3	C	V |	A
III |	A	VI	A

Fig. 5.217

Summary for Orthodontist 11			
Patients 8	NE 2	E 6	
Keys	50% or more	Less than 50%, but significant	Grade
I	8 casts		C–
II	7 3 | 3	65 | 7654	D+
III	|	21|	A–
IV	|	|	A–
V	4 casts		A–
VI		3 casts	A–

ORTHODONTIST #12

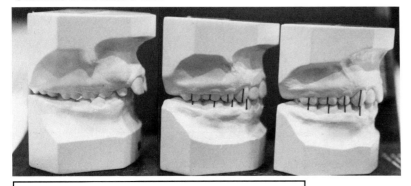

Ortho 12	Patient 1	NE	E x
Key	Grade	Key	Grade
I 2mm Cl II	C	IV |	A
II 76 3 |	C	V |	A
III 21|	B	VI	A

Fig. 5.218

106

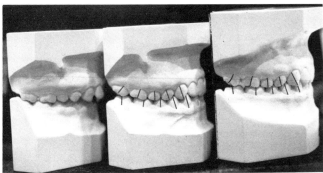

Ortho 12		Patient 2		NE x		E____	
Key		Grade		Key		Grade	
I	1.5mm Cl II	B		IV			A
II	76 43 / 7 43	E		V			A
III	21	B		VI	3mm		B

Fig. 5.219

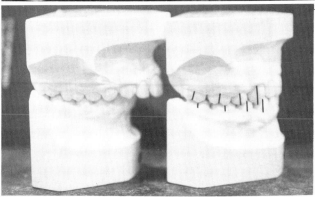

Ortho 12		Patient 3		NE____		E x	
Key		Grade		Key		Grade	
I	2mm Cl II	C		IV			A
II	76 3	C		V			A
III	21	B		VI	3mm		B

Fig. 5.220

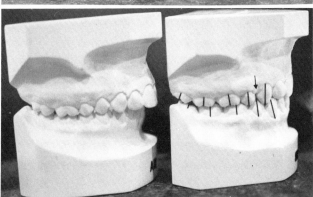

Ortho 12		Patient 4		NE____		E x	
Key		Grade		Key		Grade	
I	Cl I	A		IV			A
II	87 3 / 43	D		V	5-3		B
III	21	B		VI			A

Fig. 5.221

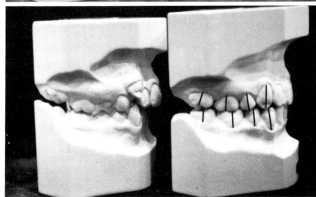

Ortho 12		Patient 5		NE____		E x	
Key		Grade		Key		Grade	
I	2mm Cl II	C		IV			A
II	76 3 / 43	D		V			A
III	21	B		VI			A

Fig. 5.222

107

Summary for Orthodontist 12			
Patients 5	NE 1	E 4	
Keys	50% or more	Less than 50%, but significant	Grade
I	4 casts		B–
II	76 3		D
	3	4	
III	21		B
IV			A
V			A
VI		2 casts	A–

ORTHODONTIST #13

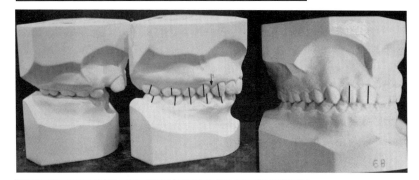

Ortho 13	Patient 1	NE x	E		
Key		Grade	Key		Grade
I	3mm Cl II	E	IV		A
II	76 21	D	V	4-3	B
	3				
III	21	B	VI	3mm	B

Fig. 5.223

Ortho 13	Patient 2	NE x	E		
Key		Grade	Key		Grade
I	2mm Cl II	C	IV	65	B
II	7 3	C	V	4-3	B
	3				
III	21	B	VI	3mm	B

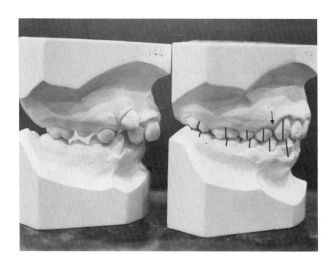

Fig. 5.224

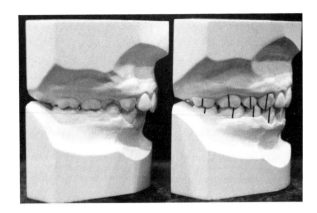

Ortho 13		Patient 3		NE ___		E x	
Key			Grade	Key			Grade
I	2mm Cl II		C	IV	65 |		B
II	7 3 |		B	V	|		A
III	21|		C	VI	_____		A
	21|						

Fig. 5.225

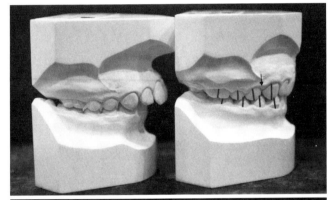

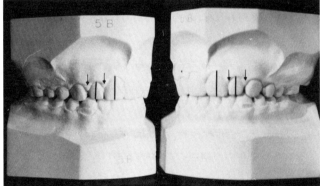

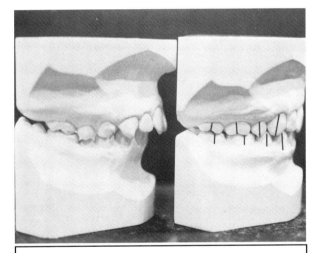

Ortho 13		Patient 4		NE x		E ___	
Key			Grade	Key			Grade
I	2mm Cl II		C	IV	|		A
II	6 321 | 12		D	V	4-3-2-1 | 1-2-3		D
	43 |						
III	21|		C	VI	3mm		B
	21|						

Fig. 5.226

Ortho 13		Patient 5		NE ___		E x	
Key			Grade	Key			Grade
I	2mm Cl II		C	IV	|		A
II	7 3 |		C	V	|		A
	3						
III	21|		B	VI	3mm		B

Fig. 5.227

109

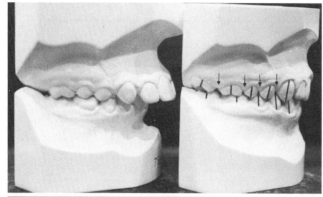

Ortho 13	Patient 6		NE x	E
Key		Grade	Key	Grade
I	1.5mm Cl II	B	IV	A
II	76543 / 43	E	V 7-6-5-4-3	E
III	21	B	VI	A

Fig. 5.228

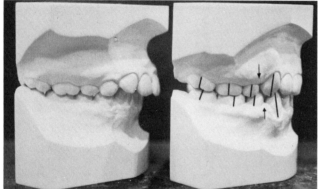

Ortho 13	Patient 7		NE	E x
Key		Grade	Key	Grade
I	2mm Cl II	C	IV	A
II	765 3 / 3	D	V 5-3 / 5-3	C
III	21	B	VI	A

Fig. 5.229

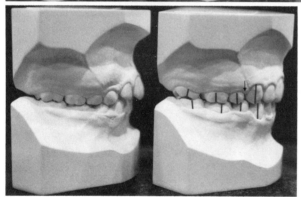

Ortho 13	Patient 8		NE	E x
Key		Grade	Key	Grade
I	2mm Cl II	C	IV 6	B
II	76 3 / 7 3	D	V 5-3	B
III	7 21 / 7	C	VI	A

Fig. 5.230

Summary for Orthodontist 13			
Patients 8	NE 4	E 4	
Keys	50% or more	Less than 50%, but significant	Grade
I	8 casts		C
II	76 3 / 3	21 / 4	D+
III	21	21	B–
IV		65	A–
V	6 casts		B–
VI	4 casts		A–

110

ORTHODONTIST #14

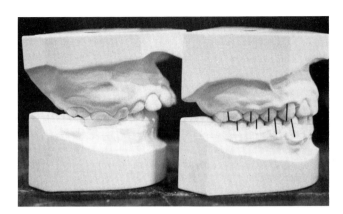

Ortho 14	Patient 1		NE x	E
Key		Grade	Key	Grade
I	2mm Cl II	C	IV	A
II	3 / 6 43	C	V	A
III		A	VI	A

Fig. 5.231

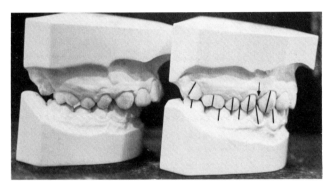

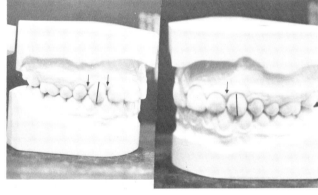

Ortho 14	Patient 2		NE x	E
Key		Grade	Key	Grade
I	1mm Cl II	B	IV	A
II	76 43 / 43 3	D	V 4-3-2 | 2-3	C
III	21	B	VI 4mm	C

Fig. 5.232

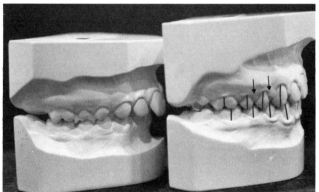

Ortho 14	Patient 3		NE x	E
Key		Grade	Key	Grade
I	2mm Cl II	C	IV	A
II	6 3 / 3	C	V 5-4-3	C
III		A	VI	A

Fig. 5.233

111

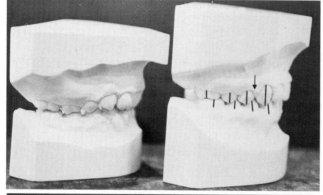

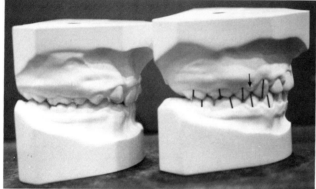

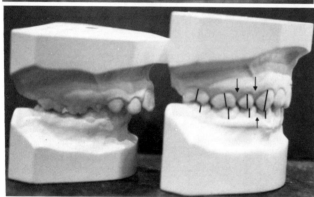

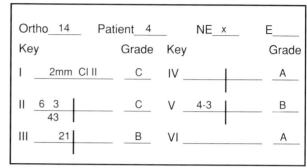

Ortho 14	Patient 4	NE x	E
Key	Grade	Key	Grade
I 2mm Cl II	C	IV ⊥	A
II 6 3 / 43	C	V 4-3 ⊥	B
III 21 ⊥	B	VI	A

Fig. 5.234

Ortho 14	Patient 5	NE	E x
Key	Grade	Key	Grade
I 1mm Cl II	B	IV ⊥	A
II 76 3 / 65 3	D	V 5-3 ⊥	B
III 6 / 21	C	VI	A

Fig. 5.235

Ortho 14	Patient 6	NE	E x
Key	Grade	Key	Grade
I 2.5mm Cl II	D	IV ⊥	A
II 7 3 / 6	C	V 6-5-3 / 5-3	D
III 21 / 21	C	VI 3mm	B

Fig. 5.236

Summary for Orthodontist 14			
Patients 6	NE 4	E 2	
Keys	50% or more	Less than 50%, but significant	Grade
I	6 casts		C
II	76 3 / 6 43		C
III	21		B
IV			A
V	5 casts		B−
VI		2 casts	A−

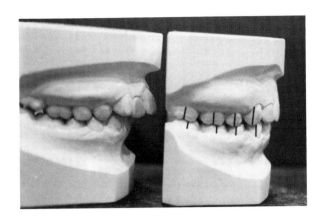

ORTHODONTIST #15

Ortho 15	Patient 1		NE		E x
Key		Grade	Key		Grade
I	3mm Cl II	E	IV	6	B
II	765 3 / 3	D	V		A
III		A	VI	3mm	B

Fig. 5.237

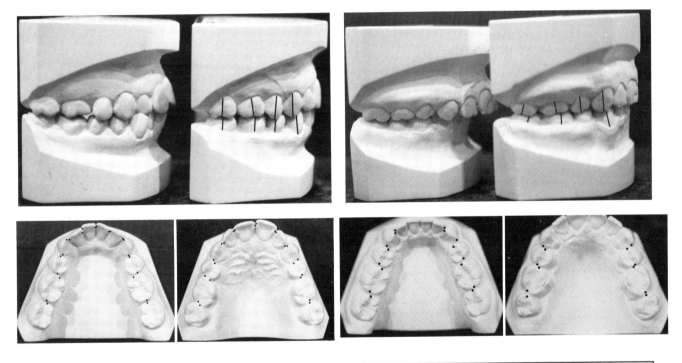

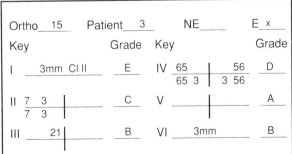

Ortho 15	Patient 2		NE		E x
Key		Grade	Key		Grade
I	3mm Cl II	E	IV	65 2 123 5 / 65 3 1 123 56	E
II	7 5 3 / 3	C	V		A
III	21	B	VI		A

Fig. 5.238

Ortho 15	Patient 3		NE		E x
Key		Grade	Key		Grade
I	3mm Cl II	E	IV	65 56 / 65 3 3 56	D
II	7 3 / 7 3	C	V		A
III	21	B	VI	3mm	B

Fig. 5.239

113

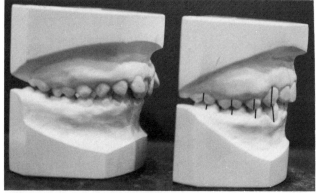

Ortho 15	Patient 4	NE	E x
Key	Grade	Key	Grade
I 3mm Cl II	E	IV	A
II 76 3 |	C	V	A
3			
III 21|	B	VI 4mm	C

Fig. 5.240

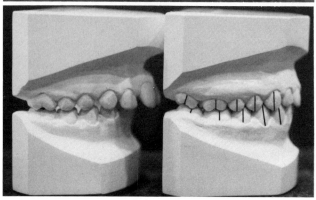

Ortho 15	Patient 5	NE x	E
Key	Grade	Key	Grade
I 2mm Cl II	C	IV 65 |	B
II 76 3 |	D	V	A
7 43			
III |	A	VI 3mm	B

Fig. 5.241

Summary for Orthodontist 15			
Patients 5 NE 1 E 4			
Keys	50% or more	Less than 50%, but significant	Grade
I	5 casts		E+
II	76 3 |	5 |	C−
	3	7	
III	21|	|	B+
IV	65 |	5 |	C
		65 3 | 3 56	
V			A
VI	4 casts		B

ORTHODONTIST #16

Ortho 16	Patient 1	NE	E x
Key	Grade	Key	Grade
I 1.5mm Cl II	B	IV 3 |	B
II 765 3 |	C	V 5-3 |	B
III 21|	B	VI 3mm	B

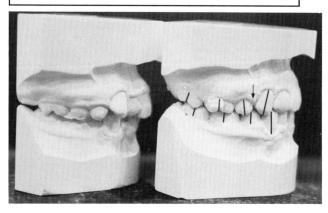

Fig. 5.242

114

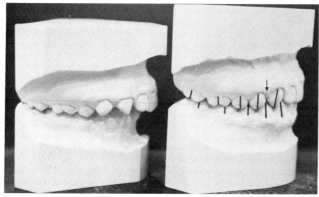

Ortho 16		Patient 2		NE x		E
Key		Grade	Key			Grade
I	Cl I	A	IV			A
II	7 3 / 43	C	V	4-3		B
III	21	B	VI	4mm		C

Fig. 5.243

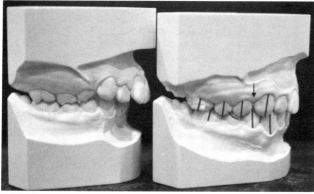

Ortho 16		Patient 3		NE x		E
Key		Grade	Key			Grade
I	1mm Cl II	B	IV			A
II	6543 / 43	D	V	4-3		B
III	21 / 21	C	VI	4mm		C

Fig. 5.244

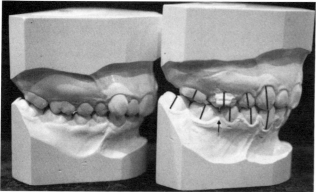
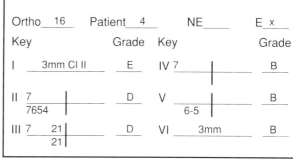

Ortho 16		Patient 4		NE		E x
Key		Grade	Key			Grade
I	3mm Cl II	E	IV	7		B
II	7 / 7654	D	V	6-5		B
III	7 21 / 21	D	VI	3mm		B

Fig. 5.245

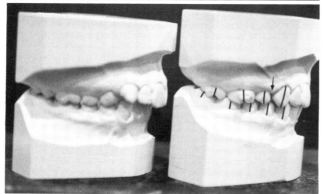

Ortho 16		Patient 5		NE		E x
Key		Grade	Key			Grade
I	2mm Cl II	C	IV	7		B
II	7 3	B	V	5-3		B
III		B	21	VI	3mm	B

Fig. 5.246

115

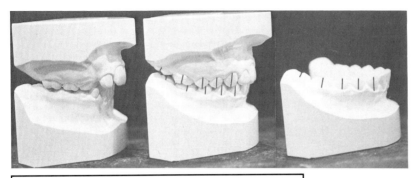

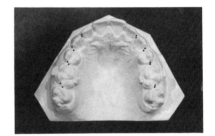

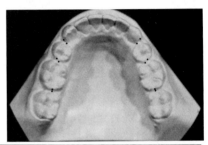

Ortho 16		Patient 6		NE x		E
Key		Grade	Key			Grade
I	1.5mm Cl II	B	IV	|		A
II	76543 |	D	V	|		A
III	21|	B	VI	4mm		C

Fig. 5.247

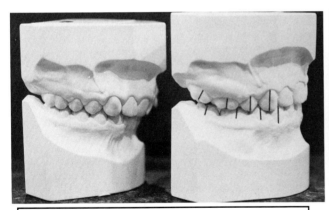

Ortho 16		Patient 7		NE		E x
Key		Grade	Key			Grade
I	Cl I	A	IV	6 |		B
II	76 3|	C	V	|		A
III	21|	B	VI	4mm		C

Fig. 5.248

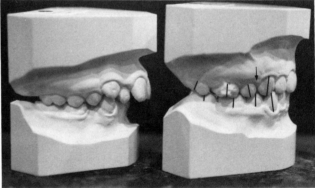

Ortho 16		Patient 8		NE		E x
Key		Grade	Key			Grade
I	2mm Cl II	C	IV	65 3 | 3 5 / 5 | 5		C
II	765 3| / 3	D	V	5-3 |		B
III	21|	B	VI	3mm		B

Fig. 5.249

116

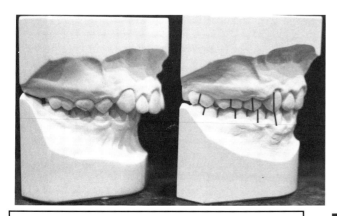

Ortho 16	Patient 9	NE	E x
Key	Grade	Key	Grade
I 2.5mm Cl II	D	IV 6	B
II 76 3 / 3	C	V	A
III 21 / 21	C	VI 3mm	B

Fig. 5.250

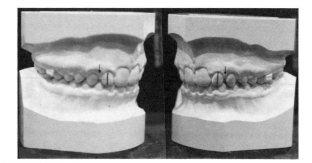

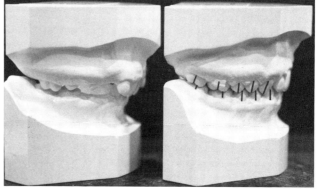

Ortho 16	Patient 11	NE x	E
Key	Grade	Key	Grade
I 2mm Cl II	C	IV	A
II 765432 / 2	D	V 3-2 / 2-3	B
III 21	B	VI 4mm	C

Fig. 5.252

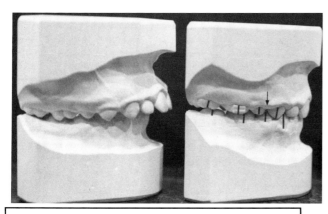

Ortho 16	Patient 10	NE	E x
Key	Grade	Key	Grade
I 2mm Cl II	C	IV 6	B
II 76 3 / 3	C	V 5-3	B
III 21	B	VI 3mm	B

Fig. 5.251

Summary for Orthodontist 16			
Patients 11	NE 4	E 7	
Keys	50% or more	Less than 50%, but significant	Grade
I	9 casts		C+
II	76 3	54 / 43	C−
III	21	21	B−
IV		6	B+
V	8 casts		B+
VI	11 casts		B−

117

ORTHODONTIST #17

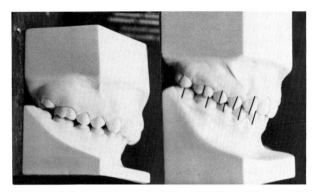
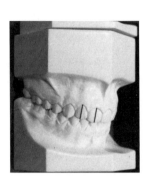

Ortho 17	Patient 1	NE x	E
Key	Grade	Key	Grade
I 1mm Cl II	B	IV	A
II 76 4321|	D	V	A
III 21| / 21|	C	VI	A

Fig. 5.253

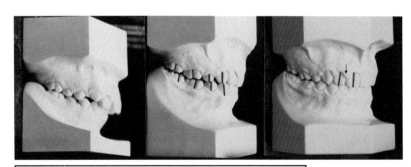

Ortho 17	Patient 2	NE	E x
Key	Grade	Key	Grade
I 2.5mm Cl II	D	IV	A
II 7 321| / 76 43	E	V 2-1	B
III 76 21|	C	VI 3mm	B

Fig. 5.254

118

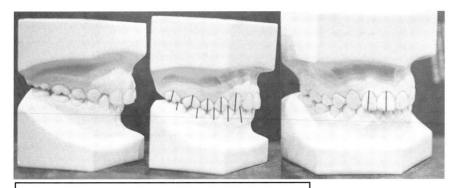

Ortho__17__		Patient__3__		NE__x__		E____	
Key		Grade	Key				Grade
I	Cl I	A	IV				A
II	76 321 / 543	E	V				A
III		A	VI	3mm			B

Fig. 5.255

Ortho__17__		Patient__4__		NE____		E_x_	
Key		Grade	Key				Grade
I	2mm Cl II	C	IV	6			B
II	7 321 / 3	D	V				A
III	21 / 21	C	VI	3mm			B

Fig. 5.256

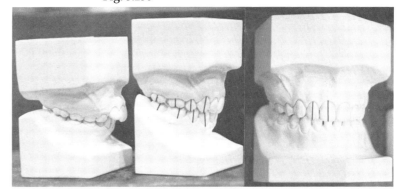

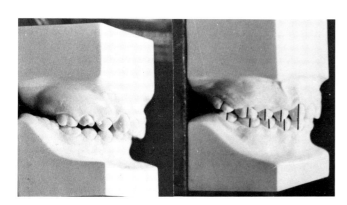

Ortho__17__		Patient__5__		NE__x__		E____	
Key		Grade	Key				Grade
I	2mm Cl II	C	IV				A
II	76 3	C	V				A
III	21	B	VI	4mm			C

Fig. 5.257

119

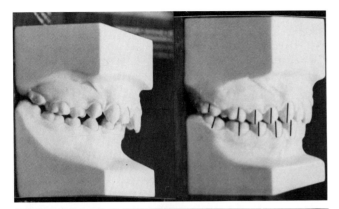

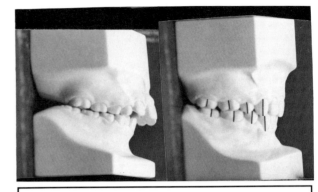

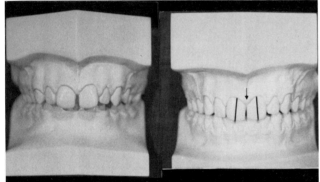

Ortho __17__   Patient __7__   NE____   E _x_

Key		Grade	Key		Grade
I	2mm Cl II	C	IV		A
II	7 3 / 3	C	V		A
III	21 / 21	C	VI		A

Fig. 5.259

Ortho __17__   Patient __6__   NE _x_   E____

Key		Grade	Key		Grade
I	2mm Cl II	C	IV	6	B
II	76543 1 / 7 ... 1	E	V	1-1	B
III	6 21	C	VI	3mm	B

Fig. 5.258

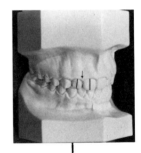

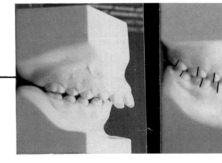

Ortho __17__   Patient __8__   NE _x_   E____

Key		Grade	Key		Grade
I	Cl I	A	IV		A
II	7 321 / 543	E	V	2-1	B
III	21	B	VI	4mm	C

Fig. 5.260

120

Summary for Orthodontist ___17___

Patients ___8___   NE ___5___   E ___3___

Keys	50% or more	Less than 50%, but significant	Grade
I	6 casts		B–
II	76 321| 3	4|	D
III	21|	7 54 6 21|	B–
IV	|	6 |	A
V		3 casts	A–
VI	6 casts		B

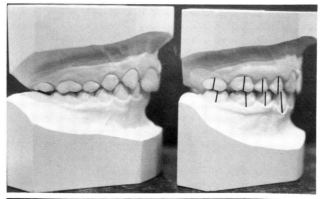

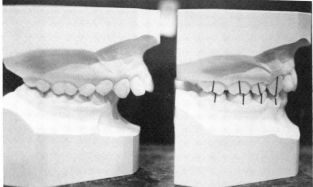

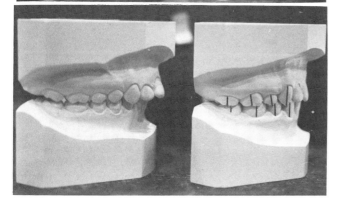

ORTHODONTIST #18

Ortho ___18___   Patient ___1___   NE_____   E _x_

Key		Grade	Key		Grade
I	3mm Cl II	E	IV	65|	B
II	7654 / 6 3 |	D	V	|	A
III	65 3 1|	C	VI		A

Fig. 5.261

Ortho ___18___   Patient ___2___   NE_____   E _x_

Key		Grade	Key		Grade
I	3.5mm Cl II	E	IV	|	A
II	7 5 3 / 5 3 |	D	V	|	A
III	|	A	VI	4mm	C

Fig. 5.262

Ortho ___18___   Patient ___3___   NE_____   E _x_

Key		Grade	Key		Grade
I	2mm Cl II	C	IV	6|	B
II	7 5 3 / 3 |	C	V	|	A
III	7 21|	C	VI		A

Fig. 5.263

121

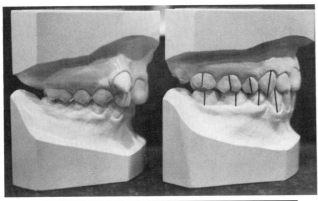

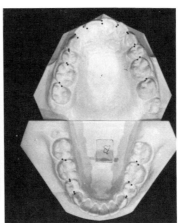

Ortho 18	Patient 4	NE	E x
Key	Grade	Key	Grade
I 2.5mm Cl II	D	IV 6 321|12 56 / 6	C
II 7 3 |	B	V |	A
III | 21	B	VI 3mm	B

Fig. 5.264

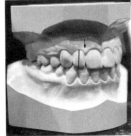

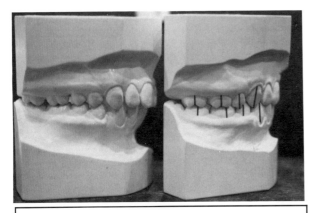

Ortho 18	Patient 5	NE	E x
Key	Grade	Key	Grade
I 2.5mm Cl II	D	IV |	A
II 76 3 | / 3	C	V |	A
III | 21 |	B	VI 3mm	B

Fig. 5.265

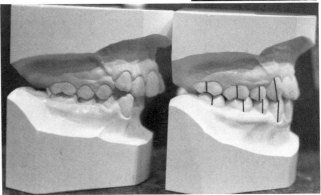

Ortho 18	Patient 6	NE	E x
Key	Grade	Key	Grade
I 2mm Cl II	C	IV |	A
II 2 |	B	V 2-1 |	B
III |	A	VI	A

Fig. 5.266

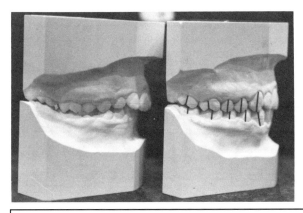

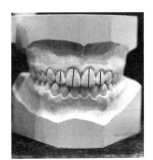

Ortho 18	Patient 7		NE x	E	
Key		Grade	Key		Grade
I	2mm Cl II	C	IV		A
II	7 54321 12 / 3	E	V		A
III	21	B	VI	3mm	B

Fig. 5.267

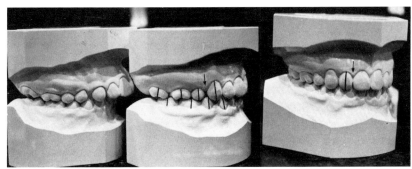

Ortho 18	Patient 8		NE	E x	
Key		Grade	Key		Grade
I	1mm Cl III	B	IV	6	B
II	7 2 / 5 3	C	V	5-3,2-1	C
III	7	B	VI	3mm	B

Fig. 5.268

Summary for Orthodontist 18				
Patients 8		NE 9	E 1	
Keys	50% or more	Less than 50%, but significant		Grade
I	8 casts			D+
II	7 3 / 3	65 2		C
III		7 21 / 21		B
IV	6			B+
V		2 casts		A–
VI	5 casts			B+

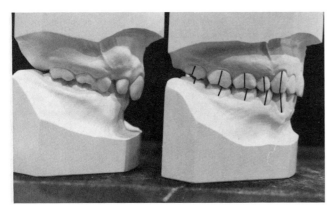

ORTHODONTIST #19

Ortho 19	Patient 1		NE	E x
Key		Grade	Key	Grade
I 3mm Cl II		E	IV	A
II 8765 3 / 765 3		E	V	A
III 21 / 21		C	VI	A

Fig. 5.269

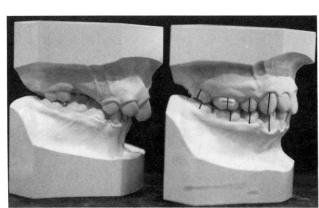

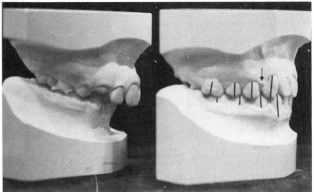

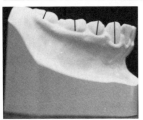

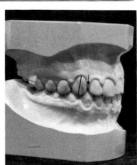

Ortho 19	Patient 2		NE	E x
Key		Grade	Key	Grade
I 3.5mm Cl II		E	IV	A
II 76 3 / 6 3		D	V	A
III / 21		B	VI 3mm	B

Fig. 5.270

Ortho 19	Patient 3		NE x	E
Key		Grade	Key	Grade
I 1.5mm Cl II		B	IV	A
II 6 3 / 543		D	V 4-3-2	C
III		A	VI	A

Fig. 5.271

124

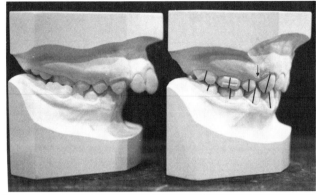

Ortho 19	Patient 4		NE	E x
Key		Grade	Key	Grade
I	2mm Cl II	C	IV	A
II	76 3 / 5 3	D	V 5-3	B
III	21	B	VI 3mm	B

Fig. 5.272

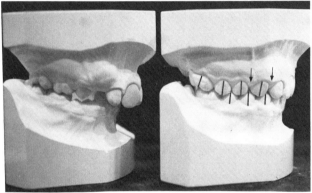

Ortho 19	Patient 5		NE	E x
Key		Grade	Key	Grade
I	1mm Cl II	B	IV	A
II	65 3	C	V 4-3-2	C
III	21	B	VI 3mm	B

Fig. 5.273

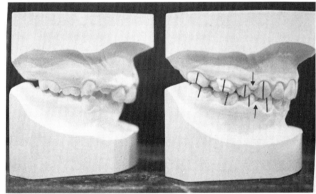

Ortho 19	Patient 6		NE	E x
Key		Grade	Key	Grade
I	2.5mm Cl II	D	IV	A
II	76 3 / 76 3	D	V 5-3 / 5-3	C
III	76 21	C	VI 3mm	B

Fig. 5.274

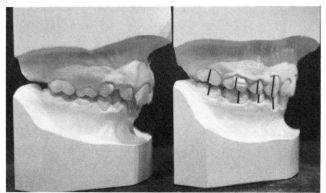

Ortho 19	Patient 7		NE	E x
Key		Grade	Key	Grade
I	3mm Cl II	E	IV 6	B
II	76 3 / 3	C	V	A
III	76 21	C	VI 3mm	B

Fig. 5.275

125

Summary for Orthodontist __19__

Patients __7__   NE __1__   E __6__

Keys	50% or more	Less than 50%, but significant	Grade
I	7 casts		D+
II	76 3 | 3	5 | 765	D
III	21	76 | 21 |	B
IV	|		A
V	4 casts		B
VI	5 casts		B+

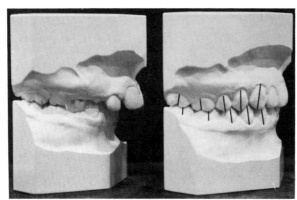

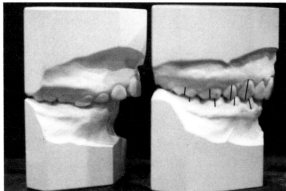

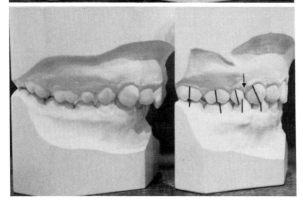

ORTHODONTIST #20

Ortho __20__   Patient __1__   NE _x_   E____

Key		Grade	Key		Grade
I	1.5mm Cl II	B	IV	5 |	B
II	7 5 3 | 543	D	V	|	A
III	|	A	VI	3mm	B

Fig. 5.276

Ortho __20__   Patient __2__   NE____   E _x_

Key		Grade	Key		Grade
I	3mm Cl II	E	IV	5 |	B
II	765 3 | 76 3	E	V	|	A
III	21 |	B	VI	3mm	B

Fig. 5.277

Ortho __20__   Patient __3__   NE____   E _x_

Key		Grade	Key		Grade
I	2.5mm Cl II	D	IV	3 |	B
II	7 5 3 | 6	C	V	5-3 |	B
III	21|	B	VI	3mm	B

Fig. 5.278

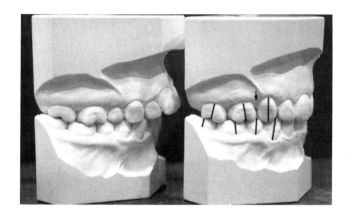

Ortho	20	Patient	4		NE		E	x
Key			Grade	Key				Grade
I	1mm Cl II		B	IV				A
II	76 3		C	V	6-3			B
	6							
III	21		B	VI				A

Fig. 5.279

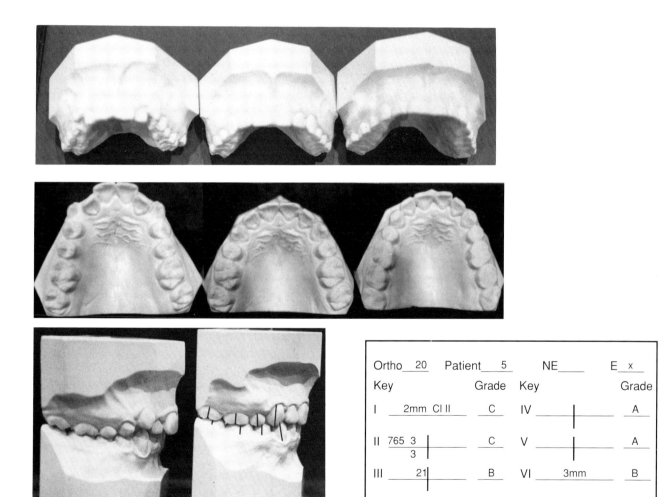

Ortho	20	Patient	5		NE		E	x
Key			Grade	Key				Grade
I	2mm Cl II		C	IV				A
II	765 3		C	V				A
	3							
III	21		B	VI	3mm			B

Fig. 5.280

127

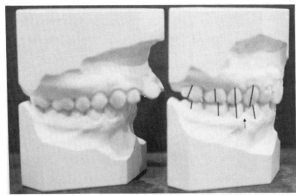

Ortho 20	Patient 6	NE	E x
Key	Grade	Key	Grade
I 3mm Cl II	E	IV	A
II 76 3 / 3	C	V 5-3	B
III 21	B	VI 3mm	B

Fig. 5.281

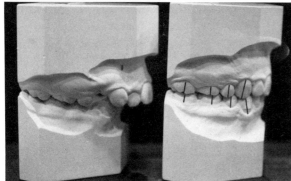

Ortho 20	Patient 7	NE	E x
Key	Grade	Key	Grade
I 3mm Cl II	E	IV	A
II 765 3 / 3	D	V	A
III 7 21	C	VI	A

Fig. 5.282

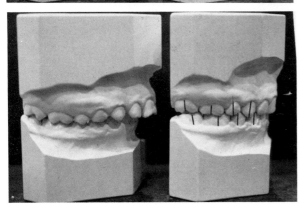

Ortho 20	Patient 8	NE	E x
Key	Grade	Key	Grade
I 1.5mm Cl II	B	IV 7	B
II 6 3 / 7	C	V	A
III 21	B	VI	A

Fig. 5.283

Summary for Orthodontist 20			
Patients 8	NE 1	E 7	
Keys	50% or more	Less than 50%, but significant	Grade
I	8 casts		C–
II	765 3 / 3		C–
III	21	6 3	B
IV		5	A–
V		3 casts	A–
VI	5 casts		B+

128

ORTHODONTIST #21

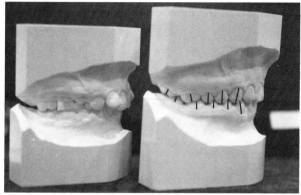

Ortho 21	Patient 1	NE x	E
Key	Grade	Key	Grade
I Cl I	A	IV	A
II 76 3 / 7 3	D	V	A
III	A	VI 3mm	B

Fig. 5.284

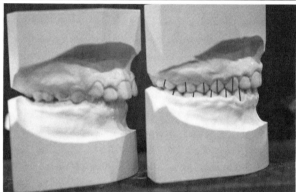

Ortho 21	Patient 2	NE x	E
Key	Grade	Key	Grade
I Cl I	A	IV	A
II 7 3 / 3	C	V	A
III 21 / 21	C	VI 3mm	B

Fig. 5.285

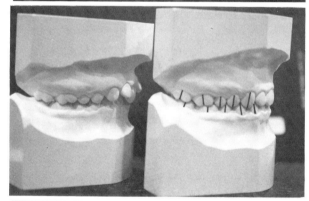

Ortho 21	Patient 3	NE x	E
Key	Grade	Key	Grade
I 1mm Cl II	B	IV	A
II 7 43 / 43	D	V	A
III 21	B	VI 3mm	B

Fig. 5.286

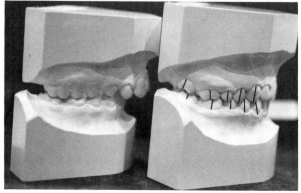

Ortho 21	Patient 4	NE x	E
Key	Grade	Key	Grade
I 2mm Cl II	C	IV 65	B
II 7 43 / 43	D	V	A
III 21	B	VI 3mm	B

Fig. 5.287

129

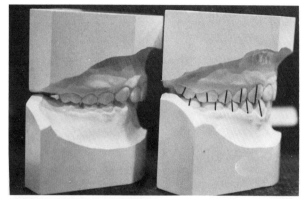

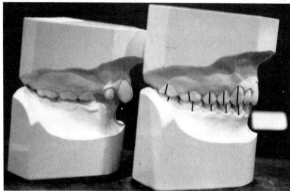

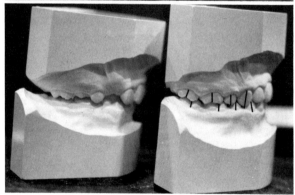

Ortho 21	Patient 5	NE x	E
Key	**Grade**	**Key**	**Grade**
I · 1mm Cl II	B	IV	A
II 7 543 / 543	E	V	A
III 21	B	VI 3mm	B

Fig. 5.288

Ortho 21	Patient 6	NE x	E
Key	**Grade**	**Key**	**Grade**
I 3mm Cl II	E	IV	A
II 7 3 / 543	D	V	A
III 21 / 21	C	VI 3mm	B

Fig. 5.289

Ortho 21	Patient 7	NE	E x
Key	**Grade**	**Key**	**Grade**
I 1.5mm Cl II	B	IV	A
II 7 3 / 3	C	V	A
III 21	B	VI 3mm	B

Fig. 5.290

Summary for Orthodontist 21			
Patients 7	NE 6	E 1	
Keys	**50% or more**	**Less than 50%, but significant**	**Grade**
I	5 casts		B
II	7 3 / 43	54 / 5	D
III	21	21	B
IV			A
V			A
VI	7 casts		B

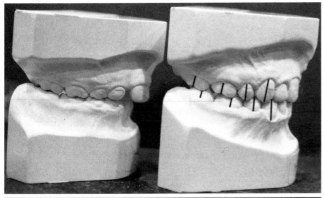

ORTHODONTIST #22

Ortho 22	Patient 1		NE	E x	
Key		Grade	Key		Grade
I	2mm Cl II	C	IV		A
II	76 3 / 3	C	V		A
III	21	B	VI	3mm	B

Fig. 5.291

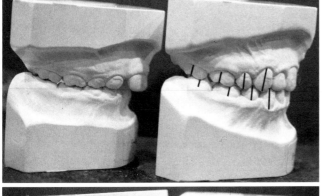

Ortho 22	Patient 2		NE	E x	
Key		Grade	Key		Grade
I	2mm Cl II	C	IV	65	B
II	76 3 / 3	C	V		A
III		A	VI		A

Fig. 5.292

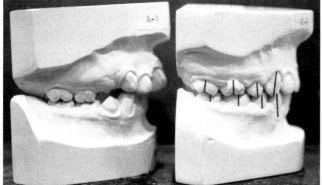

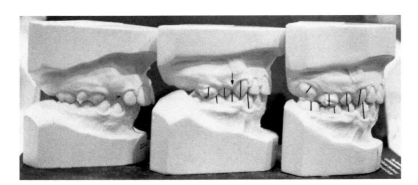

Ortho 22	Patient 3		NE	E x	
Key		Grade	Key		Grade
I	1mm Cl II	B	IV	6	B
II	6 3 / 6 3	C	V	5-3	B
III		A	VI		A

Fig. 5.293

131

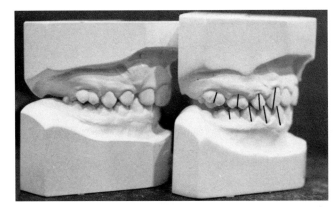

Ortho 22	Patient 4		NE	E x	
Key		Grade	Key		Grade
I	1mm Cl II	B	IV 7		B
II	76 3	E	V		A
	6543				
III	7 21	C	VI		A

Fig. 5.294

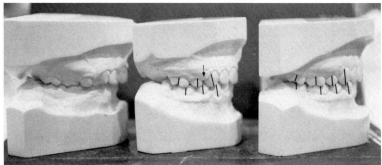

Ortho 22	Patient 5		NE	E x	
Key		Grade	Key		Grade
I	1.5mm Cl II	B	IV		A
II	6	B	V 5-3		B
	3				
III		A	VI 3mm		B

Fig. 5.295

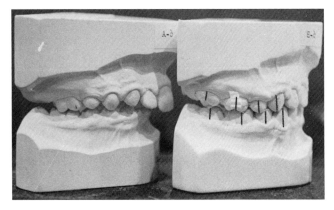

Ortho 22	Patient 6		NE	E x	
Key		Grade	Key		Grade
I	2mm Cl II	C	IV 6		B
II	76 3	D	V		A
	76 3				
III	76	B	VI 3mm		B

Fig. 5.296

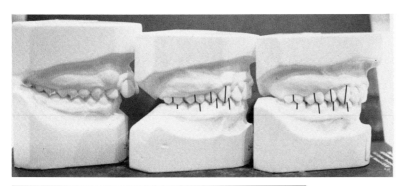

Ortho 22	Patient 7	NE	E x
Key	Grade	Key	Grade
I 1.5mm Cl II	B	IV 6		B
II 76 3	C	V		A
3				
III 21	B	VI 3mm	B

Fig. 5.297

Summary for Orthodontist 22			
Patients 7	NE	E 7	
Keys	50% or more	Less than 50%, but significant	Grade
I	7 casts		B–
II	76 3		C
	3	6	
III		7 21	B+
		21	
IV	6		B+
V		2 casts	A
VI	4 casts		B+

133

Chapter 6

Normality—Abnormality—Optimality

A quarter-century of clinical experience and research devoted to naturally optimal and treated occlusions has yielded not only the quantified Six Key objectives for orthodontic treatment, but also several principles fundamental to the concept of a fully programmed appliance. These principles, later explained in detail, can be summarized as follows.

1. Each normal tooth type is similar in shape from one individual to another.

2. The size of normal crowns within a dentition has no effect on their optimal angulation or inclination, or on the relative prominence of their facial surfaces.

3. Most individuals have normal teeth regardless of whether their occlusion is flawed or optimal.

4. Jaws must be normal and correctly related to permit the teeth to be correctly positioned and related.

5. Dentitions with normal teeth and in jaws that are or can be correctly related can be brought to optimal occlusal standards.

Normal versus Abnormal Teeth and Jaws

Wheeler [29] demonstrates that within any one normal tooth type there are important regularities, such as crown shape, number of cusps, number of grooves, and location of contact areas. No dentist would have difficulty describing a specific tooth type, or identifying each type in a large sample of extracted teeth. The measurement study (Chapter 4) demonstrated consistent angulation and inclination of the FACCs of correctly positioned tooth types. Therefore it can be inferred that there are correlations between the occlusal and facial surfaces of tooth types. This is important information for orthodontists—most of whom treat and, to some extent, assess treatment progress and results from the facial surfaces of the crowns.

Peg-shaped maxillary lateral incisors, cleft palates, crown-size discrepancies, some missing teeth, and some interjaw disharmonies are abnormalities. Patients with such characteristics present special orthodontic problems. But even in these cases, brackets programmed to guide normal teeth to specific positions can be used with less, or no more, attention than is required with an edgewise appliance that is not programmed at all.

Generally, all teeth in a single dentition are compatible in size—being either large, medium, or small. But crown size has no effect on their individual angulation, inclination, or relative facial prominence, or on interarch relationship. Abnormal size-variation within the same dentition is a problem that can be handled by the generalist. Interdental space problems caused by an isolated crown-size discrepancy (solvable by stripping, enlarging with composite, or crowning) must be differentiated from space problems induced by orthodontic treatment—for example, incorrect angulation or inclination of incisors, or insufficient closure of extraction sites. Crown size is important in appliance design in only one way: the bracket must not be too large for the crown.

Optimal Occlusion and Normal and Abnormal Malocclusions

Most of the population is afflicted with malocclusion. That fact could be interpreted to mean that occlusal deviations are "natural" characteristics for humankind, and therefore should not be tampered with. Indeed, malocclusion may be the untreated "natural" or "normal" condition for most individuals. But that does not mean it is comfortable, efficient, aesthetically pleasing, or healthful either physiologically or psychologically.

Individuals with abnormal jaws and teeth fall outside the large, basically *normal* pattern. Treatment of individuals with such differences, even with help from other specialists or from the generalist, may have to be compromised. However, within the normal group are those with normal teeth and jaws who require no treatment (naturally optimal)

and those who can be treated to optimal standards (normal malocclusions).

A cardinal axiom in biology is that the normal is always a range. Even in the naturally optimal sample (Chapters 2 and 4) there were differences in tooth positions and interarch relationships. But the ranges for those factors were smaller than in the pretreatment casts of the 1150-cast sample that, for the most part, were normal malocclusions (Chapter 5). Both the optimal occlusions and most malocclusions have normal teeth and jaws; to distinguish between the two, this text denotes preferred occlusion as "optimal," and the other as "normal malocclusion." Optimal, according to Merriam-Webster, is "most desirable or satisfactory." Dentitions that cannot be treated to optimal occlusal standards without the generalist or surgical specialist because of abnormal teeth or jaws are "abnormal."

Most patients with malocclusions have normal teeth and jaws, and can and should be treated to optimal standards. For them, the Six Keys are considered to be attainable treatment results. If, as has been proposed, normal tooth types are similar in shape, and require similar positions for occlusion to be optimal, why should clinicians spend so much of their lives making virtually identical bends in identical wires, each time striving to estimate the requirements for efficient tooth guidance? It seemed feasible to design an appliance that could be readily applied to normal teeth within dentitions with normal malocclusions, and direct them to optimal goals. When correctly sited, the brackets would be designed to correctly site slots designed to provide the guidance needed with few, if any, wire bends. The development of that appliance resulted partly from the studies already described in this book. Additional justification came from a detailed analysis of the virtues and limitations of the Angle edgewise appliance, which is discussed in the next chapter.

Chapter 7

The Nonprogrammed Appliance

The need for an improved edgewise appliance is better understood when Edward H. Angle's edgewise bracket design is examined in the light of new information about tooth shape and position, and in the light of new treatment goals concerning facial aesthetics, which may require extractions and jaw surgery. Once called by Angle "the latest and best," his appliance is now the oldest and among the least efficient of all edgewise appliances.* Extensive wire bending is required because each bracket is the same but the optimal positions differ for most tooth types in a dentition. Intended only for nonextraction treatment, his appliance requires even more wire bending when teeth have been extracted. The rectangular slot itself, however, remains an effective shape for controlling teeth in three dimensions.

Orthodontic treatment usually involves a blending of two phases. Initially the teeth in each arch are leveled and aligned, and extrac-

tion sites, if present, are closed; concurrently, the interjaw and interarch relationships may be made more harmonious. The second phase involves fine-tuning the positions of the teeth to optimal occlusal standards. The appliance and the skill of the operator determine treatment efficiency.

Removable appliances and fixed appliances without rectangular slots can deal successfully with treatment requiring tipping but are not efficient for tooth translation or fine-tuning tooth position. Fixed appliances with edgewise slots are best for those procedures because the slot permits three-dimensional control; the edgewise appliance also is effective for tipping. Perhaps with the exception of expanding the maxilla at the intermaxillary suture, the edgewise appliance is the best choice for most treatment requirements because it is the most versatile and requires the least skill and effort. Achieving optimal occlusion with other appliances requires greater skill and effort proportional to their inability to control individual tooth movement in all three planes of space.

The terminology needed to explain the

---

*There is at least one currently available edgewise appliance with some built-in guidance features that requires more wire bending.

design and effects of a nonprogrammed appliance follows. Several terms were defined earlier but are repeated because of their importance in this chapter.

Andrews plane. The surface or plane on which the midtransverse plane of every crown in an arch will fall when the teeth are optimally positioned. If the plane is concave or convex, technically it is a surface; but in all instances it will be referred to here as the Andrews plane (Fig. 3.1).

Angulated slot. A slot angled more or less than 90° to the bracket's vertical components.

Base point. The middle of the bracket base. It falls on an extension of the faciolingual axis of the bracket stem (Fig. 7.1).

Bracket base. The portion of the bracket stem intended to mate with the surface of the crown (Fig. 7.1).

Bracket siting. Any procedure that affects positioning the bracket. Bracket siting is influenced by bracket design and crown landmarks.

Bracket stem. The portion of the bracket that includes the bracket base, the lingual half of the slot, and the portions between (Fig. 7.1).

Edgewise appliance. A set of brackets, each with a rectangular slot. The slot enables three-dimensional tooth movement.

Facial plane of a crown. Any plane that is tangent to a point on the crown's face.

Fully programmed appliance. A set of brackets designed to guide teeth directly to their goal positions with unbent archwires.

Horizontal bracket components. The occlusal and gingival sides of the bracket (Fig. 7.1).

Molar offset. The angle between the crown's embrasure line and a line connecting the buccal cusps. It is measured along the crown's midtransverse plane (Fig. 4.17).

Nonprogrammed appliance. A set of brackets designed the same for all tooth types, relying totally on wire bending (except possibly for angulation if the bracket is angulated)

to achieve the optimal position for each individual tooth.

Partly programmed appliance. A set of brackets designed with some built-in features, but that always requires some wire bending (though less than is required by nonprogrammed appliances).

Slot base. The surface of the slot closest to the tooth (Fig. 7.1).

Slot point. The midpoint of the slot (Fig. 7.1).

Slot siting. Any procedure that affects positioning the bracket slot. Slot positioning is influenced by bracket design, bracket siting, and crown morphology.

Vertical bracket components. The mesial and distal sides of the bracket and tie wings (Fig. 7.1).

Edgewise Appliance Classification

In spite of the historic advances made by Angle in designing an appliance with a rectangular slot, his bracket cannot compete with

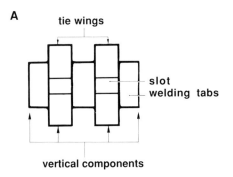

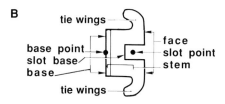

Fig. 7.1. Nonprogrammed bracket features.

some of today's brackets in terms of built-in features. The several types of edgewise appliances are best differentiated by placing them into three categories: nonprogrammed, partly programmed, and fully programmed.

The fundamental differences in the three categories can be learned from the definitions (see terminology above). Design differences cause each category to perform differently, even when all brackets are sited alike. The distinction between the categories will become clear as each is discussed in its respective chapter.

The Angle-designed edgewise brackets are "nonprogrammed" because of their bilaterally symmetrical design. If located on the FA point and the FACC and used with progressively larger unbent archwires, the brackets ultimately would cause the inclination of the facial plane of each crown to be at 90° to the occlusal plane, the occlusogingival position of each crown to be irregular, all crowns to have equal facial prominence, and the angulation of the FACC of each crown to be at 90° to the occlusal plane.

Angle recognized some consistencies in the positions of optimally occluded teeth, as shown in his directive to complete active treatment with an "ideal" archwire [7]. However, Angle did not incorporate these treatment objectives into his appliance. In fact, except for some variations in mesiodistal width, the brackets are identical for all tooth types. Yet within a dentition, optimal crown inclination, angulation, and prominence differ for almost every crown, thus making wire bending imperative.

Design Shortcomings

For tooth movement not involving translation, six factors cause the slot of nonprogrammed edgewise brackets to be sited in ways that always require archwire bends.

Each factor may cause the slot to be misdirected by more than 2° from its optimal angulation and inclination and by more than 0.5 mm occlusogingivally, mesiodistally, and faciolingually. The six factors are (1) bracket bases are perpendicular to the bracket stems; (2) bracket bases are not contoured occlusogingivally; (3) slots are not angulated; (4) bracket stems are of equal faciolingual thickness; (5) maxillary molar offset is not built in; and (6) bracket-siting techniques are unsatisfactory. How these factors affect slot siting is discussed in the following sections.

Perpendicular Bases

The base of the nonprogrammed bracket is perpendicular to the faciolingual axis of its stem (Fig. 7.2). This feature causes problems of slot inclination and occlusogingival position.

Each crown in an arch has its own optimal amount of inclination. Therefore, brackets having bases that are perpendicular to their stems, and sited base-point-to-FA-point of each crown, will target their slots to that many different inclinations and occlusogingival levels (Fig. 7.3).

Perhaps, because implementing functional goals is so new to orthodontists, the clinical significance of the occlusogingival disharmony of the slot positions has not been generally recognized. Therefore the need for second-

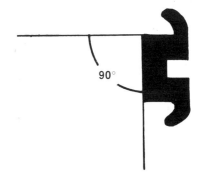

Fig. 7.2. The base of a nonprogrammed bracket is perpendicular to its stem.

order bends to deal with this slot-targeting problem has heretofore not been reported. Figure 7.4 quantifies the inclination and occlusogingival disharmony of the slots in each arch relative to the Andrews plane. The measurements are made and illustrated under the following conditions: the base points of the brackets are sited to the crowns' FA points; the distance from the base point to the slot point is 1.5 mm; and the crowns are correct in their occlusogingival position and optimally inclined. The inclination range for the maxillary arch is 16° (7° to –9°). If one subscribes to the need for 12° of FACC inclination for maxillary central incisors, the range increases to 21° (12° to –9°). If one subscribes to 25° of FACC inclination for maxillary central incisors, the inclination range for the maxillary arch is 34° (25° to –9°).

The occlusogingival disharmony range for the slots in the maxillary arch is 0.42 mm (from 0.18 mm above the Andrews plane to 0.24 mm below). If one prefers 12° of facial-axis inclination for maxillary central incisors, the occlusogingival range increases to 0.56 mm (from 0.32 mm above to 0.24 mm below the Andrews plane); for 25° of maxillary inclination, the range is 0.88 mm (from 0.64 mm above to 0.24 mm below the Andrews plane).

For the mandibular arch the inclination range for the slot is 34° (from 1° to 35° above the Andrews plane), and the occlusogingival range for the slot is 0.86 mm (from 0.01 mm to 0.87 mm above the Andrews plane) (Fig. 7.4). Figure 7.5 illustrates the effects on inclination and occlusogingival tooth position when full-size unbent archwires are used. The effects are compared with each crown's optimal position.

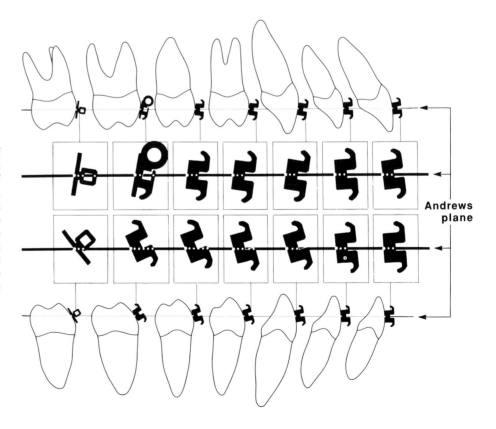

Fig. 7.3. Inclination and occlusogingival slot siting. Even when the base points of nonprogrammed brackets are sited on the FA points of optimally positioned crowns, occlusogingivally the slots are poorly aligned relative to the Andrews plane, and the inclinations of the slots are as different from each other as are the inclinations of the crowns. Enlarged bracket positions *(center)* are identical to those on teeth.

Andrews plane

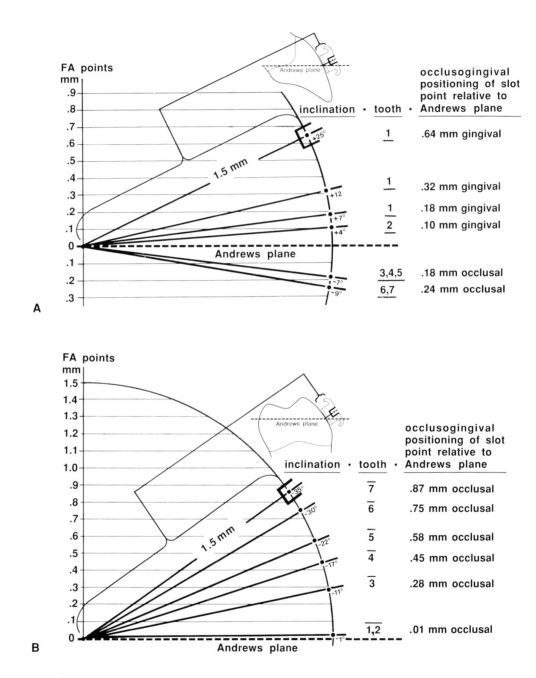

Fig. 7.4. Graphs illustrating slot inclinations and slot occlusogingival positions, relative to the Andrews plane, for non-programmed brackets: *A*, maxillary quadrant; *B*, mandibular quadrant. Heavy solid lines represent an enlarged distal perspective of the faciolingual axis for each bracket in a quadrant (a normal-size, one-tooth example is seen in each graph's upper right corner). Dashed lines represent the Andrews plane. The light horizontal lines represent .1-mm increments. The left ends of the axes are located at the FA points of optimally positioned crowns. Near the right ends of the axes are dots representing the middle of each slot, and numbers indicating each slot's inclination. The column to the far right lists data about how far each slot is occlusal to or gingival to the Andrews plane. The inside column labels the teeth.

141

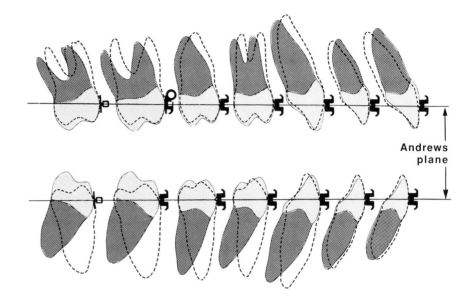

Fig. 7.5. Effects on tooth inclination and occlusogingival position when the nonprogrammed brackets sited as shown in Fig. 7.3 are aligned to receive full-size unbent archwires. Dashed lines indicate optimal tooth positions.

Andrews plane

Bases Not Contoured Occlusogingivally

Occlusogingivally, the bracket base is flat (Fig. 7.6), but the facial surface of a crown is curved (Fig. 7.7). When such a bracket is being attached to a crown, either directly or with a band, it can unintentionally be rocked occlusally or gingivally. Thus there is uncertainty as to which portion of the base will end up touching the crown once the adhesive is set. The actual portion of the bracket base that touches the crown cannot be visualized, so when an orthodontist sites the bracket, gravity, a bandpusher, or an unsteady hand can cause a different part of the base to touch the crown than was intended. When that occurs the slot inclination and occlusogingival positions may vary even more than shown in Figures 7.3 and 7.4, and the effects on tooth position when the brackets are aligned may be greater than shown in Figure 7.5. If the cementing material sets with the slot sited to a position other than the one intended, compensatory archwire bends will be required.

For each tooth, the potential inclination range for the slot, because the flat-based bracket

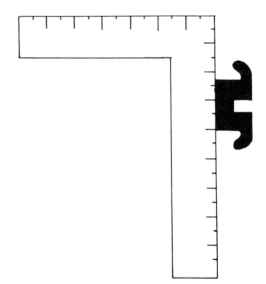

Fig. 7.6. Occlusogingivally, the base of a nonprogrammed bracket is flat.

can rock, is greater than 2°. For many teeth the potential occlusogingival range for the slot is greater than 0.5 mm. For mandibular first premolars the range for inclination of the slot is 14°; occlusogingivally it is 0.6 mm (Fig. 7.7B). For a mandibular second premolar these ranges are even larger because the radius of the vertical

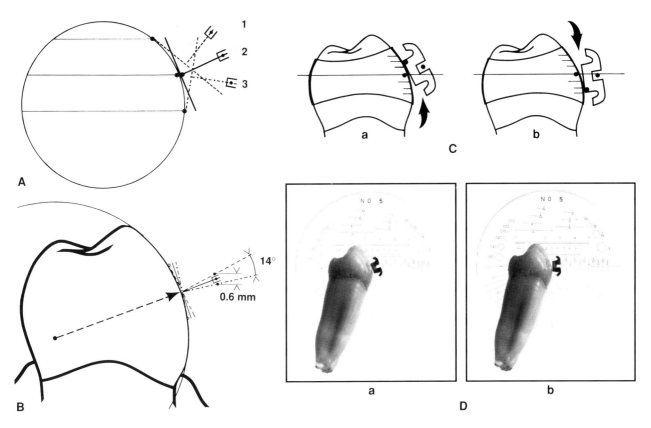

Fig. 7.7. Range of possible slot inclinations and occlusogingival positions when a flat-based bracket is sited on a curved surface. *A,* Diagrammatic example; *B,* quantified inclination and occlusogingival range for a mandibular first premolar. *C,* Range of slot positions for a mandibular first premolar: *a,* occlusal rocking; *b,* gingival rocking. *D,* Example of range of slot positions for a mandibular first premolar: *a,* occlusal rocking; *b,* gingival rocking.

crown curvature is smaller than that of the mandibular first premolar. Second- and third-order bends will be needed to deal with these visually imperceptible but clinically significant bracket-siting and slot-siting errors.

Figure 7.8 illustrates irregular slot siting in each arch caused by the many possible ways of siting a vertically flat-based bracket. Note the incongruence of the slots, in both inclination and occlusogingival position, when sited on optimally inclined crowns. In this illustration the gingival portion of the bracket base is the only part of the base touching the crown on the odd-numbered teeth; for the even-numbered teeth, the situation is just the opposite. This is a worst-case example, but even when the intent is to site the base point of flat-

based brackets to each crown's FA point there is unpredictability about what part of the base will end up touching the crown, and where the slot will be sited. Figure 7.9 illustrates the effects on crown inclination and occlusogingival position when brackets are sited as shown in Figure 7.8 and when the teeth are positioned so the slots are passive to full-size unbent archwires. The effects are compared with each crown's optimal position.

Mesiodistal Base Contour

Figure 7.10 illustrates irregular mesiodistal slot siting that can occur when the mesiodistal contour of the bracket base does not match that of the crown.

143

Fig. 7.8. Inclination and occlusogingival incongruence of slots when nonprogrammed brackets are sited alternately at opposite ends of their bases. The teeth are optimally inclined. Enlarged bracket positions *(center)* are identical to those on teeth. White dots centered in bases of enlarged brackets indicate base points. White asterisks indicate where brackets actually touch the crowns.

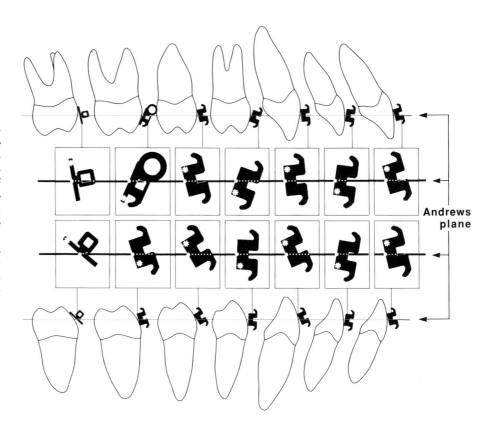

Fig. 7.9. Effects on tooth inclination and occlusogingival position when the nonprogrammed brackets sited as shown in Fig. 7.8 are aligned to receive full-size unbent archwires. Dashed lines indicate optimal tooth positions.

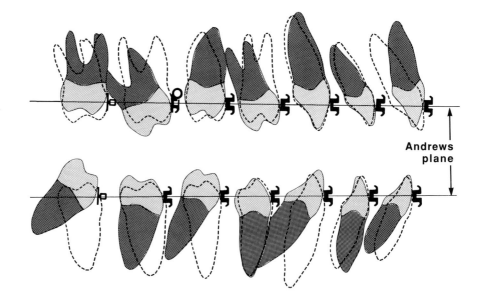

Slots Not Angulated

When the teeth in an arch are optimally positioned, each crown has its own optimal amount of angulation, and each FA point is on the Andrews plane. When the vertical components of the brackets are sited parallel to the FACC, and the base point is sited to the FA point of correctly positioned crowns, the angle of the slots will vary to that many different angulations (Fig. 7.11). Figure 7.12 illustrates the effects on angulation and occlusogingival position when teeth are positioned so the slots are passive to unbent archwires.

When the vertical components of the brackets parallel the FACC (Fig. 7.13) but the brackets are rocked as they are in Figure 7.8, the effects of a full-size wire on angulation and inclination are as shown in Figure 7.14.

To reduce or eliminate the need for second-order bends for angulation, many or-

thodontists angulate brackets. The nonprogrammed bracket, however, was not designed for such a technique, because its base curves only horizontally. If the bracket is angulated on the crown, a two-point contact is created between the tooth and the diagonally opposite corners of the horizontally contoured bracket base (Fig. 7.15a). Under these conditions, the inclination and occlusogingival ranges for slot siting are greater (Fig. 7.15b,c) than when the bracket is not angulated (Fig. 7.7, 7.8).

Stems of Equal Prominence

The distance from the bracket base to the center of the slot is the same in each bracket (Fig. 7.16). Therefore the slots are as irregular in facial prominence as are the crowns when the teeth are optimally positioned (Fig. 7.17). Figure 7.18 illustrates that the brackets are equal in prominence when the slots are aligned to receive full-size unbent archwires. The effects are compared with each crown's optimal position.

Maxillary Molar Offset Not Built-In

The midsagittal planes of the crowns and slots are coincidental except for maxillary molars (Fig. 7.17A). The mesiobuccal cusp of each optimally positioned maxillary molar is more facially prominent than the distobuccal cusp. This causes the midsagittal plane of the stem and slot to be angular to the midsagittal planes of the crown. Figure 7.18A shows the rotational effects on the maxillary molars after the slots have been aligned to receive a full-size unbent archwire. First-order offset bends must be installed into the archwire to accommodate these differences.

Unsatisfactory Landmarks

Authors of major texts on orthodontics seldom agree about which landmarks are best

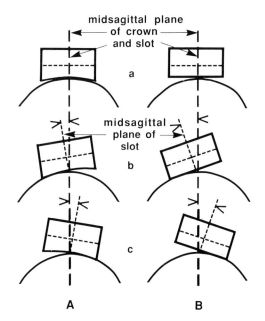

Fig. 7.10. Occlusal perspective of mesiodistal slot position range. *A,* Bracket with partly contoured base; *B,* bracket with no base contour. *a,* Midsagittal plane of slot and crown coincide; *b,* maximum mesial range for slot position; *c,* maximum distal range for slot position.

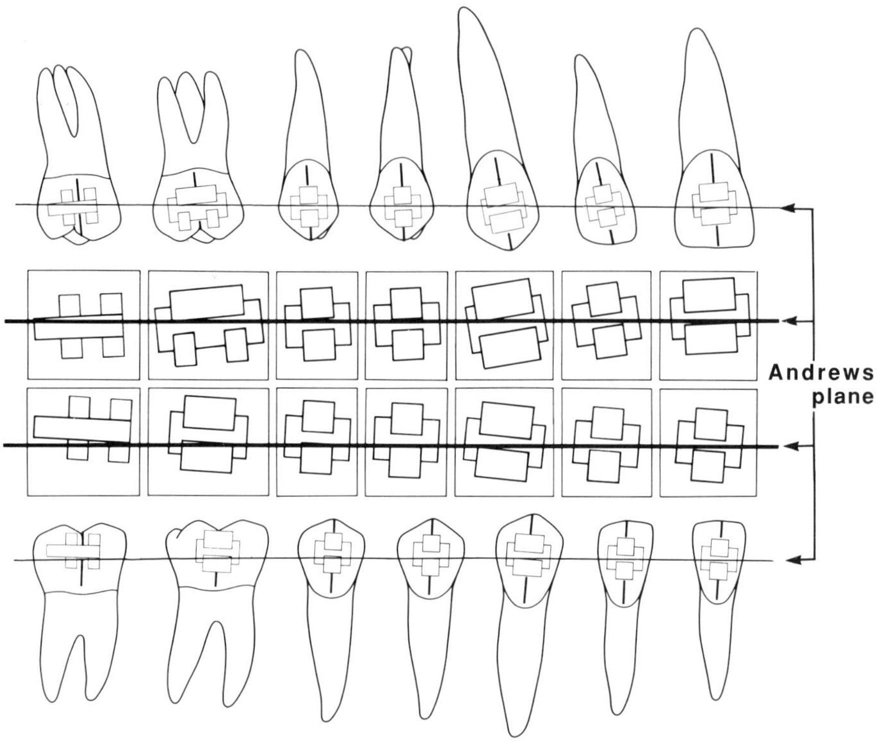

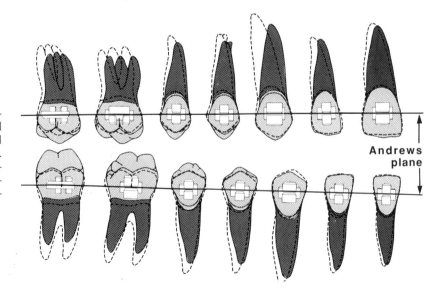

Fig. 7.11. Slot angulations and occlusogingival positions are not harmonious with the Andrews plane when nonprogrammed brackets are located on the FACCs and FA points of optimally positioned crowns.

Fig. 7.12. Effects on tooth angulation and occlusogingival position when nonprogrammed brackets sited as shown in Figs. 7.3 and 7.11 are aligned to receive full-size unbent archwires. Dashed lines indicate optimal tooth positions.

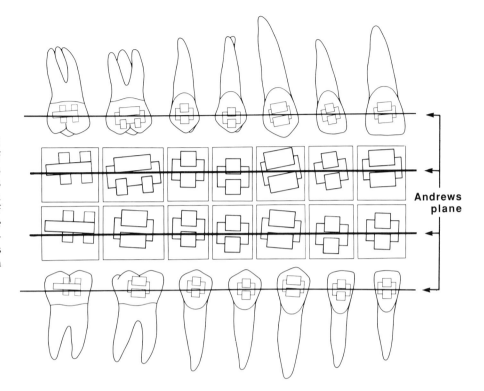

Fig. 7.13. Nonprogrammed brackets sited along the FACC of optimally positioned crowns with alternate ends of their bases touching the crowns, as shown in Fig. 7.8. The angulations of the slots match those of the crowns, but the slots' occlusogingival positions are even less harmonious than those shown in Figs. 7.3 and 7.11.

Fig. 7.14. Effects on tooth angulation and occlusogingival position when the nonprogrammed brackets sited as shown in Figs. 7.8 and 7.13 are aligned to receive full-size unbent archwires. Dashed lines indicate optimal tooth positions.

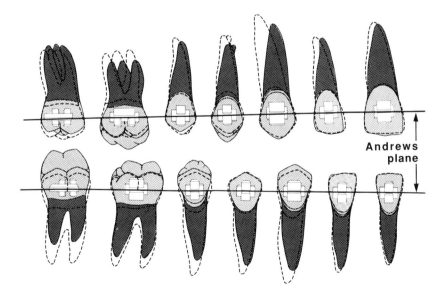

147

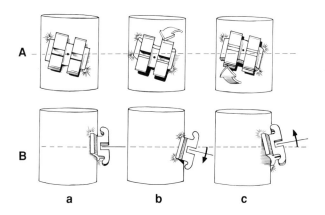

Fig. 7.15. The ranges of inclination and occlusogingival slot position for an angulated nonprogrammed bracket. *A,* Facial perspective; *B,* distal perspective. *a,* Bracket that is angulated but not rocked is perched on diagonal corners; *b,* bracket that is both angulated and rocked downward until the third corner touches; *c,* bracket that is angulated and rocked upward until the fourth corner touches. Dashed line represents Andrews plane.

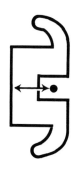

Fig. 7.16. The base-point-to-slot-point distance is the same for all nonprogrammed brackets.

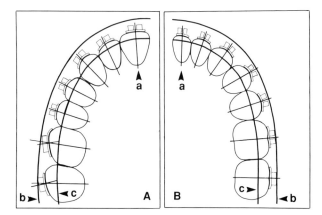

Fig. 7.17. Faciolingual and mesiodistal slot siting: base points of nonprogrammed brackets sited on the FA points of optimally positioned crowns. The midsagittal plane *(a)* of each crown and slot coincide, except in maxillary molars. The distance between each slot and a line *(b)* that touches the most facial part of the molar bracket and parallels the embrasure line *(c)* differs for most tooth types. *A,* Maxillary quadrant; *B,* mandibular quadrant.

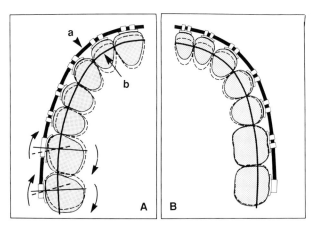

Fig. 7.18. The effects on optimal tooth position when the brackets shown in Fig. 7.17 are positioned to receive full-size unbent archwires *(a).* The facial surfaces of all crowns at the bracket sites become equidistant from the embrasure line *(b),* and the maxillary molars become rotated. *A,* Maxillary quadrant; *B,* mandibular quadrant. Dashed lines indicate optimal tooth positions.

148

for bracket siting. Each variation results in slot-siting variation. Each requires different wire bending.

The photographs of posttreatment casts shown in Chapter 5 demonstrate that the ranges of crown inclination and angulation are greater than for the optimal sample shown in Chapter 2. The ranges were similar for a given clinician, but often varied from orthodontist to orthodontist. The ranges for extraction treatment were greater than for nonextraction treatment. No two orthodontists do things quite the same, and nowhere is that more evident than in siting a nonprogrammed edgewise bracket. For those who subscribe to Angle's "ideal arch," this factor alone would explain much of the tooth-position variation found in treatment results. Most orthodontists routinely replace or reposition nonprogrammed brackets of patients transferred to them, even if they use the same kind of appliance. Why? Because brackets are so small that orthodontists cannot visually perceive where each slot is targeted or what landmarks were used for bracket siting; they would rather deal with the irregular and unpredictable slot-targeting range of their own bracketing approach than with that of someone else.

Angulation Landmarks

Just as the nonprogrammed bracket has at least six design shortcomings that affect accurate slot siting, the landmarks traditionally used for siting the bracket have their own deficiencies. For angulation, each orthodontist selects one of the five landmarks, but each of these prevents the bracket—and therefore the slot—from being positioned within the specified range. The five traditionally used angulation landmarks are the long axis of the crown, long axis of the tooth, incisal edges, marginal ridges, and contact points.

The long axes of crowns or teeth are not reliable referents because they run through the center of the teeth and cannot be observed

or marked (Fig. 7.19Aa,Ab,Ba). Brackets cannot be reproducibly sited to these internal axes with confidence in meeting the 0.5-mm and 2° constraints, let alone in siting the slot to those standards. And contact points, even though not internal, are not practical referents because they cannot be readily observed (Fig. 7.19Ac).

Incisal edges are tangible, but of limited value as an angulation landmark when brackets are bonded, because they are too far from the bracket slots. (Before brackets were direct-bonded, band rims were used as an intermediate referent.) In addition, incisal edges are unreliable because frequently they are fractured or excessively worn. In maxillary lateral incisors these edges are particularly unsuitable guides, even when virginal, because they are markedly curved (Fig. 7.19Ad). Their distoincisal corner must conform to the shape of the cusp of the mandibular canine with which with it functions during working excursions. In spite of these drawbacks, most orthodontists do use incisal edges for angulation landmarks. Thus it is not surprising that in the posttreatment occlusion study (Chapter 5), maxillary

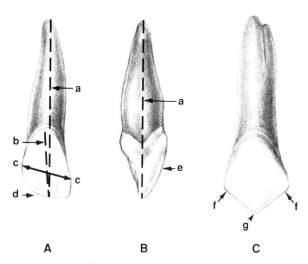

Fig. 7.19. Traditional bracket-siting landmarks and referents: facial *(A)* and distal *(B)* views of maxillary lateral incisor; *C*, facial view of maxillary first premolar. *a*, Long axis of tooth; *b*, long axis of crown; *c*, contact points; *d*, incisal edge; *e*, face of crown; *f*, marginal ridges; *g*, cusp tip.

lateral incisors were found to be among the most incorrectly angulated teeth.

Posterior teeth have cusp tips, not incisal edges. Cusp tips are ineffective as angulation landmarks, so some clinicians use marginal ridges. These, like incisal edges, are at least tangible, but they are of limited value as referents for bonding brackets because, without the rims of bands to mediate, marginal ridges are too far from the bracket slot for accurate visual orientation (Fig. 7.19Cf).

Strang [24] advises placing the band at right angles to the tooth, but orienting the bracket on the band so that its slot will later be passive to an unbent archwire when each tooth is correctly positioned. However, Strang does not specify the amount of bracket angulation this requires at the beginning of treatment. Holdaway [15], like Strang, advises placing the band at right angles to the tooth, and recommends angulating the brackets. The amount of angulation is based on the treatment plan. Tweed [27] recommends that the vertical components of all brackets parallel the long axis of the tooth. Lindquist [19] advocates using incisor edges for judging incisor bracket angulation. Saltzmann [22] positions incisor brackets parallel to incisal edges. For posterior teeth, Saltzmann recommends that the bracket parallel the contact points, but he does not provide a method for locating the contact points, which usually are hidden from view.

The landmarks used for bracket siting for angulation have little or no use in siting for inclination. Another referent must be used for that purpose, thereby introducing another potential slot-siting variable.

Inclination Landmarks

To know how much to incline the wire, an orthodontist must know the intended inclination of each crown from its inclination landmark. Equally important is how accurately the bracket is sited to the landmark, for this determines how accurately the slot represents the landmark. It is assumed that the base point of the bracket will be located at the inclination landmark, and therefore the slot will reflect the inclination of the facial plane of the crown at that site.

The inclination referent adopted by many orthodontists is the long axis of the crown or tooth. But these axes are just as unsatisfactory for inclination as for angulation, and for the same reasons. The inadequacy of the long axis of a crown or tooth is compounded by the fact that not only does the facial surface of a crown not parallel either axis, it is an arc; therefore no two sites on its surface have the same angular relationship to the long axis of the crown or tooth (Fig. 7.19Be). More important is that no two sites on a crown's facial surface have the same angular relationship to the plane of the crown's occlusal surface, to the crown's midtransverse plane, or to the occlusal plane of the arch when the teeth are optimally positioned (Fig. 7.20).

In an attempt not to compound the inclination and occlusogingival slot-targeting variables that occur from the use of the inadequate landmarks just discussed, many orthodontists use a site that is a specified number of millimeters from the incisal edge or cusp tip. Unfortunately, this approach is also unreliable, because the inclination of the slots of brackets located this way will vary from patient to patient for those with differing crown heights. The inclination of an optimally inclined short crown differs from that of a taller crown of the same type when both are measured at a given distance from the cusp tip or the incisal edge (Fig. 7.21A). When this method is used, the range of slot inclinations among patients can be larger than the 2° error limit. However, when the bracket's base point is located at the crown's FA point, the inclination of the slot maintains a constant relationship with that of the crown regardless of the crown's height (Fig. 7.21B).

The diversity of bracket-siting techniques for inclination is evident when the literature is

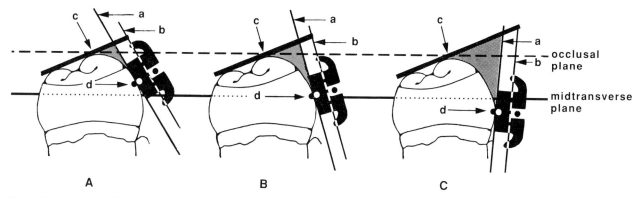

Fig 7.20. Using differing occlusogingival positions on the crown's face for bracket siting causes differing angles between the plane of the slot's base and the plane of the crown's occlusal surface, as well as differing occlusogingival slot positions. *A–C,* Optimally positioned mandibular first premolars, each with the same nonprogrammed bracket sited at a different occlusogingival position. *a,* Facial plane of crown and plane of bracket base; *b,* plane of slot base; *c,* plane of crown's occlusal surface; *d,* point of contact of bracket and crown.

reviewed. Tweed [27] recommended siting brackets a specified number of millimeters from the incisal edge or cusp tip. Saltzmann [22] recommends, except for maxillary lateral incisors, that the brackets be located in the middle one-third of the crown. As explained above, this site does have a consistent angular relationship to the plane of the crown's occlusal surface, regardless of crown size (Fig. 7.21B), but then Saltzmann goes on to say that any height is acceptable as long as it is the same throughout.

Holdaway [15] advocates that bracket siting be altered according to characteristics of the malocclusion, e.g., within the gingival one-third in open-bite malocclusions, or the occlusal one-third for deep bites. The advantages of siting nonprogrammed brackets at different occlusogingival heights on crowns to help correct such problems is questionable when the range of third-order bends required for this approach is considered.

According to Jarabak [17], bracket sites for inclination should be determined by the shape of the crown. For example, on ovoid crowns the bracket site should be in the middle third; on tapering crowns it should be 1–2 mm from the incisal edge; and on square crowns it should be as close to the incisal edge as possible. Lindquist [18] recommends that brackets on posterior teeth be located relative to the height of the marginal ridges.

Slot inclination can differ as much as 45°, depending on which portion of the crown is chosen as the bracket site (Fig. 7.22).

The extent to which the slot actually reflects the angulation and inclination landmarks of a specific crown cannot be accurately interpreted by visual inspection, nor can the position of each slot be determined relative to all other slots in the arch—not with the precision mandatory for orthodontic purposes. For transferring patients and treatment reporting, orthodontists using a nonprogrammed appliance must specify bracket siting in terms of millimeters or degrees from the landmarks or referents they use. Even then, bracket design and the unreliability of traditional landmarks make those data also unreliable.

The wide range in slot positions brought about by bracket design and the use of varied and inadequate landmarks may partly explain why treatment results differ so much among orthodontists (Chapter 5). Results are also influenced by wire bending, which does not always deliver the intended effects.

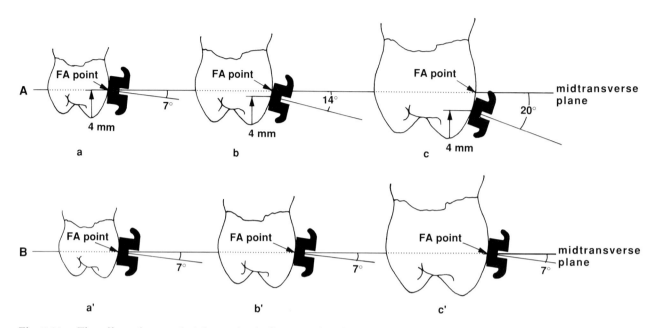

Fig. 7.21. The effect of crown height on slot inclination. *A,* When a bracket is sited the same distance from the cusp tip (e.g., 4 mm) of optimally positioned short *(a),* medium *(b),* and tall *(c)* crowns of the same tooth type, the inclination of each slot, relative to the crown's midtransverse plane, is different. *B,* When a bracket is sited on the FA point of optimally positioned short *(a'),* medium *(b'),* and tall *(c')* crowns of the same tooth type, the inclination of each slot, relative to the crown's midtransverse plane, is the same.

Wire Bending

Nonprogrammed brackets are simple in design, easily manufactured, and inexpensive. Unfortunately, they are difficult to use because considerable wire bending is needed throughout treatment. Next to the shortcomings of bracket design and landmarks, the most obvious reason for so much bending is that the brackets are all the same but the positions of most tooth types are different. All tooth guidance, beyond leveling and aligning and (possibly) angulation, must be provided by forming and bending the archwire. This must be done in all three planes of space. *First-order,* *second-order,* and *third-order* are conventional adjectives for identifying the plane in which the wire is bent, but not necessarily the plane of the effect. In this book, the terminology *primary,* *secondary,* and *tertiary* will be used to connote the effects of wire bends.

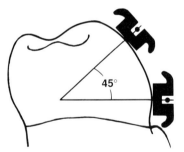

Fig. 7.22. Examples of the range for slot inclination for a mandibular molar.

With the nonprogrammed appliance there are four reasons to bend the wire in *each* of the three planes: (1) to initiate or maintain movement of a tooth; (2) to compensate for slot-siting errors caused by inadequate bracket design or incorrect bracket siting; (3) to compensate for the side effects of wire bending and wire forming, and (4) to correct for earlier "human-error" inaccuracies in wire bending.

Primary Wire Bends

A primary archwire bend is a first-order, second-order, or third-order bend intended for the most direct movement of teeth.

The slot of the bracket is intended to indirectly represent the crown landmarks chosen by the orthodontist for angulation, occlusogingival position, inclination, and facial prominence. If the slot does accurately represent these landmarks, then the primary bends required for each tooth, as well as the magnitude of the bends, can be calculated.

Picture optimally positioned teeth with the vertical components of each bracket paralleling and straddling each crown's facial axis, while at the same time the bracket's base point is sited at the FA point. Under these conditions the bracket slot indirectly represents (1) the angulation of the facial axis of the crown (Fig. 7.23); (2) a different occlusogingival position than the FA point of the crown (Fig. 7.24); (3) the inclination of the facial plane of the crown at its midpoint (Fig. 7.25); (4) maxillary molar offset (Fig. 7.26A); and (5) prominence of the crown (Fig. 7.26).

Assuming no occlusogingival or mesiodistal "rocking" (although that is clinically unrealistic), and with the brackets sited as just explained, picture the teeth in both arches optimally positioned with "ideal" rectangular archwires that passively fit all bracket slots. The number and magnitude of primary first-, second-, and third-order bends in those archwires can be quantified. For the maxillary and mandibular teeth, 26 second-order angulation bends are needed, totaling 112° (Fig. 7.23). In addition, 16 primary second-order occlusogingival bends are needed, totaling approximately 2.36 mm (Fig. 7.24). For inclination, 16 primary

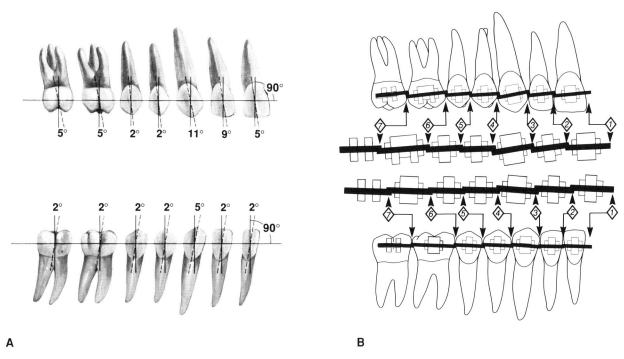

A **B**

Fig. 7.23. Second-order wire bending for angulation: *A,* optimal crown angulations; *B,* nonprogrammed brackets located along the FACCs and at the FA points of optimally positioned crowns. For the archwire to fit the slots passively, 6 second-order angulation bends *(arrows)* are required per quadrant and one at each midline. Enlarged bracket positions and wire bends shown in the middle of *B* are identical to those shown on the teeth.

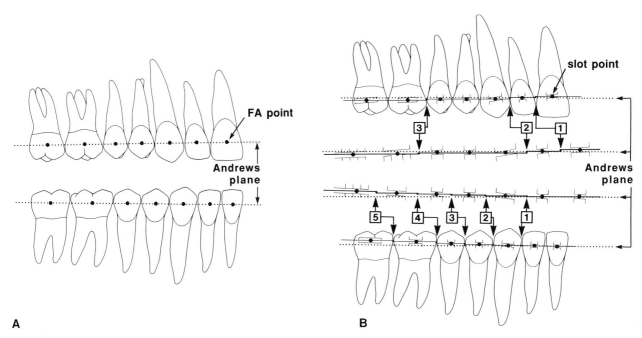

Fig. 7.24. Second-order wire bending for occlusogingival slot position: *A*, optimally positioned crowns showing harmony of FA points with Andrews plane; *B*, nonprogrammed brackets located along the FACC with base points on the FA points of optimally positioned crowns. The slots' midpoints *(large dots)* are sited above or below the Andrews plane *(dotted line)* and the FA points. To accommodate these errant slots, 3 maxillary and 5 mandibular second-order bends are needed per quadrant. Enlarged bracket slots and slot points *(large dots)* shown in the middle of the illustration are identical to those shown on the teeth.

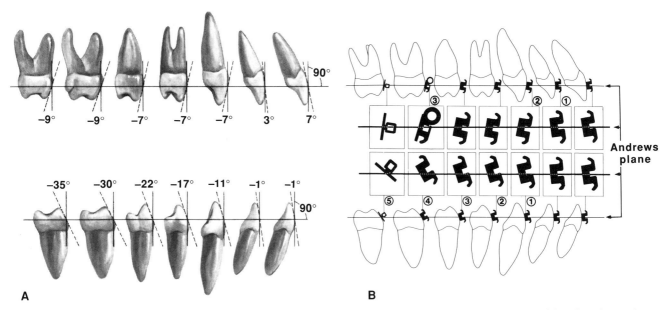

Fig. 7.25. Third-order wire bending for inclination: *A*, optimal crown inclinations; *B*, nonprogrammed brackets located along the FACC at the FA points of optimally positioned crowns. Slot inclinations differ to the extent that crown inclinations differ. To accommodate the errant slots, 3 maxillary and 5 mandibular third-order bends *(numbers)* are needed per side. Enlarged bracket positions *(center)* are identical to those shown on teeth.

154

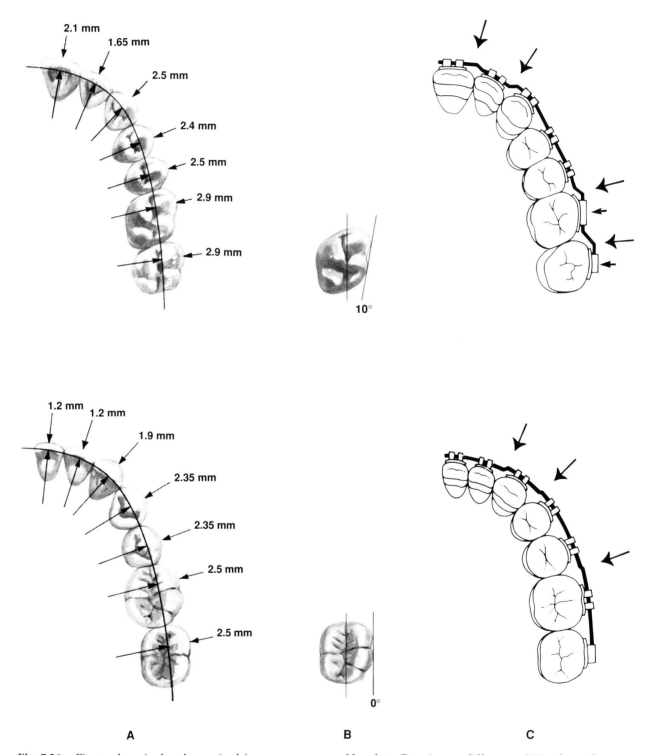

Fig. 7.26. First-order wire bends required for nonprogrammed brackets. Prominence differences *(A)* and maxillary molar offset *(B)* require 4 maxillary and 3 mandibular first-order prominence bends per quadrant *(C, large arrows)*. The maxillary molars require 2 offset bends *(C, small arrows)*.

155

third-order bends are required, totaling 215° (Fig. 7.25). For crown prominence, 14 first-order bends are needed, totaling 6.5 mm. And for maxillary molars, there must be 4 first-order offset bends totaling 40° (Fig. 7.26).

Thus when the brackets are sited on a full complement of optimally positioned teeth, the final "ideal" archwire will require 76 primary wire bends if it is to be placed passively into the slots. This number includes 46 bends (totaling 484°) for angulation, inclination, and offset; and 30 bends (totaling 24.3 mm) for prominence and occlusogingival slot-position error. These totals do not include primary bends needed for translation and for overcorrection of teeth that require translation, nor for the countless progress bends throughout the course of treatment.

Secondary Wire Bends

Secondary wire bends are any bends for tooth guidance that are not primary bends. Secondary bends are needed to compensate for slot-siting irregularities caused by bracket design and unreliable bracket-siting techniques, wire-bending and wire-forming side effects, and judgment errors in bending.

Slot-Siting Irregularities

The extent and direction of tooth movement from specific landmarks on the crown may be known in advance of treatment; what cannot be visually perceived, because of the slot's small size, is how accurately the slot reflects those landmarks. With a nonprogrammed bracket, reliable slot siting is not readily achieved—because of the bracket's design and because traditional landmarks and bracket-siting techniques are inadequate. These design and siting factors, previously discussed, often demand secondary wire bends simply because the guidance the tooth appeared to need was based on the incorrect

assumption that the slot truly reflected the landmark or referents used for siting the brackets.

Side Effects

Wire bending and wire forming required for a nonprogrammed appliance consume perhaps more operatory time per patient than any other procedures. Secondary wire bends are necessary even if the bracket slot represents each crown as intended. The reason is that the mere acts of wire bending or wire forming can generate side effects within the wire that may introduce unwanted tooth movement. When this happens, unscheduled wire adjustments are required. Such side effects are thoroughly discussed in Chapter 12.

Human Error

Archwire construction varies remarkably among clinicians, and sometimes within the work of one clinician. It is difficult or impossible to look at a bracket on a tooth and ascertain exactly what primary bends are needed. It is equally difficult to precisely execute those bends or to transfer them from one progress archwire to another. Thus it is doubtful whether archwires can be adjusted to keep tooth movement unerringly on the intended course.

Tertiary Wire Bends

A tertiary bend is one placed for any reason other than guidance. Examples are omega loops for stops, loops for increasing wire flexibility, and loops for elastics.

Discussion

The vast majority of casts shown in Chapter 5 represent treatment with a nonprogrammed edgewise appliance, and few meet Six Key standards. Treatment goals are more readily conceived than achieved. En route to their goals, orthodontists often encounter slot-siting problems caused by bracket design and bracket siting. Personal skills in wire manipulation vary. Wire bending and wire forming introduce side effects that may produce errant results. Thurow warns, "There is no such thing as an isolated orthodontic act. More effort and knowledge is required to prevent or control unwanted movements than to apply the primary forces"[26]. Some of these events cannot be perceived clinically, but any one of them can affect tooth position beyond the established 0.5-mm or 2° error limits. Therefore each can affect the quality and efficiency of treatment.

Orthodontists can cope with this complex puzzle, at least to some extent, by using scientific landmarks for bracket positioning that can be readily located within 0.5 mm and 2°; brackets designed to work with a siting system that ensures locating them within the 0.5-mm and 2° guidelines; and brackets designed so that, when correctly placed, they will automatically direct each slot to within 0.5 mm and 2° of a specified site. An appliance whose design and siting system offer these three features will reduce or eliminate the need for wire bending; it will also stimulate greater emphasis on diagnosis, treatment planning, and execution of treatment.

Chapter 8

Individualized Brackets — Bracket Siting — Slot Siting

Reducing the number of archwire bends had been thought of long before the Straight-Wire Appliance was introduced in 1970. In 1927 Angle had suggested angulating the entire bracket on the band to free the archwire of "bends in the second order"[8]. Holdaway in l952 suggested bracket overangulation for teeth on either side of an extraction site, to reduce the second-order wire bends otherwise needed to promote both translation and angulation overcorrection [15]. Bracket angulation, however, is a process—not a built-in feature. In 1957 Jarabak incorporated slot inclination to reduce the need for third-order archwire bends, so he is credited for being first to actually build guidance into the bracket [17]. Jarabak also recommended bracket angulation.

In 1958 John J. Stifter was granted a U.S. patent for an edgewise bracket comprising a male and a female component. The female part was attached to the tooth; it was designed to receive one of many interchangeable male components with various combinations of inclination, angulation, and prominence. The inserts were to be progressively selected at each visit and placed according to the guidance then needed for each tooth. This was the first edgewise bracket designed to build guidance into all three planes of space. Its lack of acceptance may be partly because it did not address optimal tooth position and because too many separate parts were needed. Had optimal position been addressed, there would have been no need for inserts. Also, the Stifter design did not attend to the quality or quantity of slot-siting features. The planes of the slot for each tooth type were not correlated with those of its crown, nor with those of other crowns when the teeth were correctly positioned. The flat base of the female component demanded a one-point contact with the crown, assuring the maximum potential range for errant slot siting, and the appliance lacked a scientific bracket-siting system, further ensuring unreliable slot siting.

But the trend was set, and the issue became focused on how much effective guidance could be built into an appliance. To clarify (although this moves ahead of the sequence of events), the ideal was perceived to be an appliance whose slots, when the brackets were correctly sited on the crowns, would be as malpositioned as the teeth. Such an appliance, when used with progressively larger unbent archwires, would flex each archwire only to the diminishing extent that the slots and teeth remained incorrectly positioned, until gradually the teeth, slots, and wires would become aligned or "straight."

This concept can perhaps best be visualized by first imagining the appliance at the conclusion of treatment, on teeth that are optimally positioned. In each arch, all bracket slots are aligned so that a full-size and unbent archwire lies passively within them. Next, imagine the archwire gone and the teeth gradually moved out of position, carrying the brackets with them until the teeth are malaligned as much as at a patient's first office visit. The slots, of course, have become just as malaligned as the teeth. (This is, in fact, the condition that actually exists when fully programmed brackets are properly sited on the crowns.)

To initiate correction, a deflected but unbent archwire is installed—one that has a small diameter relative to the dimensions of the slot. The deflection creates tension in the wire, so the wire will press against the slot walls, seeking to regain its original arch form. As it straightens, the wire will improve the alignment of the slots and the positions of the teeth. As the teeth, slots, and wire "straighten," the wire must periodically be replaced with one having a larger diameter, to maintain the tension. Each replacement requires less flexing, because the malalignment of the teeth and slots has been reduced. This procedure is repeated with progressively larger wires until ultimately the teeth and slots are optimally positioned, and the final full-size archwire is straight.

Returning to the chronology: by the early 1960s, there were individualized bands for each tooth type, but not individualized brack-

ets. Edgewise brackets with inclined slots were available in 5° increments from 5° to 25°. But except for the amount of inclination and, perhaps, mesiodistal size, these brackets were alike and could be used for any tooth type. However, they seldom were used other than for maxillary incisors. Orthodontists began to realize the advantage of angulating the bracket and of inclining the slot, but there was no consensus about the amount of angulation and inclination appropriate for each tooth type, nor about which landmark on the tooth should be used for siting the bracket.

Little progress was made thereafter, in terms of building more treatment into the appliance, until the next evolutionary step was considered—that of designing individual brackets for each tooth type to work without wire bending. This involved (1) deciding whether the brackets could be individualized or had to be customized,* (2) developing a scientific bracket-siting technique, and (3) determining where the slot must be sited for each tooth type. Not until these problems were dealt with could the designing of a fully programmed appliance proceed.

Individualized or Customized Brackets

Can individualized brackets be sufficiently programmed to work without wire bending for most patients? The answer depends partly on the clinical significance of patient-to-patient variations in the shape and optimal position of each tooth type. These issues can be viewed from two perspectives.

The first perspective recognizes that for

---

*As the terms are used in this book, an *individualized appliance* is one whose design tailors each bracket to morphological and positional norms of its tooth type, and to the most widely used treatment plans. A *customized appliance* is one designed and fabricated to precisely match the unique morphology and guidance needs of a specific patient.

each tooth type, both shape and optimal position are similar among nearly all individuals with normal teeth. This view suggests that the slots of individualized brackets, correctly designed and sited, can use flexed but unbent archwires to guide the teeth of most patients with normal teeth and normal malocclusions to the Six Key goals.

In contrast, the second perspective assumes that the shape and optimal position of each tooth type vary sufficiently among individuals to require a customized bracket for each tooth for each patient. This approach requires one-of-a-kind brackets that can be constructed only after the treatment plan is decided and the teeth in a patient's pretreatment dental casts have been positioned to meet treatment objectives, as in a diagnostic setup.

In the broadest sense, if occlusal results from an individualized appliance should prove significantly better than the results observed in the 1150 posttreatment samples (Chapter 5), the first perspective should be clinically justifiable. One disadvantage of the individualized approach, compared to customizing, might be the occasional need for some wire bending at the end of treatment for individuals whose teeth differed from the shape or intended position programmed into the brackets. But the alternative—a customized appliance—would require a second set of casts to construct each patient's customized appliance; deciduous teeth and broken or lost brackets could require additional impressions and casts.

After careful consideration of both views, the first perspective was adopted for testing. If individualized brackets could produce satisfactory results without any wire bending for a high percentage of patients, then customized brackets would not have to be constructed for each person. This proved to be the situation.*

---

*This fact has extensive ramifications. In addition to its more direct significance for patients, it presented orthodontists with consequences of many kinds—technological, economic, and pedagogical.

Examples of such treatment are shown in the photographs of pretreatment and posttreatment casts in Chapter 9 (nonextraction) and Chapter 10 (extraction).

Bracket Siting

Siting the brackets of an appliance designed for use with unbent archwires is critical. Reliable bracket siting depends on a suitable bracket site, dependable landmarks for locating the site, features for locating the bracket on that site, and a reliable technique. A discussion of each of these vital factors follows.

Bracket Site

A suitable bracket site has three criteria. First, a bracket located there will not interfere with either the gingiva or with the opposing teeth during occlusion. Second, the angulation and inclination of the crown at the site will have a consistent angular relationship to the plane of each tooth's occlusal surface at all times and to the occlusal plane of the arch when the teeth are optimally positioned. Finally, the middle of each bracket site must share the same plane or surface when the teeth in an arch are optimally positioned. The site that meets these requirements is the area in immediate proximity to the crown's FA point.

The area around the FA point is neutral enough in location so that properly designed brackets positioned there are generally free of occlusal and gingival interference. The angulation and inclination of the site are consistently related to the plane of the crown's occlusal surface at all times, and to the occlusal plane of the arch when the teeth are optimally positioned. The center of the site, the FA point, always falls on the Andrews plane when the teeth are optimally positioned (Fig. 8.1).

Landmarks

The criteria for the landmarks used to locate the bracket site and to position the bracket are that the landmarks be accurately and readily visible by all orthodontists, and that the same landmarks be valid for both the anterior and posterior teeth.

The landmarks that meet these requirements are the same as those used for the mea-surement study (Chapter 4): the facial axis of the clinical crown (FACC), and the occlusogin-gival extremities of each clinical crown (the gingiva and incisal edge or cusp tip) for locating the midpoint of the FACC—the FA point. The FACC and its gingival extremities meet the stated specifications in the following ways.

Unlike the long axes of teeth or crowns, the FACC is a practical landmark for orienting the bracket for angulation because it can be

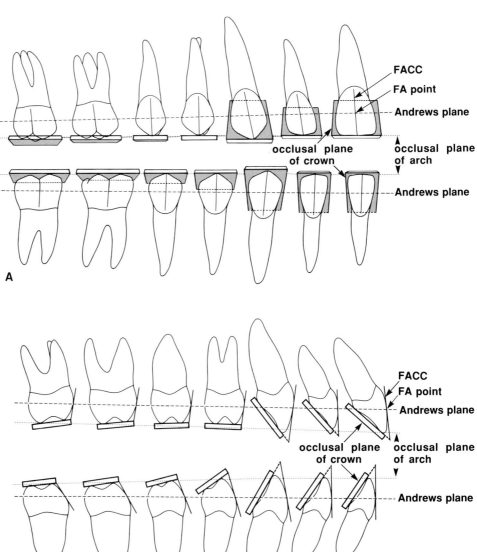

Fig. 8.1. For each tooth type the angulation and inclination of the FACC to the plane of the crown's occlusal surface is consis-tent at all times, and con-sistent with the arch's oc-clusal plane when the teeth are optimally posi-tioned—at which time the FA points fall on the An-drews plane. *A*, Angula-tion; *B*, inclination.

seen and marked. The FACC also makes it easy to inspect the angulation of a crown before treatment. During treatment, the FACC can be observed indirectly via the bracket's vertical components, which are designed to parallel and straddle the FACC. Unlike traditional bracket-siting landmarks, the FACC can be used for angulation and inclination for both the anterior and the posterior teeth.

The landmarks used for locating the FA point are also practical for locating the bracket occlusogingivally, because they too are tangible and can be observed before and during treatment and can be used for both anterior and posterior teeth.

All in all, it would be difficult to exaggerate the advantages in using the FACC and the occlusal and gingival extremities of each clinical crown as the landmarks for the bracket site. Bracket siting is an important link in the chain of requirements for accurate slot siting. Accuracy in this matter requires a technique for siting the bracket to within 2° of the FACC, and the base point of the bracket to within 0.5 mm of the FA point.

Bracket-Siting Technique

To explore whether a parallel-and-midpoint technique for bracket siting can be accurate within 2° and 0.5 mm, several experiments were conducted. The participants were 54 orthodontists who had various levels of experience with fixed appliances, mostly edgewise. Each orthodontist was asked to use a straightedge to draw two vertical lines, approximately one centimeter long and two millimeters

apart, and parallel (Fig. 8.2). Erasing was permitted, but no measuring. This was a test of the ability to estimate parallelism; the reader may wish to try this experiment at test space B in Figure 8.2.

Next, the participants were asked to draw four vertical lines about one centimeter long. Another line was then drawn to each vertical line at a specified angle, as shown in Figure 8.3A. The four angles to be estimated are 2°, 5°, 9°, and 11°. A straightedge was allowed, but no measuring instruments. This exercise was to test the ability to judge angulation as one does when angulating a bracket on a crown. The four vertical lines in Figure 8.3B are to be used for trying this test. After the estimated angles are drawn, the results should be measured with a protractor.

Finally, the participants were instructed to draw a vertical line approximately one centimeter long and to mark its estimated midpoint (Fig. 8.4A). This was a test of ability to judge the midpoint of a line about as long as that of the FACC. Use Figure 8.4B for this test.

The findings showed remarkable accuracy in drawing parallel lines. The average error was 0.194°. Ninety-two percent of the results were within the arbitrary 2° error range. Only four orthodontists exceeded this error limit, and only one of the four erred by as much as one additional degree.

The results of estimating angulation were not satisfactory: the angles drawn at an estimated 2° ranged from 1.5° to 12°, averaging 4°. One-third of the efforts fell outside the

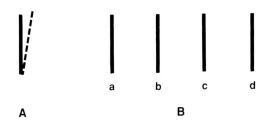

a   b   c   d

A   B

Fig. 8.3. Angulation test: *A,* example; *B,* test space—vertical lines to which estimated angles are to be drawn: *a,* 2°; *b,* 5°; *c,* 9°; and *d,* 11°.

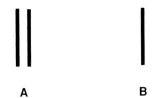

A   B

Fig. 8.2. Paralleling test: *A,* example; *B,* test space.

allowable 2° error range. The estimated 5° angles ranged from 5° to 18° and averaged 8°; 46% of the participants were outside the arbitrary 2° range. The attempts to draw 9° angles ranged from 6° to 34°, averaging 13°; 61% erred by more than 2°. When estimating an 11° angle, the participants produced angles as small as 7° and as large as 26°; the average was 15°. Nearly three out of four results (74%) exceeded the 2° tolerance (Fig. 8.5). It is important to note that the vertical lines used were visible, as is the FACC, so even the poor results of this test in estimating angulation from a tangible line may be better than can be expected from clinical use of the invisible axes of crown or tooth.

In selecting the midpoint of a line representing the height of a normal maxillary central crown, 91% of the participants missed the center by less than 0.5 mm. The average error was 0.165 mm; only one error exceeded 1 mm.

These test results showed that (1) without instruments, two lines can be drawn parallel more accurately than at a specified angle, and (2) the midpoint of a line approximately as long as the FACC can be identified almost exactly. It was concluded that more than 90% of the time the precision of the parallel-and-midpoint technique for bracketing is within the allowable 2° and 0.5-mm guidelines.

Bracket-Siting Features

A suitable bracket site is of limited value if the bracket is not compatibly designed. A bracket will be accurately sited when it parallels and straddles the FACC and when it is equi-

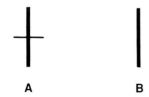

A   **B**

Fig. 8.4. Midpoint test: *A*, example; *B*, test space.

distant from the gingiva and the most occlusal portion of the crown's face. This automatically locates the midpoint of the bracket base squarely on the crown's FA point (Fig. 8.6).

Slot Siting

Accurate bracket siting is of limited value unless each bracket positions its slot with equal accuracy at a site that would allow it to passively receive an unbent archwire when the teeth are optimally positioned. Reliable slot siting depends on a suitable slot site, dependable landmarks for locating that site, and brackets designed to locate the slots on that site. A discussion of each of these vital factors follows, but first the terminology required for this new concept will be introduced.

Note: Terms that refer to the transverse, sagittal, and frontal planes of individual teeth or brackets are referenced from the facial aspects of individual teeth or brackets, not from the planes of the head. Several of the following definitions appear in earlier chapters, but because of their importance in this chapter they are repeated.

Andrews plane. The surface or plane on which the midtransverse plane of every crown in an arch will fall when the teeth are optimally positioned. If the plane is concave or convex, technically it is a surface, but in all instances here it will be referred to as the Andrews plane (Fig. 3.1, 8.1).

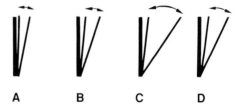

A   **B**   **C**   **D**

Fig. 8.5. Results of angulation study. *A*, The estimated 2° angle ranged from 1.5° to 12°. *B*, The estimated 5° angle ranged from 5° to 18°. *C*, The estimated 9° angle ranged from 6° to 34°. *D*, The estimated 11° angle ranged from 7° to 26°.

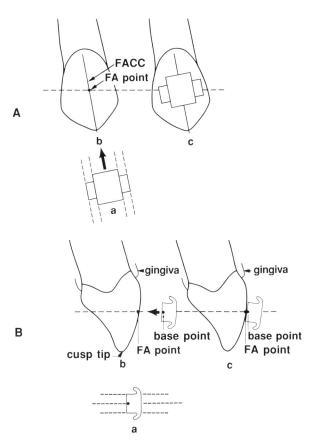

Fig. 8.6. Bracket design for siting. *A,* Facial perspective of a crown and a bracket. *B,* Distal perspective of a crown and a bracket. The bracket's vertical landmarks (*Aa*) should parallel and straddle the crown's vertical landmark (*Ab*), as shown at *Ac.* The bracket's horizontal landmarks (*Ba*) should be equidistant from the crown's horizontal landmarks (*Bb*). This will place the bracket's base point on the crown's FA point as shown at *Bc.*

Embrasure line. An imaginary line, at the level of the Andrews plane, that would connect the most facial portions of the contact areas of a single crown, or of all crowns in an arch when they are optimally positioned (Fig. 4.4).

Midfrontal plane of the crown. The plane that separates the facial from the lingual half of a clinical crown.

Midsagittal plane of the crown. The plane that separates the mesial and distal portions of a crown at its facial axis (Fig. 8.7C).

Midtransverse plane of the crown. The

plane that separates the occlusal portion of a clinical crown from its gingival portion (Fig. 8.7D).

Prominence plane of the crown. A plane that is at right angles to each crown's midtransverse and midsagittal planes and is 1 mm farther facially from each crown's embrasure line than is the most facially prominent cusp of the first molar in that arch (Figs. 8.7B, 8.8).

Slot-target point. The midpoint of the slot site for a tooth type. It is located at the junction of the crown's prominence plane and facial extensions of the crown's midsagittal and midtransverse planes (Fig. 8.7A).

Slot site. The area that the slot must occupy if it is to passively receive an unbent archwire when the teeth are optimally positioned.

The criterion for the slot site is that it be passive to an unbent archwire when the teeth are optimally positioned. For this condition to occur, the planes of each slot must be harmonious with those of the crown at all times, and with all other slots in an arch when the teeth are optimally positioned.

Landmarks and Referents

The center of the slot site—the slot-target point—is located where the crown's prominence plane meets facial extensions of the crown's midsagittal and midtransverse planes (Fig. 8.7A). The landmarks and referents used for locating these planes are explained below.

Midsagittal Plane
The mesiodistal position of the slot-target point is determined by a facial extension of the crown's midsagittal plane. The midsagittal plane of each crown separates the crown mesiodistally at the FACC (Fig. 8.7C).

Midtransverse Plane
The occlusogingival position of the slot target point is determined by a facial extension of the crown's midtransverse plane. The

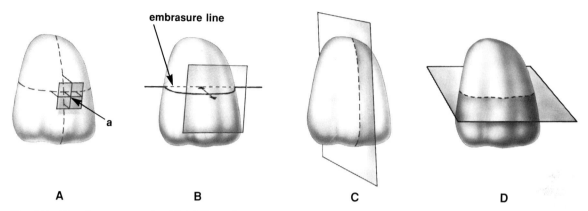

embrasure line

A   B   C   D

Fig. 8.7. The slot-target point (*Aa*) falls at the junction of the crown's prominence plane (*B*) with facial extensions of the crown's midsaggital (*C*) and midtransverse (*D*) planes.

crown's midtransverse plane separates the occlusal half of the crown from the gingival half (Fig. 8.7D). When the teeth are optimally positioned, every crown's midtransverse plane and FA point will fall on the Andrews plane of the arch (Fig. 8.1), and therefore so will every crown's slot-target point.

Prominence Plane

The faciolingual position of the slot-target point is determined by the crown's prominence plane. The prominence plane for each crown is measured from the embrasure line (Fig. 8.7B).* This distance is the sum of the molar prominence in that arch and the bracket-stem prominence (Fig.8.8), and is equal for all crowns in an arch. The prominence plane is at right angles to facial extensions of the crown's midtransverse and midsagittal planes (Fig. 8.7A). Bracket stems for teeth other than molars are more prominent than the molar brackets' stems—in inverse proportion. This approach compensates for the unequal prominence of crowns in an arch and eliminates first-order bends for most arches.

Molar prominence. To obviate the need for first-order wire bends it is essential for all the slot-target points in an arch to be equidistant from the embrasure line. The distance, in part, is dictated by the first permanent molars, which are the most facially prominent crowns in the arch. The remaining distance is determined by the distance required for constructing the least prominent molar bracket possible. Molar prominence is illustrated in Figure 8.8; the amount is shown in Figures 4.24 and 4.28; the method of measurement is shown in Figure 4.20. The fact that molar prominence may vary from individual to individual is not important. This approach works because the relative prominence for tooth types within an

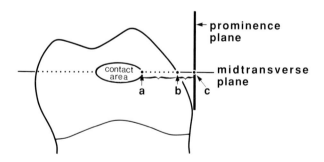

Fig. 8.8. The molar prominence plane (distal view) is as far from the embrasure line (*a*) as is the molar's most facially prominent site along its midtransverse plane (*b*) plus one millimeter (*b–c*).

---

*The embrasure line was selected over the crowns' midfrontal plane to avoid excessive bracket prominence for incisors and canines.

arch varies little between individuals with large teeth or small teeth.

Stem prominence. If brackets are to be clinically unobtrusive for crowns that are less facially prominent than the molars, it is essential that the molar brackets have minimum prominence. Thus the slot point must be as close to the molar as bracket design will allow. For the molars that distance is 1 mm. The base-point-to-slot-point distance for the molar bracket can be thought of as the sum of three parts:

1. The facial surface of a molar crown is inclined relative to its midtransverse plane, but the base of the bracket slot is at 90° to its midtransverse plane. Therefore, if the slot base were located as close to the crown's face as possible, only the gingival portion of the base would actually touch the crown. There would be a gap of ap-

proximately 0.25 mm between the most prominent portion of the crown and the base of the slot when measured along the midtransverse plane (Fig. 8.9A). This 0.25 mm constitutes the first portion of the molar bracket stem.

2. An additional 0.25 mm is added to the first portion (Fig. 8.9B) to ensure that, during manufacturing, the slot will not penetrate the base of the bracket. This tolerance factor, though present in all other brackets, is critical only for molar brackets, because in them the base of the slot is closer to the crown's facial surface than in brackets for any other tooth.

3. The midfrontal plane of a slot is facial to the base of the slot by half the faciolingual size of the slot. This distance will vary with slot size. It is shown in Figure 8.9C as 0.50 mm.

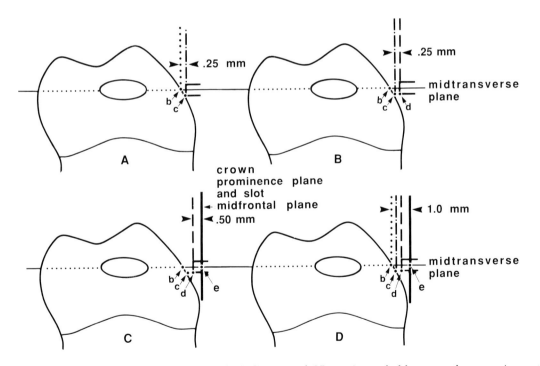

Fig. 8.9. Linear components of the bracket stem. *A,* A distance of .25 mm is needed between the crown's most facially prominent point along its midtransverse plane *(b)* and the base of the slot *(c)* because the crown face is inclined but the slot base is not. *B,* The slot base moved facially a distance of .25 mm from *c* to *d* to provide space for manufacturing tolerance. *C,* A distance of .50 mm is needed between the base of the slot *(d)* and the slot point *(e)* for the lingual half of the slot. *D,* A composite of *A, B,* and *C.*

This distance must then be added to portions one and two. Totaled, they establish the faciolingual location of the prominence plane, the slot-target point for the molars, and the midfrontal plane of the slot when the slot is correctly sited (Fig. 8.9D).

For each arch, the distance from each crown's embrasure line to its slot-target point is equal (Fig. 8.10). However, the distance between the slot-target point and the face of each crown varies inversely with the facial prominence of each tooth type (Fig. 8.10). It is this distance that establishes the stem's faciolingual thickness. In other words, the prominence of the stem for each tooth type is the same as for the molars *plus* the difference by which the facial prominence of the molars exceeds that of the tooth type.

* * *

To understand how the slots will passively receive an unbent rectangular wire, imagine such a wire embedded within all crowns, with its center coincident with the embrasure line of optimally positioned crowns. Then imagine the wire removed and relocated at the slot sites, altering only its form to match the larger circumference. Under these conditions the wire will fit the slot sites passively, because the planes of the crown and slot site are harmonious. A one-

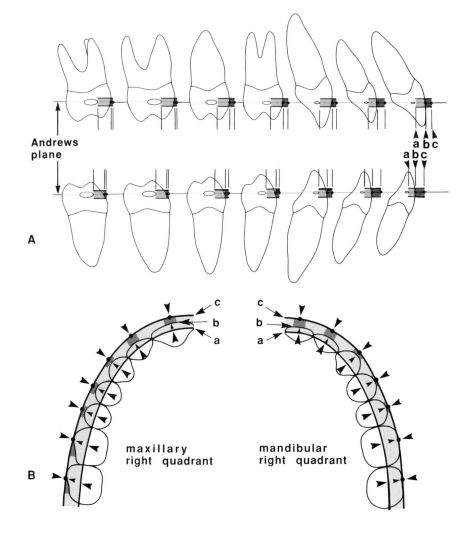

Fig. 8.10. The distance between the embrasure line (*a*) and the slot-target point (*c*) is the same for each crown in an arch. The distance between the embrasure line (*a*) and the most facially prominent portion of the crown (*b*) is the greatest for the molars, and is less, and different, for most other crowns in an arch. The distance between *b* and *c* is inversely proportional to the *ab* distance. *A*, Distal view; *B*, occlusal view. Ovals in the centers of crowns indicate the contact areas.

tooth example of this condition is shown in Figure 8.11.

By contrast, in the nonprogrammed bracket (assuming best possible bracket siting) only the midsagittal plane of its slot matches the planes of the crown (Fig. 8.12).

Once the location of the slot site has been

defined, each bracket can be designed so that when it is correctly sited the planes of its slot will automatically match those of the crown's slot site. The design of each bracket can be completed by filling in the space between the slot site and the bracket site, then adding convenience and auxiliary features.

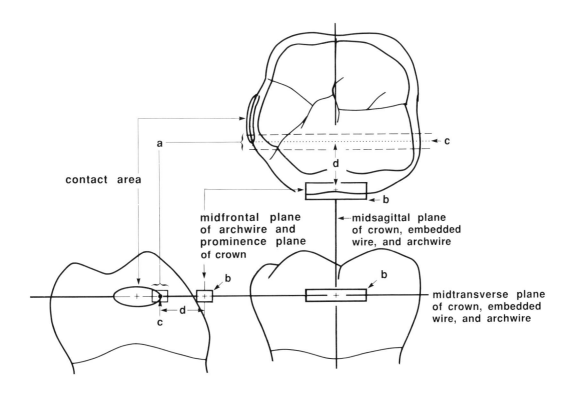

Fig. 8.11. The midsagittal, midtransverse, and prominence planes of the crown, the embedded wire (*a*), and the archwire (*b*) are harmonious. The crown's prominence plane and the midfrontal plane of the archwire are the same and equidistant (*d*) from the embrasure line (*c*).

169

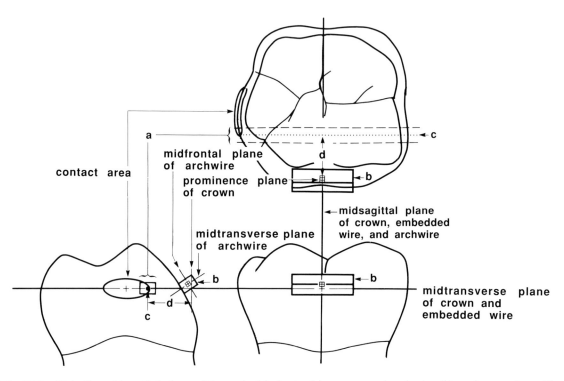

Fig. 8.12. Only the midsagittal plane of the embedded wire (*a*), crown, and archwire (*b*) are harmonious. The distance (*d*) between the embrasure line (*c*) and the prominence plane is not the same as for the midfrontal plane of the archwire.

Chapter **9**

Fully Programmed Standard Brackets

The concept of programming tooth guidance into the bracket rather than into the wire is based on the recognition that extensive similarities prevail in the morphology of normal tooth types, and in their positions when they are optimally occluded. A fully programmed appliance puts these similarities to work, accomplishing all or nearly all tooth guidance with flexed but unbent archwires.

The simplest version of a fully programmed appliance consists of brackets designed to guide teeth that do not require translation. In this book such brackets are referred to as standard brackets. There is one standard bracket for each tooth type except for the incisors and maxillary molars: for incisors there are three, for maxillary molars, two. To eliminate archwire bending, more slot-siting features are required than just the correct amount of slot angulation, inclination, and facial prominence. Brackets with only these three features are only partly programmed, because they will not target the slot within 2° and 0.5 mm of the slot site. To explain the design of fully programmed standard brackets, the following terminology is required. (Several of these terms have been defined in earlier chapters, but are repeated here because of their importance in this chapter.)

Auxiliary feature. A design feature that contributes to the biological aspect of treatment but is not involved in targeting the slot.

Convenience feature. A design feature that facilitates use by the orthodontist or promotes comfort for the patient but does not contribute to the biological aspects of treatment or to targeting the slot.

Embrasure line. An imaginary line, at the level of the crown's midtransverse plane, that would connect the most facial portions of the contact areas of a single crown, or of all crowns in an arch when they are optimally positioned.

Facial plane of a crown. Any plane that is tangent to a point on the crown's face.

Fully programmed appliance. A set of brackets designed to guide teeth directly to their goal positions with unbent archwires. The term *straight-wire appliance* is used as a synonym in this book.

Inclined base. A bracket base that is angled more or less than 90° to the midtransverse plane of the bracket stem.

Inclined slot. A slot whose midtransverse plane is inclined relative to the midtransverse plane of the bracket stem.

Maxillary molar offset. The angle between the crown's embrasure line and a line connecting the buccal cusps of a maxillary molar. It is measured along the crown's midtransverse plane.

Mesiodistal base contour. The horizontal contour of the bracket's base.

Occlusogingival base contour. The vertical contour of the bracket's base.

Slot point. The junction of the midtransverse, midsagittal, and midfrontal planes of the bracket slot.

Slot site. The area that the bracket slot must occupy if it is to passively receive a full-size and unbent archwire when a tooth is optimally positioned.

Slot-siting feature. A design feature for positioning the bracket slot.

Slot-target point. The midpoint of the slot site for a tooth. It is located at the junction of a crown's prominence plane and facial extensions of the crown's midtransverse and midsagittal planes.

Standard bracket. A fully programmed bracket designed for teeth that do not require translation.

Stem prominence. Distance from the base point of the bracket to its slot point.

Straight-wire appliance. A set of brackets designed to guide teeth directly to their goal positions with unbent archwires: used synonymously for *fully programmed appliance.*

Straight-Wire Appliance. The registered name of a fully programmed appliance manufactured by a specific orthodontic company.

Translation bracket. A fully programmed bracket for teeth that require translation. It is designed to promote bodily movement during mesial or distal movement, and to overcorrect in proportion to the distance moved.

Design Features

The design of fully programmed brackets emanates from the slot site (Chapter 8). Fully programmed standard brackets include slot-siting features, convenience features, and auxiliary features.

Slot-Siting Features

Fully programmed standard brackets provide slot-siting features of the quality required—and in the number required—for treatment with unbent archwires. One slot-siting feature for each of the three planes of space is not sufficient; eight in all are needed. These essential elements will be explained from the perspectives of the planes of individual teeth and brackets, not in relation to the planes of the patient's head.

Midtransverse Plane

The midtransverse plane of the slot must coincide with a facial extension of the crown's midtransverse plane (Fig. 9.1). To achieve this objective, siting features 1, 2, and 3, discussed below, are required.

Feature 1. The midtransverse planes of the slot, stem, and crown must be the same (Fig. 9.1).

Feature 2. The base of the bracket for each tooth type must have the same inclination as the facial plane of the crown at the FA point (relative to the crown's midtransverse plane; see Fig. 9.1). For the method of measurement see Figures 4.15 and 4.16; for the amount of inclination for each tooth type see Figures 4.23 and 4.27.

Feature 3. Each bracket's inclined base must be contoured occlusogingivally to match the curvature of the crown (Fig. 9.2). Occlusogingivally contoured bracket bases eliminate the potential for the many slot-siting variations inherent in brackets whose bases are occlusogingivally flat (Figs. 7.6, 7.7). For the method of determining this contour see Figure 4.10.

* * *

Features 1 through 3 are of little value if the midpoint of the bracket base (base point) is not sited on the corresponding crown landmark (FA point). The bracket's base point is as readily determined as the crown's FA point. The parallel-and-midpoint technique for placing the base point on the FA point of the crown is easily and accurately accomplished, as discussed in Chapter 8 and illustrated in Figure 8.6.

If features 1 through 3 are incorporated into the bracket design and the brackets are sited correctly, each slot's midtransverse plane will be aligned with that of the crown, regardless of the crown's position. When the teeth are optimally positioned, the midtransverse planes of all the crowns, stems, and slots in an arch will coincide with the Andrews plane (Fig. 9.3). The three midtransverse slot-siting features eliminate the need for several kinds of bends—second-order bends to deal with occlusogingival disharmony in slot siting, third-order bends for inclination (Chapter 7), and other bends to deal with inherent side effects of wire bending (Chapter 12).

Midsagittal Plane

The midsagittal plane of each slot must superimpose on a facial extension of the crown's midsaggital plane (Fig. 9.4). To achieve this objective, siting features 4 through 7 are required.

Feature 4. The midsagittal plane of the slot, stem, and crown must be the same (Fig. 9.4).

Feature 5. The plane of the bracket base at its base point must be identical to the facial plane of the crown at the FA point. In maxillary molars the angle is 100° (Fig. 9.4A). In all crowns other than maxillary molars, this plane bears 90° to the midsagittal plane (Fig. 9.4B). In the maxillary molars the extra 10° prosthetically equalizes the unequal facial prominence of the molar buccal cusps, while directing the midsagittal plane of the bracket stem and slot to that of the crown. For the method of measurement see Figures 4.17 and 4.18. For the number of degrees see Figure 4.25.

Feature 6. The base of each bracket must be contoured to match the mesiodistal radius of the area of the crown it is designed to fit (Fig. 9.5). Conformity of crown and bracket-base curvature prevents any play between the base and crown that might cause the midsagittal plane of the bracket to be directed mesially or distally to the crown's midsagittal plane. For the method of measuring contour see Figure 4.19.

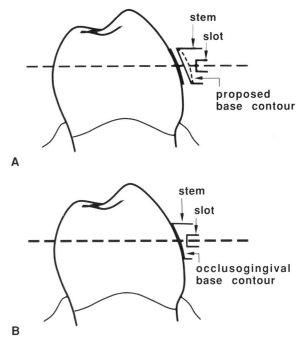

Fig. 9.2. Occlusogingival contour of the bracket base and the crown are the same: *A*, flat-based bracket, with proposed change; *B*, contoured bracket mated with crown.

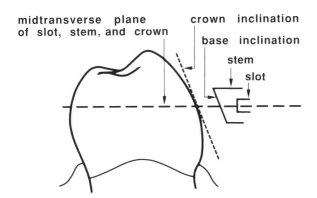

Fig. 9.1. The midtransverse planes of the slot, stem, and crown are the same. The base of the bracket and the facial plane of the crown have the same inclination.

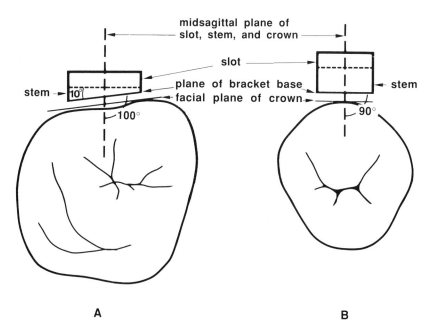

Fig. 9.3. When fully programmed brackets are correctly sited, the midtransverse planes of the crowns, stems, and slots coincide with the Andrews plane. Enlarged bracket positions (*center*) are identical to those on teeth. Dots indicate base points of brackets.

Andrews plane

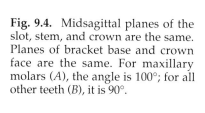

midsagittal plane of slot, stem, and crown

slot

stem

plane of bracket base

facial plane of crown

stem

100°

90°

Fig. 9.4. Midsagittal planes of the slot, stem, and crown are the same. Planes of bracket base and crown face are the same. For maxillary molars (*A*), the angle is 100°; for all other teeth (*B*), it is 90°.

A

B

Feature 7. In each fully programmed bracket, the vertical components (in this example the mesial and distal borders of the bracket stem and tie wings) are designed to parallel one another (Fig. 9.6Aa, Ba). These components, when the parallel-and-midpoint bracket-siting technique is used (see Chapter 8), are to parallel and straddle the vertical landmark of the crown—the FACC (Fig. 9.6Ac, Bc)—as shown in Figure 9.6Ad, Bd. The horizontal components of the bracket are the superior and inferior sides of the bracket stem (Fig. 9.6Ab,Bb). When these components are sited equidistant from the crown's gingiva and cusp tip the base point of the bracket will mate with the crown's FA point. The slot point, base point, and FA point will all be on a plane that coincides with the crown's mid-transverse plane (Fig. 9.6Ae, Be).

From the facial perspective the occlusal and gingival borders of some brackets are perpendicular to their vertical components (Fig. 9.6Aa), and others are more or less than 90° (Fig. 9.6Ba). Bracket siting or slot siting is not affected by the angle between the bracket's occlusal or gingival borders and its vertical components (Fig. 9.6Ad,e, Bd,e).

Once the midtransverse and midsagittal features are incorporated, the slot is angular to each bracket's vertical components (Fig. 9.7Aa, Ba) to the same extent that the midtransverse plane of the crown is angular to the crown's FACC and midsagittal plane (Fig. 9.7Ab, Bb). These features make it unnecessary to angle the bracket to align the slot with the crown's midtransverse plane (Fig. 9.7Ac, Bc), a procedure that can misdirect the slot in several ways (Fig. 7.15). The occlusogingival borders of some brackets do not parallel the slots (Fig. 9.7Aa); others do (Fig. 9.7Ba). If otherwise identical, either will target the slot correctly if the parallel-and-midpoint technique is used (Fig. 9.7Ac,d, Bc,d). For the method of measurement see Figure 4.13; for the amount of angulation for each tooth type see Figures 4.22 and 4.26.

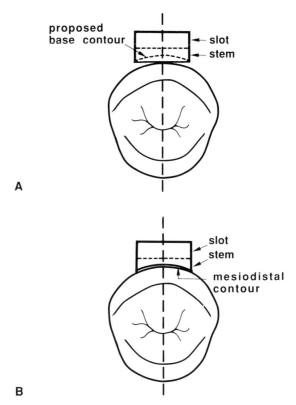

Fig. 9.5. The mesiodistal contour of the bracket base and the crown are the same: *A*, proposed change in flat-based bracket to match crown contour; *B*, contoured bracket mated with crown.

Midsagittal slot-siting features 4–7, when brackets are correctly sited, eliminate the need for first-order maxillary molar offset bends (Fig. 7.26C). They also eliminate first-order bends to deal with errant mesiodistal slot siting (Fig. 7.10), second-order bends for angulation (Fig. 7.23), and errant occlusogingival slot siting (Fig. 7.24) caused by bracket design (Fig. 7.3) and by angulated brackets (Fig. 7.15). The same features eliminate side effects related to those wire bends.

Midfrontal Plane

The midfrontal plane of each slot must superimpose on its crown's prominence plane.

Feature 8. Within an arch, all slot points must have the same distance between them

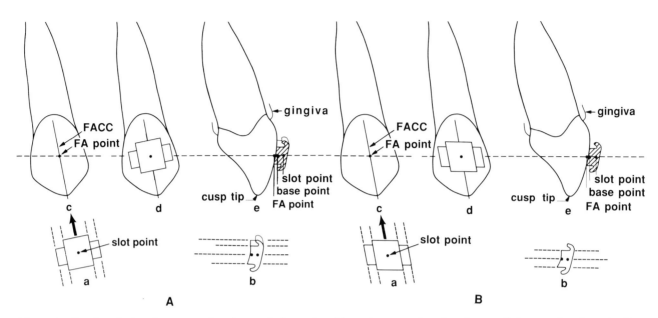

Fig. 9.6. Bracket design for correct bracket and slot-point siting: *A,* square bracket; *B,* parallelogram bracket. *Aa, Ba,* From the facial perspective the vertical components of a bracket are parallel. *Ab, Bb,* From the distal perspective the horizontal components of a bracket are parallel. *Ac, Bc,* The landmark for siting the bracket vertically is the FACC. *Ae, Be,* Landmarks for siting the bracket horizontally are the gingiva and cusp tip. *Ad, Bd,* The vertical components of a bracket should parallel and straddle the crown's FACC. *Ae, Be,* The bracket's horizontal components should be equidistant from the gingiva and cusp tip, which automatically locates the base point of the bracket to the crown's FA point. *Aa, Ad, Ba, Bd,* Bracket siting and slot-point siting are not affected by the angle between the bracket's horizontal and vertical borders. Dashed line indicates midtransverse plane of crowns.

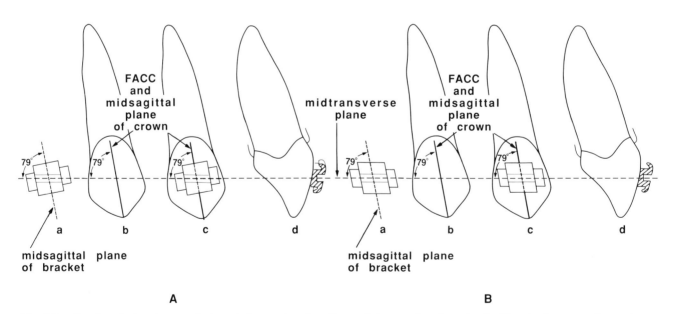

Fig. 9.7. Bracket design for angulation. *A,* Square bracket; *B,* parallelogram bracket. *Aa, Ba,* The slot is as angular to the midsagittal plane of the bracket as the midtransverse plane of the crown is angular to the FACC and midsagittal plane of the crown (*Ab, Bb*). When the bracket is correctly sited, the respective midsagittal and midtransverse planes of the bracket and crown are the same (*Ac, d, Bc, d*).

176

and the crown's embrasure line (Fig. 9.8). At the same time, the distance between the slot points and the face of each crown, when measured along their respective midtransverse planes, must be inversely proportional to the distance between each crown's face and its embrasure line (Fig. 9.8). Feature 8 eliminates first-order wire bends to accommodate for varying crown prominence (Fig. 7.26). For the method of measuring crown prominence see Figure 4.20. For the amount see Figures 4.24 and 4.28. For the method of computing slot prominence see Chapter 8.

Convenience Features

Machining procedures suitable for manufacturing bilaterally symmetrical nonprogrammed brackets are not efficient for producing fully programmed brackets. For such a complex design, casting or molding is the practical manufacturing process. Casting or molding can also be used to include both convenience and auxiliary features.

Convenience features do not play a role in slot siting, but they make the appliance easier for the orthodontist to use and sometimes

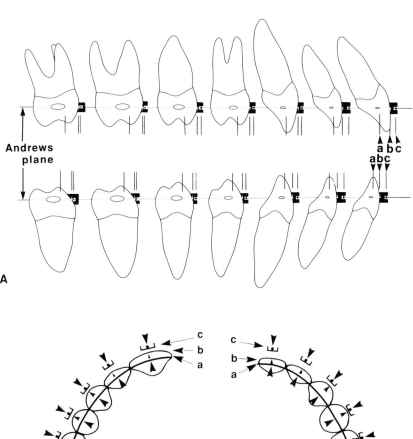

Fig. 9.8. Bracket design for prominence: the distance from the embrasure line (*a*) to the slot point (*c*) is the same for all brackets in an arch. The distance between each crown's most prominent point on its midtransverse plane (*b*) and the bracket's slot point (*c*) is inversely proportional to the *ab* distance. *A*, Distal view; *B*, occlusal view. Ovals in the centers of crowns indicate the contact areas.

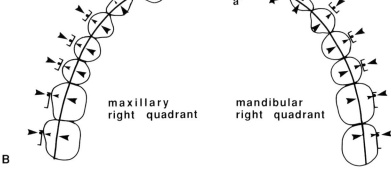

more comfortable for the patient. The gingival tie wings on posterior brackets, for example, are designed to extend farther laterally than they do on nonprogrammed brackets (Figs. 9.9, 9.10). This facilitates ligation and eliminates gingival impingement. The bases of fully programmed brackets are inclined, so on mandibular premolars and molars the stem and tie wings are directed more gingivally than they are in nonprogrammed brackets. This slot-siting feature eliminates or reduces occlusal interference that often occurs with brackets whose bases are not inclined (Fig. 9.10). In this example a slot-siting feature doubles as a convenience feature.

The facial surfaces of incisor and canine brackets are designed to parallel their bases,

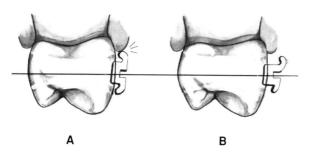

A   **B**

Fig. 9.9. Convenience feature: *A,* symmetrical tie wings. *B,* Asymmetrical tie wings.

which in turn parallel the crowns' faces. This feature is for lip comfort (Fig. 9.11). For the mandibular canine it also reduces some of the potential for occlusal interference with opposing teeth. Consequently, these brackets' faces have been altered from being flat and perpendicular to the midtransverse plane of the slot and stem to being curved and parallel to the crown face (Fig. 9.12). The inclined bracket face gives the impression that the slot is inclined in the bracket face. Close inspection reveals that the midtransverse planes of the crown, stem, and slot are the same. Any inclination intended for the crown is restricted to the base of the bracket, as in all other fully programmed brackets. The contour and inclination of the face of these brackets are convenience features and do not affect slot siting. In the most facially prominent of all the brackets—those for the mandibular incisors—the occlusal tie wings are designed with the least amount of occlusofacial prominence, to reduce the potential for occlusal interference with the opposing incisors (Fig. 9.11Bb, Bc).

Another convenience element provides bracket identification. Slot-siting features for all nonprogrammed brackets are the same, so identification is not required. Fully programmed brackets are as different as are tooth

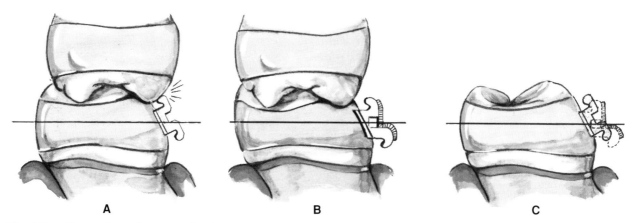

A   **B**   **C**

Fig. 9.10. Convenience feature: A bracket base perpendicular to the stem (*A*) positions the bracket stem and tie wings more occlusally than does an inclined bracket base (*B*). (*C*), Superimposed brackets with inclined (*dashed lines*) and perpendicular (*solid lines*) bases.

types. However, because they are so much smaller than teeth, their differences are not always readily visible without special marking. Thus brackets that cannot be easily identified relative to tooth type are marked in one or more ways. The markings enable one to look at a bracket and tell (1) which arch it is for; (2) which quadrant; (3) which class; (4) which type; (5) whether it is a standard or a translation bracket; (6) for incisors, the category of inclination; and (7) for maxillary molars, whether it is for a Class I or Class II relationship. The markings or features used in the Straight-Wire Appliance for these purposes are explained and illustrated in Figure 9.13.

Auxiliary Features

Unlike convenience features, auxiliary features contribute to the biologic aspect of treatment, even though they are not involved in siting the slot. Examples are power arms, hooks, face-bow tubes, utility tubes, and rotation wings. Casting permits these features to be integral parts of the bracket rather than separate elements that must be added later.

Incisor Brackets

As reported in the measurement study (Chapter 4), the inclination range for the incisors was greater than for other teeth. This presumably does not reflect differing tooth morphology, but differing skeletal patterns

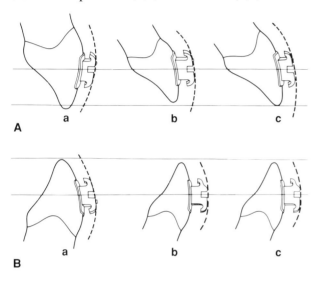

Fig. 9.11. The faces of canine and incisor brackets are contoured to parallel their bases. *A,* Maxillary: canine (*a*), lateral incisor (*b*), and central incisor (*c*). *B,* Mandibular: canine (*a*), lateral incisor (*b*), and central incisor (*c*).

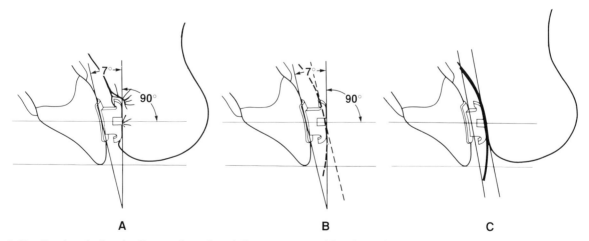

A   **B**   **C**

Fig. 9.12. Bracket design for lip comfort: *A,* a fully programmed bracket whose face is angular to its base and not contoured. *B,* Dashed lines show proposed matching of inclination and contour of the bracket's face with its base. *C,* Bracket with matching contour and inclinations.

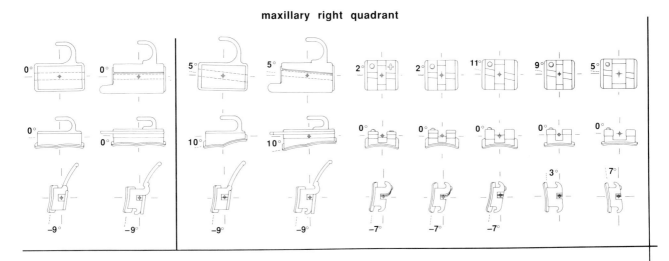

maxillary right quadrant

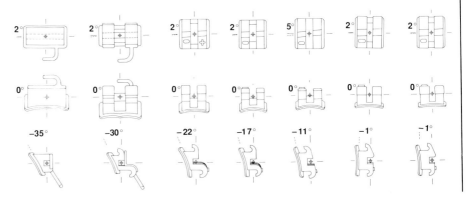

mandibular right quadrant

Fig. 9.13. Bracket identification for incisors, canines, and premolars.

Factor to be identified	Identifying feature
Arch	
Maxillary	Dot on bracket face
Mandibular	Dash on bracket face
Quadrant	
Maxillary	Dot on distogingival portion of bracket face
Mandibular	Dash on distogingival portion of bracket face
Class	
Maxillary	
Incisors	Least base contour
Canine	Most slot angulation (11°)
Premolars	Prominent gingival tie wings
Mandibular	
Incisors	Greatest faciolingual thickness, least base contour
Canine	Most slot angulation
Premolars	Prominent gingival tie wings

Factor to be identified	Identifying feature
Type	
Central from lateral	
Maxillary	Central less faciolingual thickness
	Central 5° slot angulation, lateral 9°
Mandibular	Left central and lateral alike
	Rights mirror images of lefts
Canines	
Maxillary	Most slot angulation (11°)
Mandibular	Most slot angulation (5°)
First from second premolar	
Maxillary	Second has + sign on mesiogingival tie wing
Mandibular	Second has + sign on mesiogingival tie wing
Incisor inclination	
Category I	One (or no) notch on occlusal portion of base
Category II	Two notches at occlusal portion of base
Category III	Three notches at occlusal portion of base

that exist even in patients with exemplary occlusion. There must be at least three standard brackets, each with a different base inclination to accommodate one of the three acceptable but different posttreatment interjaw relationships.

To some extent, orthodontists can predict the posttreatment interjaw relationship for any patient. Certainly, little change will occur in adults unless they have surgery, and the effect of jaw surgery can be accurately planned. Orthopedic treatment for a growing patient is to some extent predictable with the application of orthopedic forces. The base inclination for incisor brackets selected at the beginning of treatment should conform to the crown inclinations that are harmonious with the anticipated interjaw relationship. Of the three brackets designed for maxillary central incisors, one is to be used when the interjaw relationship is anticipated to be Class I; another is for Class II interjaw tendencies; and the third is for Class III tendencies.

A problem associated with prescribing these brackets, even when the posttreatment interjaw relationship is known, is that most cephalometric analyses deal with the inclination of the long axes of the central incisors, whereas prescription of fully programmed brackets is based on the inclination of the crowns' facial axes. Since tooth axes and crown facial axes are not parallel, a study was undertaken to ascertain whether there was a predictable relationship between the two.

For the maxillary central incisor, an unpublished study by Andrews (1968) of 100 cephalograms showed an average difference of 18° between the inclination of the *facial axis of the crown* and that of the *long axis of the tooth* (Fig. 9.14A). The correct maxillary incisor bracket can be selected by subtracting 18° from the projected posttreatment inclination of the tooth's long axis, relative to a line 90° to the occlusal plane. For example, if the posttreatment long axis is projected to be 20° from a line 90° to the occlusal plane, 18° subtracted from 20° indi-

cates that a bracket with 2° of base inclination should be prescribed. This inclination applies when the interjaw relationship tends to be Class II. For Class I interjaw conditions the inclination of the maxillary incisor must be approximately 25°; this, minus 18°, converts to a bracket-base inclination of 7°. When the tooth's long-axis inclination is 30°, the bracket-base inclination should be 12° (Fig. 9.15). This prescription is for Class III interjaw tendencies.

In the measurement study (Chapter 4), the maxillary lateral incisor's inclination was found to average 4° less than that of the maxillary central incisor, regardless of the latter's inclination. So whatever bracket-base inclination is prescribed for the maxillary central incisor, the lateral's bracket-base inclination should be 4° less. For example, the maxillary lateral bracket that is the mate for the 2° central bracket has a base inclination of –2°; for the 7° central bracket the inclination is 3°; and for the 12° central bracket the inclination is 8° (Fig. 9.16).

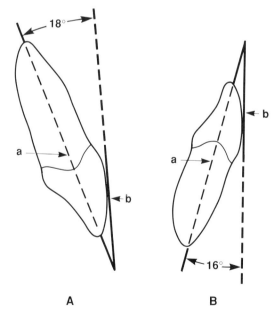

Fig. 9.14. The angle of the central incisor's long axis (*a*) and its FACC (*b*) is 18° for maxillary central incisors (*A*), and 16° for mandibular central incisors (*B*).

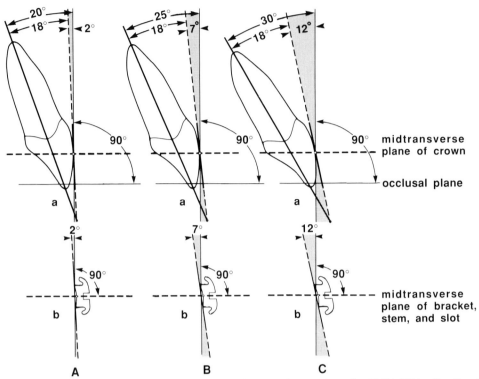

Fig. 9.15. Bracket prescription for maxillary central incisors: for a 20° long axis and a 2° FACC inclination (*Aa*) a bracket base inclination of 2° is required (*Ab*). For a 25° long axis and a 7° FACC inclination (*Ba*) a bracket base inclination of 7° is required (*Bb*). For a 30° long axis and a 12° FACC inclination (*Ca*) a bracket base of 12° is required (*Cb*).

The same 100-cephalogram sample indicated that the mandibular central incisor has an average difference of 16° between the FACC and the long axis of the tooth (Fig. 9.14B). The correct mandibular incisor bracket can be determined by subtracting 16° from the projected posttreatment inclination of the tooth's long axis, relative to a line 90° to the occlusal plane. For Class II interjaw tendencies the posttreatment mandibular incisor's long axis should be approximately 20° from a line 90° to the occlusal plane. Subtracting 16° from 20° indicates that a bracket with 4° base inclination should be prescribed. For a Class I interjaw condition, a mandibular incisor's long axis should be inclined approximately 15°, requiring a bracket-base inclination of –1° (15° less 16° = –1°). For Class III interjaw tendencies the incisor's long axis should be inclined approximately 10°; subtracting 16°

from 10° indicates the base inclination of –6° (Fig. 9.17). The measurement study (Chapter 4) indicated that the crown inclinations of the mandibular central and lateral incisors are approximately equal, so whatever inclination is prescribed for mandibular centrals would also be prescribed for the laterals.

The angulation and prominence remain the same for each incisor tooth type, for each of the three differing base inclinations.

Posterior Brackets

Except for maxillary molars, only one standard bracket is needed for each tooth type. Maxillary molars require two brackets: one for a Class I interarch relationship and one for Class II.

A limited exception to the molar portion of

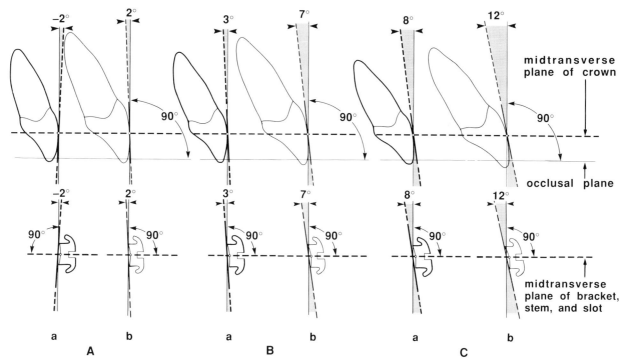

Fig. 9.16. Inclination prescription for the maxillary lateral incisor bracket is 4° less than for the central. A lateral bracket with –2° of base inclination (*Aa*) is used with a 2° central bracket (*Ab*). A lateral bracket with 3° of base inclination (*Ba*) is used with a 7° central bracket (*Bb*). A lateral bracket with 8° of base inclination (*Ca*) is used with a 12° central bracket (*Cb*).

Key I is permissible when the treatment plan calls for the molars and maxillary second premolars to be left in a Class II relationship while treating the rest of the dentition to Class I, for example, after first or second premolar extraction in the maxillary arch only. Under that condition the mesiobuccal cusp of the maxillary molar articulates in the embrasure between the mandibular first molar and premolar. The distobuccal cusp of the maxillary molar articulates with the mandibular molar's mesiobuccal groove, which extends farther occlusally than does the distobuccal groove (Fig. 9.18).

For a Class II molar relationship, the angulation of the maxillary molar crowns should be upright (Fig. 9.19); for Class I, it should be approximately 5° (Fig. 9.20).

Relative to the embrasure line, the mesiobuccal groove of a mandibular first molar is more facially prominent than its distobuccal

groove (Fig. 9.21). The mandibular second molar generally does not have a distobuccal groove, but its buccal groove, like that of the first molar, is more facially prominent than the distal portion of its distobuccal cusp (Fig. 9.21). Therefore, when the interarch relationship is Class I, the mesiobuccal cusps of the maxillary molars should be more facially prominent than the distobuccal cusps (Fig. 9.22). The mesiolingual cusps occlude within the central fossae of the mandibular molars (Fig. 9.22).

When molars are treated to a Class II interarch relationship, the buccal cusps of the maxillary molars should be equal in facial prominence. This is because they now occlude in grooves and embrasures that also are equal in facial prominence (Fig. 9.23).

The mesiolingual cusp of a maxillary molar treated to a Class II relationship generally requires equilibration, because it occludes

183

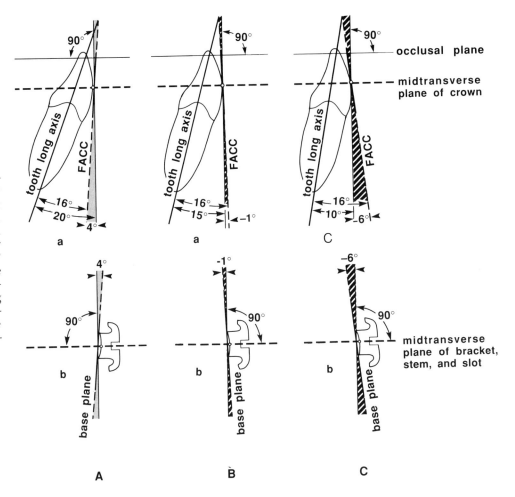

Fig. 9.17. Bracket prescription for mandibular incisors: for a 20° long axis and a 4° FACC (*Aa*) a bracket base inclination of 4° is required (*Ab*). For a 15° long axis and a –1° FACC (*Ba*) a bracket base inclination of –1° is required (*Bb*). For a 10° long axis and a –6° FACC inclination (*Ca*) a bracket base inclination of –6° is required (*Cb*).

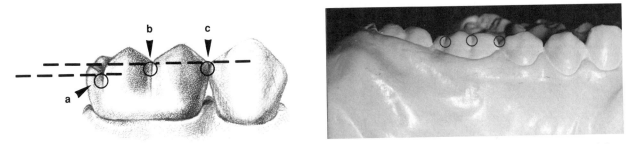

Fig. 9.18. The articular portion of the molar's distobuccal groove (*a*) is less occlusal than the mesiobuccal groove of the mandibular first molar (*b*) and the embrasure formed by the molar and premolar cusps (*c*). Circles indicate articular areas.

with marginal ridges, and they are more oc-clusal than the fossae (Fig. 9.23).

Inventory

Illustrations and vital statistics of all stan-dard brackets are shown in Figures 9.24 to 9.38.

Treatment Sample

Fifteen pretreatment and posttreatment casts are shown in Figures 9.39 to 9.53 to dem-onstrate treatment with fully programmed standard brackets. Treatment required no ex-tractions and little or no translation.

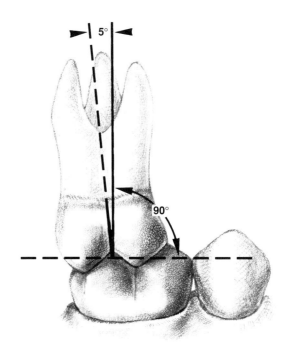

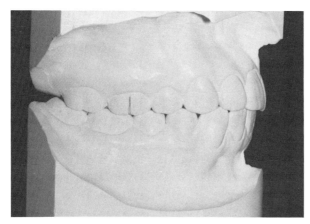

Fig. 9.19. For Class II molars, the FACC of maxillary molars should be approximately 90° to the occlusal plane (*horizontal dashed line*).

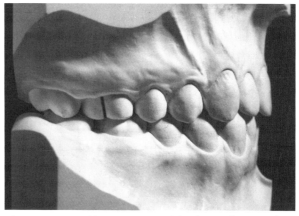

Fig. 9.20. For Class I, the FACC of maxillary molars should be approximately 5° to a line perpendicular to the occlusal plane (*horizontal dashed line*).

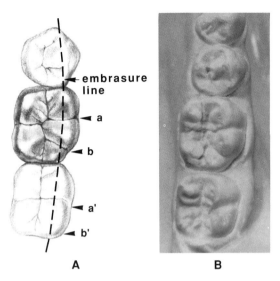

Fig. 9.21. Relative to the embrasure line, the mesiobuccal groove of a mandibular first molar (*a*) is more facially prominent than the distobuccal groove (*b*). The buccal groove of the mandibular second molar (*a'*) is more prominent than the distal portion of its distobuccal cusp (*b'*).

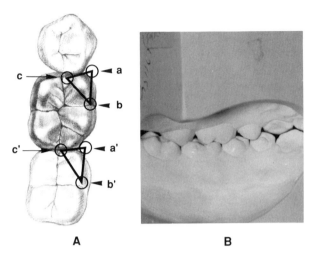

Fig. 9.23. For Class II, the buccal cusps of maxillary molars (*circles Aa, a' and b, b'*) should have equal facial prominence. The mesiolingual cusps of the maxillary molars should occlude with marginal ridges (*circles Ac, c', and B*).

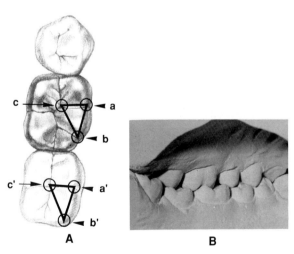

Fig. 9.22. When Class I, the mesiobuccal cusps of maxillary molars (*circles Aa, a'*) should be more facially prominent than the distobuccal cusps (*circles Ab, b'*). The mesiolingual cusps should occlude within the central fossae of the mandibular molars (*circles Ac, c', and B*).

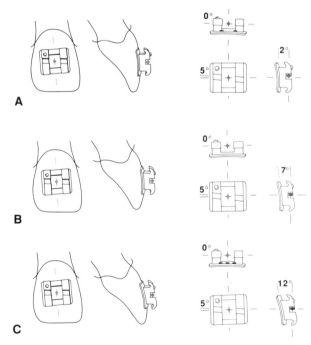

Fig. 9.24. Maxillary central incisor standard brackets: *A*, for Class II jaws, Category II; *B*, for Class I jaws, Category I; *C*, for Class III jaws, Category III:
Angulation: 5°
Inclination: *A*, 2°; *B*, 7°; *C*, 12°
Prominence: 1.8 mm

186

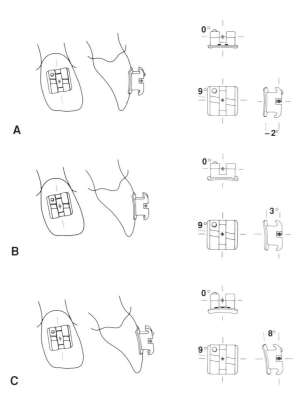

Fig. 9.25. Maxillary lateral incisor standard brackets: *A*, for Class II jaws, Category II; *B*, for Class I jaws, Category I; *C*, for Class III jaws, Category III:

Angulation: 5°
Inclination: *A*, –2°; *B*, 3°; *C*, 8°
Prominence: 2.25 mm

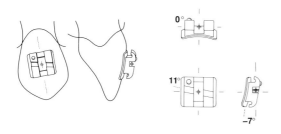

Fig. 9.26. Maxillary canine standard bracket:

Angulation: 11°
Inclination: –7°
Prominence: 1.4 mm

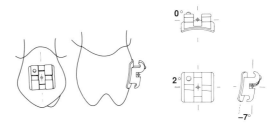

Fig. 9.27. Maxillary first premolar standard bracket:

Angulation: 2°
Inclination: –7°
Prominence: 1.5 mm

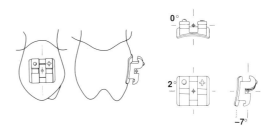

Fig. 9.28. Maxillary second premolar standard bracket:

Angulation: 2°
Inclination: –7°
Prominence: 1.5 mm

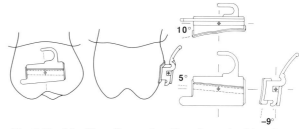

Fig. 9.29. Maxillary first molar, Class I standard bracket:

Angulation: 5°
Inclination: –9°
Prominence: 1 mm
Offset: 10°

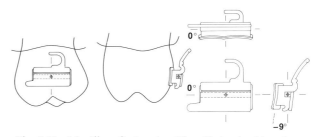

Fig. 9.30. Maxillary first molar, Class II standard bracket:

Angulation: 0°
Inclination: –9°
Prominence: 1 mm

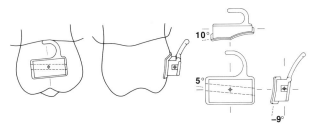

Fig. 9.31. Maxillary second molar, Class I standard bracket:
Angulation: 5°
Inclination: –9°
Prominence: 1 mm
Offset: 10°

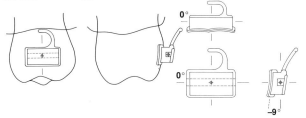

Fig. 9.32. Maxillary second molar, Class II standard bracket:
Angulation: 0°
Inclination: –9°
Prominence: 1 mm

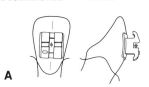
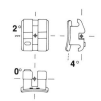

A

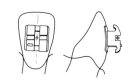
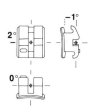

B

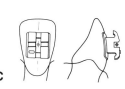
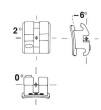

C

Fig. 9.33. Mandibular central and lateral incisor standard brackets: *A,* for Class II jaws, Category II; *B,* for Class I jaws, Category I; *C,* for Class III jaws, Category III:
Angulation: 2°
Inclination: *A,* 4°; *B,* –1°; *C,* –6°
Prominence: 2.3 mm

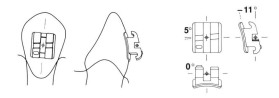

Fig. 9.34. Mandibular canine standard bracket:
Angulation: 5°
Inclination: –11°
Prominence: 1.6 mm

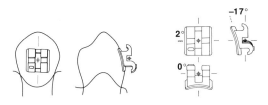

Fig. 9.35. Mandibular first premolar standard bracket:
Angulation: 2°
Inclination: –17°
Prominence: 1.15 mm

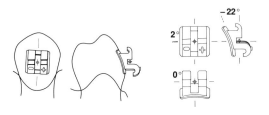

Fig. 9.36. Mandibular second premolar standard bracket:
Angulation: 2°
Inclination: –22°
Prominence: 1.15 mm

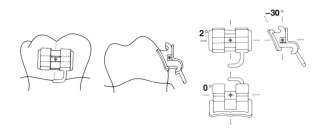

Fig. 9.37. Mandibular first molar standard bracket:
Angulation: 2°
Inclination: –30°
Prominence: 1 mm

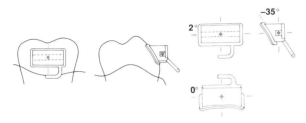

Fig. 9.38. Mandibular second molar standard bracket:
Angulation: 2°
Inclination: –35°
Prominence: 1 mm

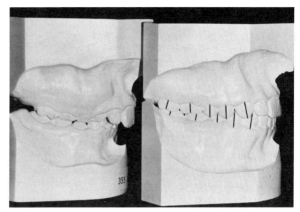

Fig. 9.41

Treatment Sample

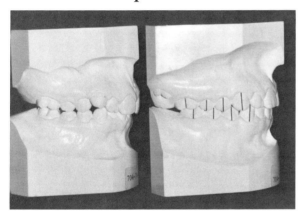

Fig. 9.39

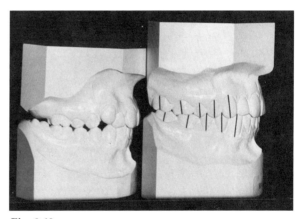

Fig. 9.42

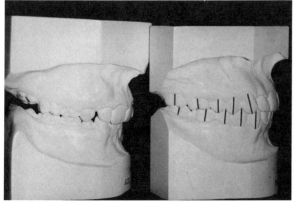

Fig. 9.40

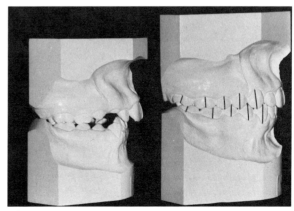

Fig. 9.43

189

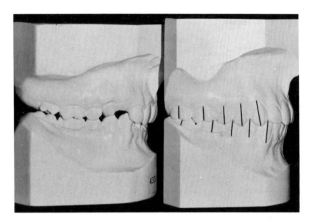

Fig. 9.44

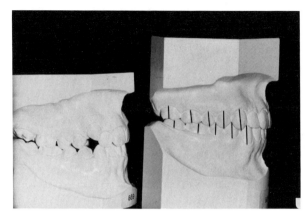

Fig. 9.47

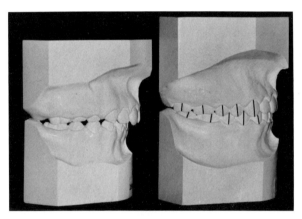

Fig. 9.45

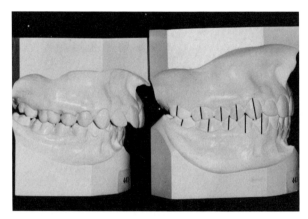

Fig. 9.48

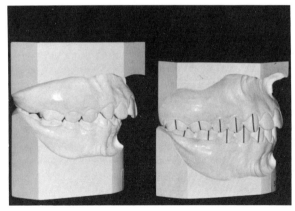

Fig. 9.46

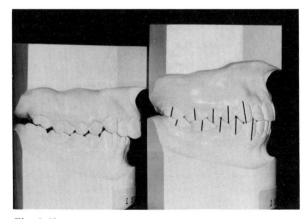

Fig. 9.49

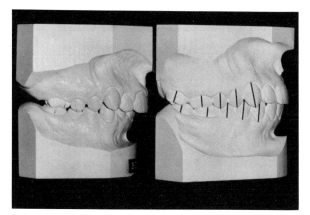

Fig. 9.50

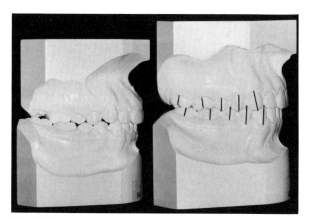

Fig. 9.51

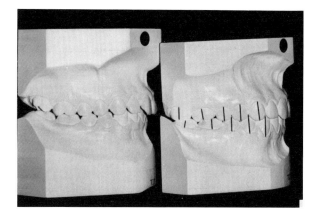

Fig. 9.52

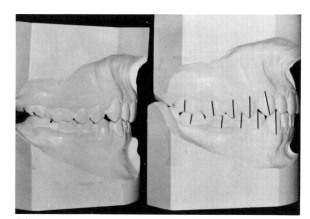

Fig. 9.53

Chapter 10

Fully Programmed Translation Brackets

A fully programmed appliance must offer more than just one standard or basic version. When teeth require bodily movement, translation brackets have significant advantages over standard brackets. If they are not available, the teeth will not be within 2° and 0.5 mm of where they should be at the conclusion of treatment without loss of efficiency or wire bending.

Translation brackets have all the qualities of standard brackets plus a power arm and two additional slot-siting features: "countermesiodistal tip" and "counterrotation." Maxillary molar brackets include a third feature, "counterbuccolingual tip." These features, along with the archwire and mesial or distal force, provide countermoments for translation and the guidance needed for overcorrection in all three planes of space. The formulae for the mesiodistal length of the brackets, length of the levers, and the amounts of countertip (mesiodistal and buccolingual) and counterrotation are based on moments and distances.

The terminology needed to explain these new brackets follows.

Counterbuccolingual tip. A slot-siting feature for maxillary molars that counteracts buccolingual tip during translation and then overcorrects.

Countermesiodistal tip. A slot-siting feature that counteracts mesial or distal tipping during translation and then overcorrects.

Counterrotation. A slot-siting feature that counteracts rotation during translation and then overcorrects.

Maximum translation bracket. A translation bracket for posterior teeth that require more than 4 mm of translation.

Medium translation bracket. A translation bracket for teeth that require more than 2 mm but not more than 4 mm of translation.

Minimum translation bracket. A translation bracket for teeth that require 2 mm or less of translation.

Power arm. A lever arm extending gingivally from the bracket, and used for delivering force toward the crown's center of resistance.

Translation bracket. A fully programmed bracket for teeth that require translation. It is designed to promote bodily movement during mesial or distal movement, and to overcorrect in proportion to the distance moved.

Translation Problems

Translation is defined as "uniform motion of a body in a straight line"[28]. For such movement to occur, the force must actually or effectively be applied to the object's center of resistance. Unfortunately, a tooth's center of resistance is in its root. From the standpoint of physics, a bracket located on a crown's face is in the "wrong" place in two ways: (1) the bracket is occlusal to the tooth's center of resistance, so when a mesial or distal force is applied, the tooth, instead of translating, will tend to tip around its horizontal center of rotation (Fig.10.1A). (2) The bracket is also located laterally to the tooth's center of resistance, so instead of translating when a mesial or distal force is

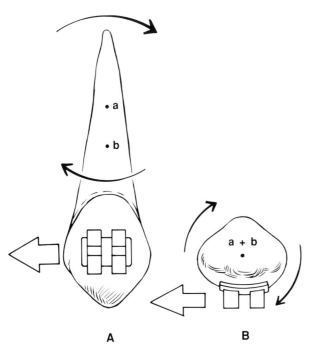

A   B

Fig. 10.1. A mesial or distal force applied at the bracket will cause a tooth to rotate around its center of rotation (*a*) because the bracket is displaced from the tooth's center of resistance (*b*). *A*, Facial view; *B*, occlusal view.

applied, the tooth will tend to rotate around its vertical center of rotation (Fig. 10.1B).

A bracket with an edgewise slot is better than other kinds of brackets for directing forces to a tooth's center of resistance. However, if an edgewise bracket is not fully programmed it is still inefficient for this purpose, as well as for overcorrection. The need for overcorrection became apparent in the study of the posttreatment positions of teeth that had required translation. As discussed and illustrated in Chapter 5, translated teeth invariably were rotated, and their angulation and inclination often differed from those in the optimal sample.

Posttreatment casts seldom are made on the day appliances are removed, so there is no way to know from casts alone whether, on that day, any teeth were rotated or incorrectly angulated or inclined. To what extent the incorrect posttreatment tooth positions resulted from rebound between the day the braces were removed and the day the casts were made is speculative. However, there is a correlation between the distance teeth were translated and their posttreatment positional discrepancies. Teeth have an inherent tendency to migrate—crowns more than roots, and buccal surfaces more than lingual surfaces. These inherent tipping and rotational tendencies often contribute to posttreatment positional problems.

With nonprogrammed brackets it is not easy to translate and overcorrect teeth to prevent unsatisfactory posttreatment positions. Standard amounts of first-order, second-order, and (if the brackets are not angulated) third-order wire bends usually are needed. In addition, first-order counterrotation bends or rotation springs, second-order countermesiodistal tip bends (if the brackets are not overangulated), and third-order counterbuccolingual tip bends for maxillary molars are needed.

When fully programmed standard brackets are used for translation and overcorrection, the standard amounts of first-, second-, and third-order bends needed for nonprogrammed brackets are *not* required, but procedures for countering rotations and tip are still needed.

The extent to which an edgewise bracket will assist in translation and overcorrection without wire bending, rotation springs, or bracket angulation depends on how effectively the bracket is designed to deliver force to the tooth's center of resistance, and to overcorrect when translation is complete.

Translation Solutions

There are two fundamental methods of moving a tooth mesially or distally, and they involve different amounts of force, bone, and efficiency. The two methods are translation (Fig. 10.2A), and tipping and then angulating (Fig. 10.2B). Tipping and then angulating compels a portion of the root to go through the same bone twice (Fig. 10.2C); such a waste of energy, movement, and efficiency is avoided if the tooth is translated (Fig. 10.2D).

Levers

Before discussing the design of translation brackets, we must consider a few principles concerning levers. One has to do with length. Archimedes said, "Give me a lever long enough and a place to stand and I can move the world." For tooth translation, optimal lever lengths are dictated by the distance between the bracket site and the tooth's center of resistance. An optimal length is one in which a force of any amount capable of moving a tooth in one plane of space can be applied without causing the tooth to rotate in that plane. Principles concerning the potential effectiveness of levers for tooth translation are illustrated in Figure 10.3. It is recommended that the reader try the illustrated experiment; all it takes is two pencils and a paper clip.

The slot of an edgewise bracket should be thought of as three levers. This is in contrast to the slot of a Begg bracket, which performs only as a fulcrum. The levers that all edgewise brackets have in common are contained within the slot and are activated by the wire. The mechanical advantage they provide in each of the three planes of space is based on their length in each plane (Fig. 10.4). Translation brackets confer still other benefits: two of the three levers are of optimal length; and, assuming that the brackets are correctly sited, the slots are automatically sited to provide the needed guidance with unbent archwires.

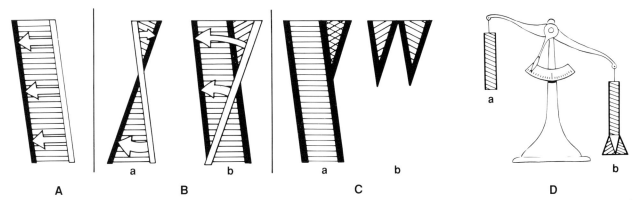

Fig. 10.2. Two methods for moving a tooth (*broad white line*) distally (*arrows*), and the amount of tooth movement and bone involvement (*shaded areas*) for each. *A*, Translation. *B*, Tipping and then angulating: *a*, first the crown moves distally while the root moves mesially; *b*, then only the root moves distally. *Ca*, Summary of total bone involvement for tipping and then angulating; *Cb*, total excess bone involvement for tipping and then angulating. *D*, Comparing bone mass involved for translation (*a*), and tipping and then angulating (*b*).

Slot-Siting Features

Counterrotation and countermesiodistal tip are two slot-siting features common to all translation brackets; in addition, maxillary molar translation brackets have counterbuccolingual tip. The criteria for locating the slot-target point for each translation bracket remain the same as for the standard bracket, except that the planes of the crown that the bracket slot represents comply with the tooth's overcorrected goal position. The criterion for the amount of counterrotation, countermesiodistal tip, and counterbuccolingual tip is distance, because the farther the tooth needs to be translated the greater the rebound potential. For counter-

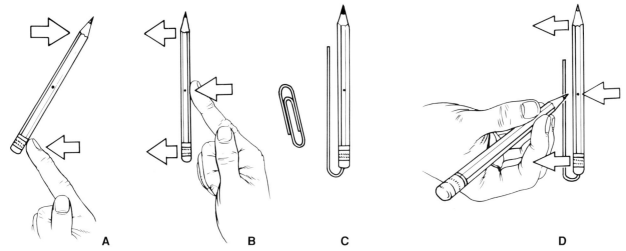

Fig. 10.3. Effects of an optimal lever. *A,* Like a tooth, a pencil rotates around its center of rotation (*dot within pencil*) when a horizontal force is applied at one end; *B,* the pencil translates if a force is applied at its center of resistance (*dot within pencil*). *C,* A lever constructed from a metal paper clip inserted into the pencil's eraser, extending at least to the pencil's center of resistance. *D,* Another pencil is used to apply a horizontal pulling force to the lever at a point opposite the center of resistance. The effect is the same as that illustrated in *B.*

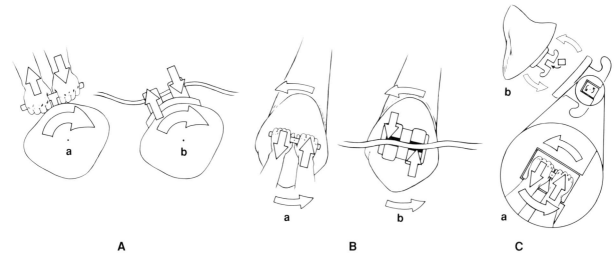

Fig. 10.4. Levers common to all edgewise brackets. The slot's mesiodistal length, when activated with a wire, is the lever that controls rotation (*Ab*) and mesiodistal tipping (*Bb*). The slot's faciolingual length is the lever that controls buccolingual tipping (*Cb*). The mechanical advantage for each is equal to an activated handlebar of equal length (*Aa, Ba, Ca*).

196

rotation the slot is rotated in the direction of translation. For countermesiodistal tip the standard amount of slot angulation is increased if the movement is distal, decreased if mesial. For counterbuccolingual tip the standard amount of slot inclination is always increased.

The features of translation brackets work as described when a tooth to be translated is first directed to the standard amounts for angulation, inclination, and prominence before translation is initiated.

Counterrotation

The slot-siting feature for counterrotation involves rotating the slot in one of three specified amounts around its vertical axis (Figs. 10.5A, 10.6). This feature, coupled with the flex of the archwire, counteracts tooth rotation caused by the mesial or distal force during mesial or distal movement (Fig. 10.5B) and overcorrects when the mesial or distal movement is complete (Fig. 10.5C). To transfer force efficiently from the bracket slot to the center of the crown, the mesiodistal length of a bracket should equal the distance from the slot point to the tooth's vertical axis. For example, if that distance is approximately 4 mm, then the mesiodistal bracket length should be 4 mm (Fig. 10.5D).

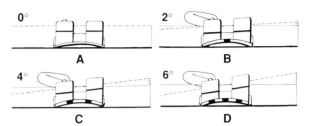

Fig. 10.6. Occlusal views of a standard bracket (*A*), which has no slot rotation, and of the three categories of translation brackets (*B–D*), which have rotated slots: the amount of rotation is indicated by the angle between the slot's mesiodistal axis (*dashed line*) and the line representing 0° rotation (*solid line*). *B*, Minimum translation bracket with 2° of slot rotation. *C*, Medium translation bracket with 4° of slot rotation. *D*, Maximum translation bracket with 6° of slot rotation.

The rationale for the three increments of slot rotation is that the farther a tooth must be translated, the greater is the amount of rotation overcorrection needed. The counterrotation formulae are as follows: 2° of slot rotation for teeth requiring 2 mm or less of translation, 4° of slot rotation for more than 2 mm but not more than 4 mm of translation, and 6° of slot rotation for more than 4 mm of translation (Fig. 10.6). The slot is rotated in the direction of translation. *Slot rotation plus mesiodistal slot length plus archwire flex plus mesial or distal force equals counterrotation and rotation overcorrection.*

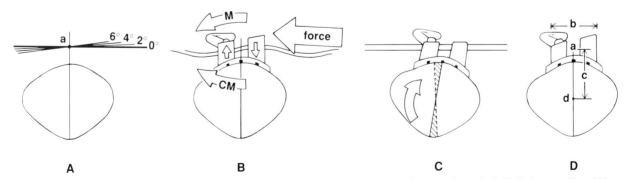

Fig. 10.5. Bracket design for controlling rotation and for rotation overcorrection (occlusal view). *A*, Relative to a line 90° to the crown's midsagittal plane, the mesiodistal axis of a standard slot is not rotated (*0° line*); for translation brackets the slot's mesiodistal axis is rotated 2°, 4°, or 6° around the slot point (*a*). *B*, When a mesial or distal force is applied, the resulting rotation moment (*M*) is controlled by the countermoment (*CM*) produced by the rotated slot and the flexed archwire. *C*, When translation is complete, the rotated slot provides rotation overcorrection (*shaded area*). *D*, For efficient rotation control the mesiodistal bracket length (*b*) should equal the distance (*c*) from slot point (*a*) to the tooth's vertical axis (*d*).

Countermesiodistal Tip

The slot-siting feature for countermesiodistal tip involves rotating the slot in one of three specified amounts around its faciolingual axis (Fig. 10.7A). The mesiodistal length of the slot is not as long as the distance from the slot point to a tooth's center of resistance (Fig. 10.7B). The countermoment produced by the angulated slot and flexed archwire counters some—but not all—of the tendency for the root to lag behind the crown when a mesial or distal force is applied (Fig. 10.7C). For translation, a lever as long as the distance from the slot point to a tooth's center of resistance is needed (Fig. 10.7D), and for every tooth this distance is greater than the mesiodistal length of the slot.

For example, the center of resistance of a typical maxillary canine is approximately 9 mm from the bracket's slot point (Fig.10.7B). For translation to occur, the angulation lever must also be 9 mm long (Fig. 10.7D). If the mesiodistal length of the slot of a canine translation bracket is 4 mm it will provide only 4/9 of the needed length (Fig. 10.7B,C). To increase the length of the lever, a gingival extension (called a power arm) of 5 mm is added to the bracket (Fig. 10.7E,F), in effect increasing the length of the slot by that amount, if both the slot and power arm are activated. If only the power arm is activated, the moment and countermoment will still be out of balance (Fig. 10.7E). Together the power-arm length and the mesiodistal slot length provide the 9-mm lever needed for the countermoment to equal the moment, a condition needed for translation (Fig. 10.7F).

The portion of the countermesiodistal tip provided by angulating the slot more than the standard amount also provides the right amount of overangulation at the end of translation (Fig. 10.7G). Ultimately the tooth assumes the desired degree of angulation after rebound. Translation brackets, because they encourage translation, are more effective than other brackets in keeping the occlusal surface of each arch from becoming concave during extraction-site closure. Without translation brackets the crowns tend to precede the roots (Fig. 10.8). Correcting such an effect adds measurably to energy requirements, and reduces treatment efficiency.

The rationale for adding slot angulation to provide for countermesiodistal tip and overangulation is the same as for counterrotation—the farther a tooth is translated, the greater the need for angulation overcorrection. However, the rebound from angulation overcorrection has been observed to be less than that for rotation overcorrection, so the countermesiodistal tip increment for every 2 mm of translation is 1° rather than 2° (after starting with a minimum of 2°).

The amount is added to the standard amount of angulation for distal translation, or subtracted from the standard amount for mesial translation. The amounts are as follows: Add or subtract 2° for 2 mm or less of translation; add or subtract 3° for more than 2 mm but not more than 4 mm of translation; and add or subtract 4° for more than 4 mm of translation (Fig. 10.9).

The optimal power-arm length for each tooth type is the distance from the bracket slot point to the tooth's center of resistance, minus the mesiodistal slot length. The power arm for a molar bracket is shorter than for a canine because the mesiodistal length of a molar bracket is longer, and the molar's center of resistance is more occlusal (Fig. 10.10). The power arm for a premolar is shorter than it is for a canine (assuming equal mesiodistal slot lengths) because the premolar is a shorter tooth. *Slot angulation plus mesiodistal slot length plus power arm length plus activated archwire and power arm equals countermesiodistal tip and angulation overcorrection.* The power arm extends from the gingival tie wing that is on the side of the intended direction of movement.

An auxiliary lever is not new to orthodontics, nor is the term *power arm*. In 1921 Calvin

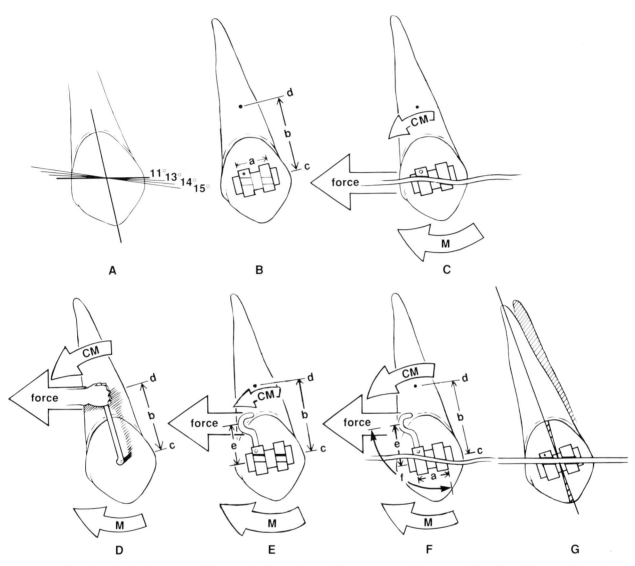

Fig. 10.7. Bracket design for controlling mesiodistal tip and for overcorrecting angulation (maxillary right canine is used as the example).

A, Standard slot angulation for a maxillary canine is 11°; for canine translation brackets the standard slot angulation is increased 2°, 3°, or 4°, to 13°, 14°, or 15°.

B, Mesiodistal slot length (*a*) is less than the distance (*b*) from the bracket (*c*) to the tooth's center of resistance (*d*).

C, When a mesiodistal force is applied to a bracket, the countermoment (*CM*) and moment (*M*) are out of balance, and the tooth tends to tip.

D, Optimal lever length for translating a tooth equals the distance (*b*) from the tooth's bracket site (*c*) to the tooth's center of resistance (*d*). Optimal lever length produces a balanced countermoment and moment.

E, Countermoment and moment are out of balance when the countermoment is produced from the power arm alone (without assistance from wire and slot), because the power arm length (*e*) is shorter than is the distance (*b*) from the bracket (*c*) to the tooth's center of resistance (*d*).

F, Translation occurs when both the slot and power arm are activated; together they provide a countermoment equal to the moment. The combined lengths (*f*) of the slot (*a*) and power arm (*e*) equal the distance (*b*) between the bracket (*c*) and the tooth's center of resistance (*d*).

G, When translation is complete the extra slot angulation provides angulation overcorrection (*shaded area*).

199

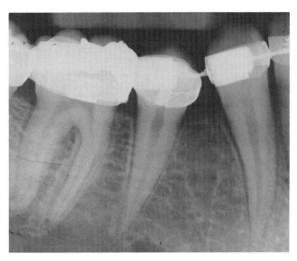

Fig. 10.8. Without translation brackets, crowns tend to precede roots when closing extraction-site space.

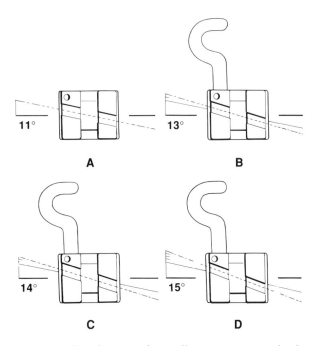

Fig. 10.9. Facial view of maxillary canine standard bracket and the three categories of translation brackets. *A,* Standard slot angulation is 11°; *B,* minimum translation bracket is 13° (11° + 2°); *C,* medium translation bracket is 14° (11° + 3°); and *D,* maximum translation bracket is 15° (11° + 4°). Dashed line represents slot angulation relative to a horizontal solid line. Angled solid line represents standard angulation (11°) in *B, C,* and *D.*

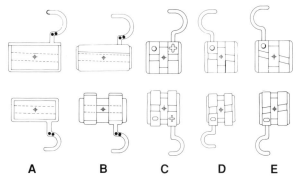

Fig. 10.10. Relative power-arm lengths for molars (*A, B*), premolars (*C, D*), and canines (*E*).

Case referred to extensions soldered to bands as "power arms"[11]. They were for controlling tip (mesiodistal and buccolingual). The first fully programmed translation brackets (1972) had countertip and counterrotation but were without such extensions. These brackets worked better than standard brackets for moving teeth mesially or distally, but more leverage than just the mesiodistal length of the slot was found (clinically as well as mathematically) to be needed. The extended levers have proven to be an excellent solution; they are named power arms in honor of Dr. Case.

Counterbuccolingual Tip

The slot-siting feature for counterbuccolingual tip involves rotating the base of the bracket in one of three specified amounts around its mesiodistal axis (Fig. 10.11A). This feature is needed only for maxillary molar translation brackets. Because maxillary molars are the only three-rooted teeth, their translation requires special consideration. Mesially directed force, applied to a nonprogrammed or a fully programmed standard bracket, predisposes this tooth to tip mesially and to rotate just like other teeth. But it also tips buccally because of the drag imposed by the tooth's dominant lingual root. Clinically this results in the buccal cusps becoming more gingivally oriented and the lingual cusps more occlusally positioned.

During mesial or distal tooth movement, the rotation and mesial or distal tipping tendencies are overcome by counterrotation and countermesiodistal tip. Buccolingual tipping is resolved by the counterbuccolingual tip feature. This feature targets the slot to provide more negative base inclination than would a standard bracket (Fig. 10.11B). The increased negative base inclination positions the slot so that a flat, rectangular archwire will provide both the counterbuccolingual tip moment needed during translation, and inclination overcorrection at the end of the translation stage (Fig. 10.11C).

Again, the rationale for the amount of counterbuccolingual tip is that the farther a tooth is translated, the greater is the amount of overcorrection needed. The formula is as follows: 4° of negative base inclination more than the standard amount when translation is to be 2 mm or less; 5° more of negative base inclination when translation is to be more than 2 mm but not more than 4 mm; 6° more of negative base inclination for translation of more than 4 mm (Fig. 10.12). *Base inclination plus faciolingual slot length plus rectangular archwire deflection plus mesial or distal force equals counterbuccolingual tip and inclination overcorrection.*

The proportionally greater amount of counterbuccolingual tip compared to countermesiodistal tip compensates for the slot's suboptimal faciolingual lever length. (The faciolingual length of the slot is not equal to the distance from the slot point to the tooth's center of resistance for inclination.) Inclination can also be supplemented with wire forming, as discussed and illustrated in Chapter 12.

The counterbuccolingual tip feature combines with the counterrotation and countermesiodistal tip features to allow each translation bracket to accomplish a prescribed amount of translation and overcorrection in all three planes of space.

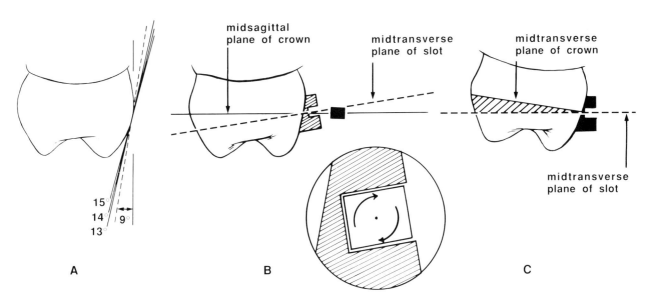

Fig. 10.11. Bracket design for controlling buccolingual tip and for overcorrecting inclination for maxillary molars:
A, standard bracket inclination for maxillary molars is –9° (*dashed line*); the bases of translation brackets are additionally inclined 4°, 5°, or 6° to minus 13°, 14°, or 15°.
B, Counterbuccolingual tip is induced by the increased negative base inclination, which cants the slot's midtransverse plane (*dashed line*) relative to the crown's midtransverse plane.
C, When translation is complete the additional negative slot inclination provides for inclination overcorrection (*hatched lines*).

Translation Bracket Categories

To stay within the specified 2° and 0.5-mm positional constraints, a different translation bracket is needed for each of three ranges of translation, whether mesial or distal. The ranges are 0.1 to 2 mm, 2.1 to 4 mm, and more than 4 mm. The translation brackets that satisfy these incremental distance requirements are called minimum, medium, and maximum.

Minimum Translation Brackets

A minimum translation bracket is recommended for teeth requiring 2 mm of translation or less. To the standard amount of angulation shown in Figure 10.9A, 2° of countermesiodistal tip and a power arm are added to the distogingival tie wing if the tooth is to be translated distally (Fig. 10.9B); 2° is subtracted if translation is to be mesial; and the power

arm is added to the mesiogingival tie wing. In both cases 2° of counterrotation in the direction of intended movement is also added (Fig. 10.6B).

Minimum translation brackets are also recommended for a tooth bordering an extraction site but not itself scheduled for translation. Such use further assures long-term harmonious proximity with the tooth that has been translated.

Minimum translation brackets for maxillary molars have, in addition to countermesiodistal tip and counterrotation, 4° of counterbuccolingual tip added to the standard amount of negative inclination (Fig. 10.12B).

Medium Translation Brackets

A medium translation bracket is recommended for teeth to be translated more than 2 mm but not beyond 4 mm. For this bracket, a power arm is added; 3° of countermesiodistal tip is added or subtracted (Fig. 10.9C); and 4° of counterrotation is incorporated (Fig. 10.6C).

Medium maxillary molar translation brackets have, in addition to countermesiodistal tip and counterrotation, 5° of counterbuccolingual tip added to the standard amount of negative inclination (Fig. 10.12C).

Maximum Translation Brackets

A maximum translation bracket is recommended for teeth to be translated more than 4 mm. For this bracket, a power arm is added; 4° of countermesiodistal tip is added or subtracted (Fig. 10.9D); and 6° of counterrotation is incorporated (Fig. 10.6D).

Maximum translation brackets for maxillary molars have, in addition to countermesiodistal tip and counterrotation, 6° of counterbuccolingual tip added to the standard amount of negative inclination (Fig. 10.12D).

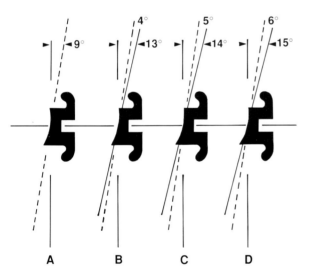

Fig. 10.12. Distal view of maxillary molar standard bracket (*A*) and the three categories of translation brackets (*B* –*D*): Standard maxillary molar bracket (*A*) with 9° base inclination. *B,* Minimum translation bracket with 13° (9° + 4°) of base inclination; *C,* medium translation bracket with 14° (9° + 5°) of base inclination; *D,* maximum translation bracket with 15° (9° + 6°) of inclination. Dashed line indicates standard base inclination relative to vertical line. Angled solid line indicates actual base inclination relative to vertical line.

Identification

Each translation bracket for the Straight-Wire Appliance is identified for arch and quadrant, for class, and for type in the same way as standard brackets (Fig. 9.13). For category identification (minimum, medium, or maximum), all translation brackets other than those for molars have one, two, or three notches at the occlusal surface of the base (Fig. 10.6). For molars, category is indicated by one, two, or three raised dots on the power arms (Fig. 10.13). One notch or dot indicates minimum translation; two, medium; three, maximum.

Inventory

Without further consideration it would appear necessary to inventory six translation brackets for each tooth type—a different bracket for each of the three ranges of mesial and distal distance. Such an inventory would be amply justified by the benefits derived from treating with unbent archwires. However, that number is excessive in view of the usual and customary treatment needs for each tooth type in normal arches. The translation brackets actually needed to solve normal malocclusions are shown in Figure 10.14. As a general rule, no tooth type requires both mesial and distal translation brackets. Instead, molars and second premolars require only mesial translation brackets, whereas first pre-

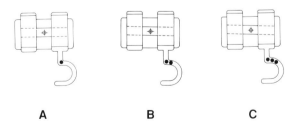

Fig. 10.13. Identification marks on molar translation brackets: *A,* minimum—one dot on power arm; *B,* medium—two dots; *C,* maximum—three dots.

molars and canines require only distal translation brackets. Fortunately, not every tooth even needs all three categories of either mesial or distal translation brackets. This further reduces the hypothetical inventory of six translation brackets per tooth type to three or fewer.

Molars and second premolars generally need only mesial translation brackets, and they need all three categories (Fig. 10.14). Any attempt to *translate* maxillary molars distally usually proves disappointing. When such distal treatment is tried—for example, to correct a Class II interarch relationship (Fig. 10.15A)—interdental spacing and changes in the inter-arch relationship of the molars frequently occur (Fig. 10.15B); but when posttreatment results are scrutinized cephalometrically, inter-arch change is most often found to be not distal translation but the result of one or more other factors. These include mesial movement of mandibular teeth, interjaw change, and distal tipping of maxillary posterior teeth. What appeared to be a Class III intermolar tendency during treatment (Fig. 10.15B) becomes a Class II tendency after space closure and rebound (Fig. 10.15C).

In the mandibular arch, when the crowns of the molars and second premolars are mesial to their roots, usually there is room to tip them distally, but seldom is there room to move them any farther. If there is such space, these teeth can be translated distally, but because of the difficulty of the procedure, most orthodontists elect to extract premolars if the molars have to be tipped distally more than 3 mm per side. Therefore, mandibular molars and second premolars do not need distal translation brackets but do need mesial translation brackets in the minimum, medium, and maximum categories (Fig. 10.14).

Maxillary and mandibular first premolars generally require only distal translation brackets in the medium category. Canines require distal translation brackets in only the medium and maximum categories. Neither

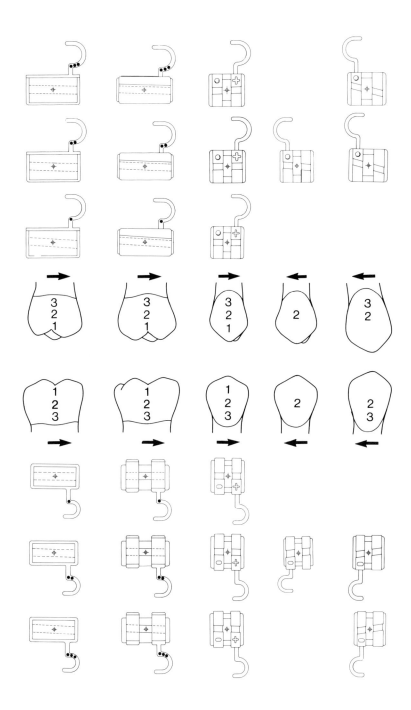

Fig.10.14. Summary inventory (by tooth) of all translation brackets required to treat normal mal-occlusions without wire bends. Arrows indicate the direction of movement; numbers on teeth indicate the categories of translation brackets each tooth requires (1 = minimum, 2 = medium, 3 = maximum). The maxillary brackets are shown above the maxillary teeth, the mandibular brackets below the mandibular teeth.

204

the first premolars nor canines require mesial translation, because teeth mesial to them are seldom extracted.

Examples of the inventory of translation brackets needed for correcting normal malocclusions are shown in three dimensions in Figures 10.16–10.39.

Discussion

The amount of translation a tooth needs should be judged from its center of rotation. One example is a canine whose crown needs to be retracted 7 mm but whose root needs no retraction. This treatment requires only tipping; any slot engagement by a straight wire would be counterproductive. Another example is a canine in which only the root needs to be retracted 7 mm. A maximum translation bracket is needed, but early in treatment the slot angulation for such a condition can undesirably extrude incisors. To avoid this side effect the archwire should not engage incisor slots until the canine angulation is correct. *The angulation and inclination of teeth being translated must be nearly optimal before translation is begun.*

For example, if the root of a maxillary canine is mesial to a crown that needs to be retracted 7 mm, translation should not begin until the crown angulation is nearly optimal. During this initial distal root-posturing procedure, the bracket slot should be the center of rotation. The crown should be tied back to prevent it from reciprocally moving mesially as the roots move distally. Again, to avoid unwanted incisor movement during canine retraction, the archwire should not engage incisor slots until the crown angulation is correct.

Assigning brackets, whether standard or translation, can be done on a tooth-by-tooth basis. However, a more efficient method is to prescribe brackets by the arch according to the treatment plan. This approach requires a coordinated system for coding bracket sets and treatment plans. Such a system is explained in Chapter 13.

Fifteen pretreatment and posttreatment casts are shown in Figures 10.40–10.54 to demonstrate treatment with fully programmed translation brackets. In each example, treatment required extractions and tooth translation.

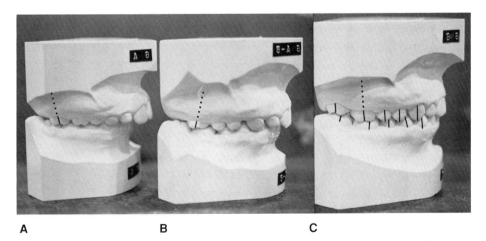

A   **B**   **C**

Fig. 10.15. *A,* Pretreatment casts with a 7-mm Class II interarch relationship. *B,* Progress casts showing a maxillary first molar that has been tipped distally and that has a cusp-embrasure molar relationship and maxillary interdental space. *C,* Posttreatment casts showing a correctly angulated maxillary molar with a 2-mm Class II relationship.

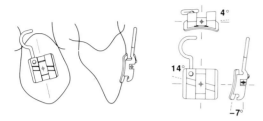

Fig. 10.16. Maxillary canine medium translation bracket:
Angulation: 14° (standard 11° + countermesiodistal tip 3°)
Rotation: 4° (standard 0° + counterrotation 4°)
Inclination: –7° (standard –7°)

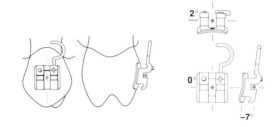

Fig. 10.19. Maxillary second premolar minimum translation bracket:
Angulation: 0° (standard 2° + countermesiodistal tip –2°)
Rotation: 2° (standard 0° + counterrotation 2°)
Inclination: –7° (standard –7°)

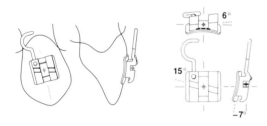

Fig. 10.17. Maxillary canine maximum translation bracket:
Angulation: 15° (standard 11° + countermesiodistal tip 4°)
Rotation: 6° (standard 0° + counterrotation 6°)
Inclination: –7° (standard –7°)

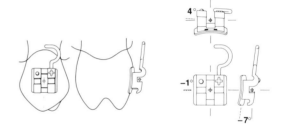

Fig. 10.20. Maxillary second premolar medium translation bracket:
Angulation: –1° (standard 2° + countermesiodistal tip –3°)
Rotation: 4° (standard 0° + counterrotation 4°)
Inclination: –7° (standard –7°)

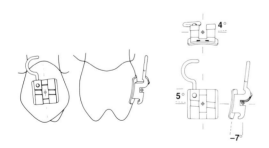

Fig. 10.18. Maxillary first premolar medium translation bracket:
Angulation: 5° (standard 2° + countermesiodistal tip 3°)
Rotation: 4° (standard 0° + counterrotation 4°)
Inclination: –7° (standard –7°)

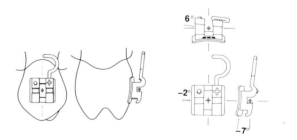

Fig. 10.21. Maxillary second premolar maximum translation bracket:
Angulation: –2° (standard 2° + countermesiodistal tip –4°)
Rotation: 6° (standard 0° + counterrotation 6°)
Inclination: –7° (standard –7°)

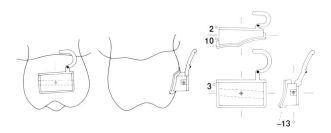

Fig. 10.22. Maxillary first molar minimum translation bracket:
Angulation: 3° (standard 5° + countermesiodistal tip –2°)
Rotation: 12° (standard 10° + counterrotation 2°)
Inclination: –13° (standard –9° + counterbuccolingual tip –4°)

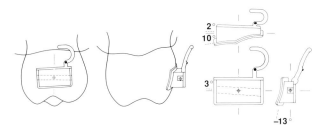

Fig. 10.25. Maxillary second molar minimum translation bracket:
Angulation: 3° (standard 5° + countermesiodistal tip –2°)
Rotation: 12° (standard 10° + counterrotation 2°)
Inclination: –13° (standard –9° + counterbuccolingual tip –4°)

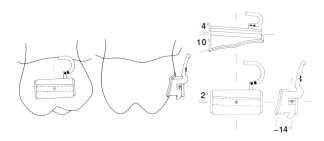

Fig. 10.23. Maxillary first molar medium translation bracket:
Angulation: 2° (standard 5° + countermesiodistal tip –3°)
Rotation: 14° (standard 10° + counterrotation 4°)
Inclination: –14° (standard –9° + counterbuccolingual tip –5°)

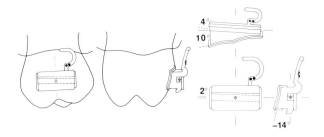

Fig. 10.26. Maxillary second molar medium translation bracket:
Angulation: 2° (standard 5° + countermesiodistal tip –3°)
Rotation: 14° (standard 10° + counterrotation 4°)
Inclination: –14° (standard –9° + counterbuccolingual tip –5°)

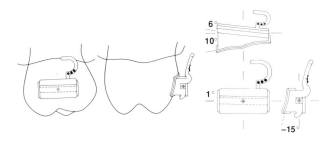

Fig. 10.24. Maxillary first molar maximum translation bracket:
Angulation: 1° (standard 5° + countermesiodistal tip –4°)
Rotation: 16° (standard 10° + counterrotation 6°)
Inclination: –15° (standard –9° + counterbuccolingual tip –6°)

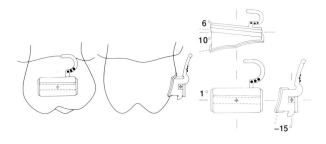

Fig. 10.27. Maxillary second molar maximum translation bracket:
Angulation: 1° (standard 5° + countermesiodistal tip –4°)
Rotation: 16° (standard 10° + counterrotation 6°)
Inclination: –15° (standard –9° + counterbuccolingual tip –6°)

207

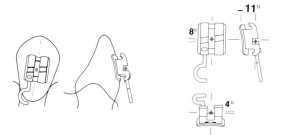

Fig. 10.28. Mandibular canine medium translation bracket:
Angulation: 8° (standard 5° + countermesiodistal tip 3°)
Rotation: 4° (standard 0° + counterrotation 4°)
Inclination: –11° (standard –11°)

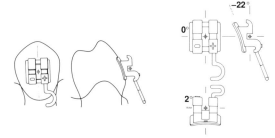

Fig. 10.31. Mandibular second premolar minimum translation bracket:
Angulation: 0° (standard 2° + countermesiodistal tip –2°)
Rotation: 2° (standard 0° + counterrotation 2°)
Inclination: –22° (standard –22°)

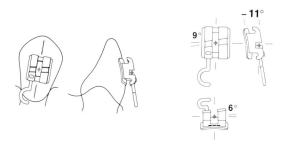

Fig. 10.29. Mandibular canine maximum translation bracket:
Angulation: 9° (standard 5° + countermesiodistal tip 4°)
Rotation: 6° (standard 0° + counterrotation 6°)
Inclination: –11° (standard –11°)

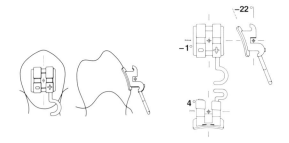

Fig. 10.32. Mandibular second premolar medium translation bracket:
Angulation: –1° (standard 2° + countermesiodistal tip –3°)
Rotation: 4° (standard 0° + counterrotation 4°)
Inclination: –22° (standard –22°)

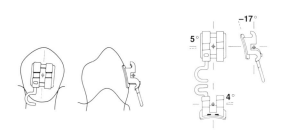

Fig. 10.30. Mandibular first premolar medium translation bracket:
Angulation: 5° (standard 2° + countermesiodistal tip 3°)
Rotation: 4° (standard 0° + counterrotation 4°)
Inclination: –17° (standard –17°)

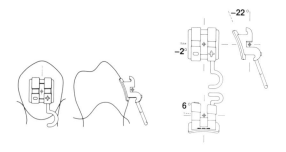

Fig. 10.33. Mandibular second premolar maximum translation bracket:
Angulation: –2° (standard 2° + countermesiodistal tip –4°)
Rotation: 6° (standard 0° + counterrotation 6°)
Inclination: –22° (standard –22°)

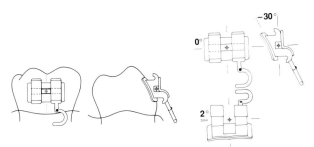

Fig. 10.34. Mandibular first molar minimum translation bracket:
Angulation: 0° (standard 2° + countermesiodistal tip –2°)
Rotation: 2° (standard 0° + counterrotation 2°)
Inclination: –30° (standard –30°)

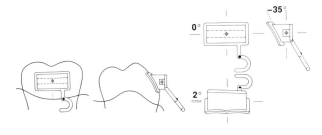

Fig. 10.37. Mandibular second molar minimum translation bracket:
Angulation: 0° (standard 2° + countermesiodistal tip –2°)
Rotation: 2° (standard 0° + counterrotation 2°)
Inclination: –35° (standard –35°)

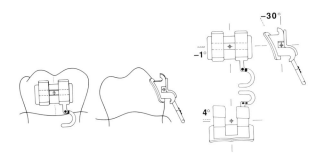

Fig. 10.35. Mandibular first molar medium translation bracket:
Angulation: –1° (standard 2° + countermesiodistal tip –3°)
Rotation: 4° (standard 0° + counterrotation 4°)
Inclination: –30° (standard –30°)

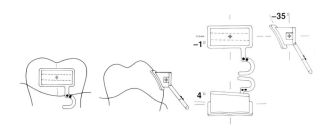

Fig. 10.38. Mandibular second molar medium translation bracket:
Angulation: –1° (standard 2° + countermesiodistal tip –3°)
Rotation: 4° (standard 0° + counterrotation 4°)
Inclination: –35° (standard –35°)

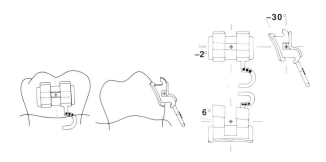

Fig. 10.36. Mandibular first molar maximum translation bracket:
Angulation: –2° (standard 2° + countermesiodistal tip –4°)
Rotation: 6° (standard 0° + counterrotation 6°)
Inclination: –30° (standard –30°)

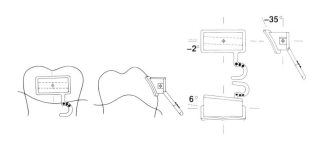

Fig. 10.39. Mandibular second molar maximum translation bracket:
Angulation: –2° (standard 2° + countermesiodistal tip –4°)
Rotation: 6° (standard 0° + counterrotation 6°)
Inclination: –35° (standard –35°)

209

Treatment Sample

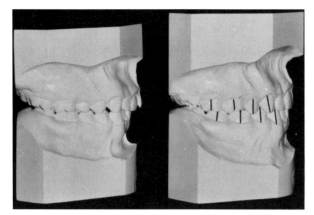

Fig. 10.40

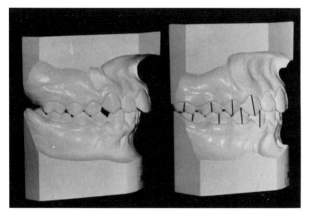

Fig. 10.41

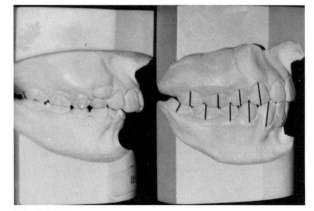

Fig. 10.42

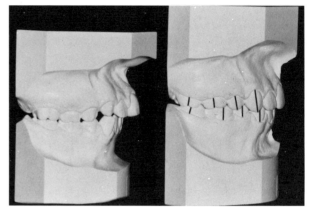

Fig. 10.43

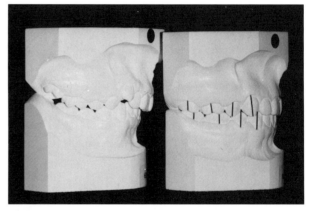

Fig. 10.44

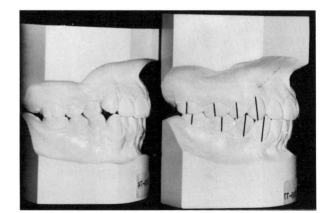

Fig.10.45

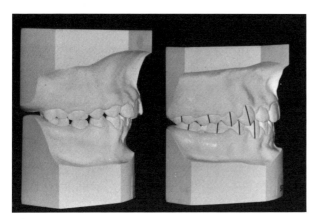

Fig. 10.46

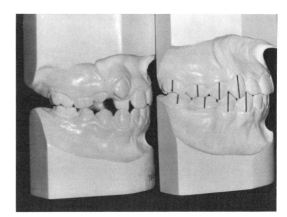

Fig. 10.49

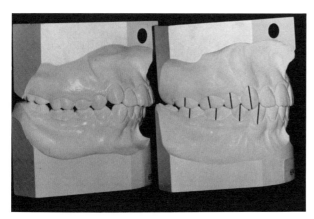

Fig. 10.47

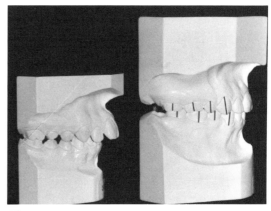

Fig. 10.50

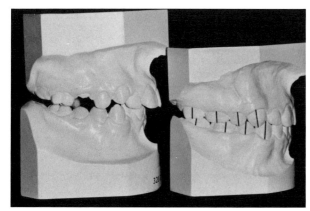

Fig. 10.48

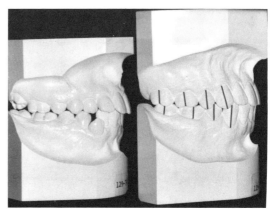

Fig.10.51

211

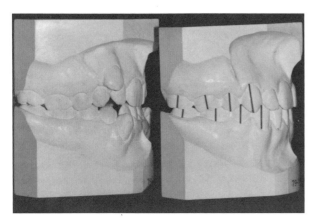

Fig. 10.52

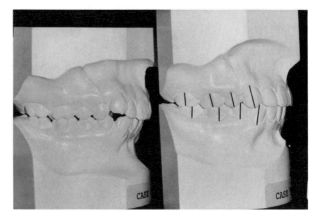

Fig. 10.54

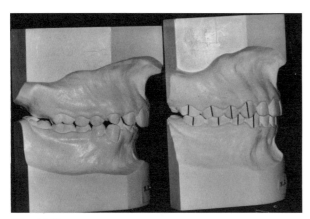

Fig. 10.53

Chapter 11

Partly Programmed Appliances

By 1988 about 30 percent of all American orthodontists were using the Straight-Wire Appliance, currently the only fully programmed appliance (David Webb, "A"-Company, Inc. personal communication). Another 50 percent were using partly programmed edgewise appliances [14]. Of the partly programmed appliances, all with more than one programmed slot-siting feature were developed after the introduction of the Straight-Wire Appliance in 1970. Patent restrictions allowed them to reproduce no more than four of the eight vital features that appear in fully programmed brackets (there are eleven features in translation brackets); of these features only one is copied correctly.

It seems logical to expect that as years pass and patents expire, all of the partly programmed appliances will be redesigned to offer the quality and quantity of features needed to locate the slots correctly. Meanwhile, the effects of such mechanisms used with unbent archwires differ from those achieved with a fully programmed appliance.

Despite their major design divergences from the Straight-Wire Appliance, partly pro-

grammed appliances are being loosely called straight-wire appliances. This chapter describes some of the variations in design, and illustrates their varying effects when used with unbent archwires, thus documenting the need for separate categories to distinguish between nonprogrammed, partly programmed, and fully programmed (straight-wire) appliances.

One apparent rationale for the unitary, simplistic labeling is that all the new appliances profess to reduce the need for wire bending. Another is that the measurements used for their limited number of slot-siting features are the same as or nearly the same as those proposed by Andrews in 1968 [2] and built into the original Straight-Wire Appliance made available in December 1970. (See measurement study, Chapter 4.)

On the surface, it might seem logical to assume that appliances with corresponding amounts of angulation, inclination, prominence, and horizontal bracket-base contour would produce similar results. Such an inference would fail to recognize the differences in (1) the quantity of the slot-siting features; (2) the quality of the design features that correctly position the slot; (3) the separate design concepts of the standard and translation brackets; (4) the system for siting each bracket; and (5) the effects when used with unbent archwires.

By definition, a partly programmed appliance lacks at least one slot-siting feature; for this reason alone, it would fail to fully direct each slot to its tooth's slot site. In actuality, the inadequacy in both quantity and quality of slot-siting features makes wire bending necessary.

Slot-Siting Features

The partly programmed appliance discussed and illustrated in this chapter is most representative of those available at the time of publication of this book. Its brackets have four slot-siting features: slot inclination, slot angulation, prominence, and horizontal base curvature. This is in contrast to the nonprogrammed appliance, which has none, and the fully programmed appliance, which has eight for standard brackets (Chapter 9) and eleven for translation brackets (Chapter 10). The measurements adopted for these four features are the same as those built into the Straight-Wire Appliance; however, the effects differ. Assuming that each partly programmed bracket is correctly sited on the crown's FACC at the FA point, the effects of the design features

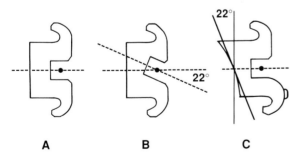

A   **B**   **C**

Fig. 11.1. Design comparison of the three categories of edgewise brackets. *A,* Nonprogrammed bracket without slot or base inclination; *B,* partly programmed bracket with 22° of *slot* inclination; *C,* fully programmed bracket with 22° of *base* inclination.

on slot siting and on tooth position, when used with unbent archwires, can be compared with those of nonprogrammed (Chapter 7) and fully programmed appliances (Chapters 9 and 10).

Slot Inclination

In the partly programmed appliance, patents have restricted inclination to the face of the bracket (Fig. 11.1B). Nonprogrammed brackets have no inclination (Fig. 11.1A). In fully programmed brackets the inclination is built into the base (Fig. 11.1C). The amount of slot inclination for each partly programmed bracket is the same as the base inclination for each fully programmed standard bracket. However, when examples of all three brackets are sited alike, only the slot of the fully programmed bracket is targeted correctly on the crown's midtransverse plane (Fig. 11.2).

Nonprogrammed and partly programmed brackets have bases that are at right angles to the stem (Fig. 11.1A,B); thus when they are similarly sited, they site their slot points identically (Fig. 11.2A,B). In contrast, the inclined base of a fully programmed bracket locates the slot point on the crown's midtransverse plane (Fig. 11.2C). Figure 11.3 illustrates optimally inclined teeth and a partly programmed appliance with the same amount of slot inclination as for a fully programmed appliance. The base point of each bracket is sited on the crown's FACC and FA point. The slot points of the brackets are directed to as many occlusogingival heights as there are differences in optimal crown inclination, just as they are for the nonprogrammed brackets (Fig. 7.3). If unbent archwires are used, the occlusogingival effect will be as shown in Figure 11.4; it is exactly the same as with the nonprogrammed appliance (Fig. 7.5). The slot points of a fully programmed appliance, however, are sited precisely on the Andrews plane (Fig. 9.3).

Patents have restricted the design of partly programmed brackets. For example, bracket

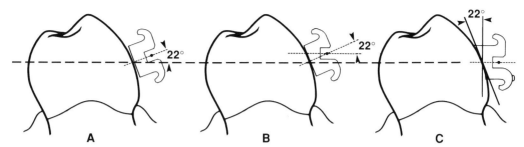

Fig. 11.2. Slot-siting comparison for the three categories of edgewise brackets on an optimally positioned lower second premolar. *A,* Nonprogrammed bracket without slot or base inclination; *B,* partly programmed bracket with 22° of slot inclination; *C,* fully programmed bracket with 22° of base inclination. Heavy dashed line is crown's midtransverse plane.

bases may not be both inclined and vertically contoured. Clinically, there is little chance of consistently positioning vertically flat-based brackets on curved tooth surfaces so that the base point touches the FA point. The vertically flat bases of partly programmed brackets are subject to the same rocking as the vertically flat bases of nonprogrammed brackets (Figs. 7.7, 7.8). With rocking shown at its full potential, the effects on slot siting for the partly programmed appliance can be seen in Figure 11.5. The occlusogingival disharmony of the slots is the same as for similarly sited nonprogrammed brackets; the inclination differs, but the amount of variability in the slots' inclination is also the same as for similarly sited nonprogrammed brackets (Fig. 7.8). The effects of an unbent archwire on tooth positions, when the partly programmed brackets are so rocked, are illustrated in Figure 11.6.

Slot Angulation

Some partly programmed brackets use both slot angulation and slot inclination, so if such brackets are sited on the FACC and the FA point of optimally positioned crowns (Figs. 11.3, 11.7), the full and correct amount of angulation and inclination should be attained. However, the occlusogingival position of the slot is not directed to the Andrews plane. The occlusogingival effects from using an unbent archwire are shown in Figures 11.4

and 11.8. When the bracket is rocked, as shown in Figures 11.5 and 11.9, the occlusogingival effect on tooth position is likely to be as shown in Figures 11.6 and 11.10.

Slot Prominence

In their literature, manufacturers of most partly programmed appliances indicate that the prominence of their brackets varies in step with the intention to eliminate or reduce the need for first-order bends. Among those who specify the amounts of prominence, none cites the same amount as used in the Straight-Wire Appliance. Several indicate faciolingual prominence that is "thicker" or "thinner" than in their nonprogrammed brackets. Because of the lack of consistency in how prominence data are reported, a consensus is not evident. If the reader wants this information for a particular appliance, it can be obtained by contacting the manufacturer or by measuring the distance from base point to slot point. A difference of more than 0.5 mm from the amount in the Straight-Wire Appliance can be considered clinically significant.

Horizontal Base Contour

Most partly programmed and some nonprogrammed brackets have horizontal base contour. The measurements used for this slot-siting feature are not generally published by

Fig. 11.3. Partly programmed bracket siting and slot siting: even when the base points of partly programmed brackets are sited on the FACCs and FA points of optimally positioned crowns, the slots are poorly aligned. Enlarged bracket positions (*center*) are identical to those shown on teeth.

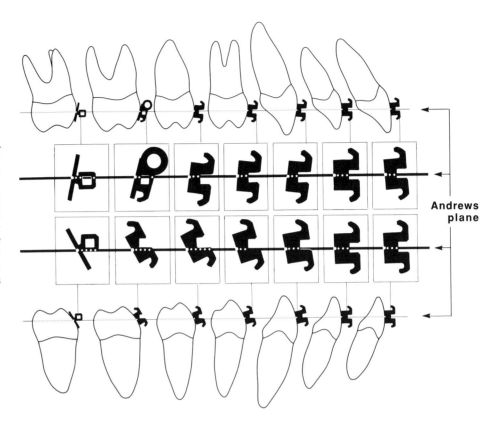

Fig. 11.4. Effect on occlusogingival position when the incorrectly sited slots of the correctly sited partly programmed brackets shown in Fig. 11.3 are made passive to full-size unbent archwires. Dashed lines represent optimal positions.

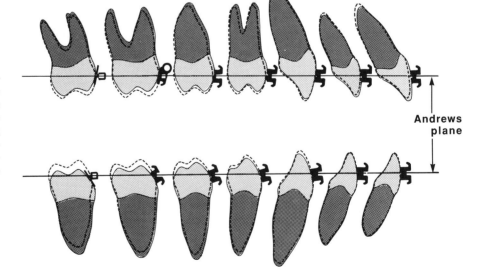

216

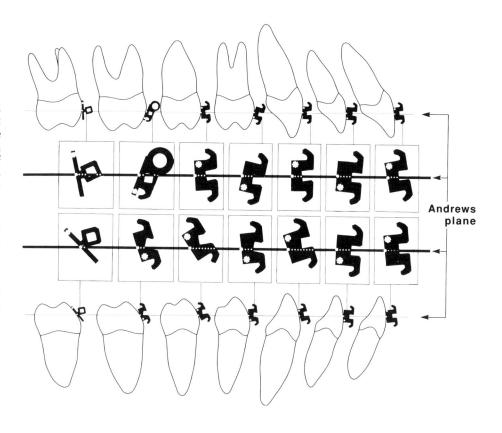

Fig. 11.5. Partly programmed bracket siting and slot siting: slot positions are even more incongruent than shown in Fig. 11.3 when the bases of partly programmed brackets contact the teeth alternately at opposite ends. The teeth are optimally inclined. Enlarged bracket positions (*center*) are identical to those shown on teeth. White asterisks indicate where bracket bases touch the crowns. White dot at the center of each bracket base indicates the base point.

Andrews plane

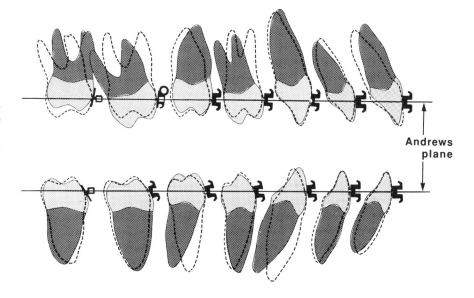

Fig. 11.6. The effects on tooth inclination and occlusogingival position when the slots of partly programmed brackets sited as shown in Fig. 11.5 are made passive to full-size unbent archwires. Dashed lines represent optimal positions.

Andrews plane

217

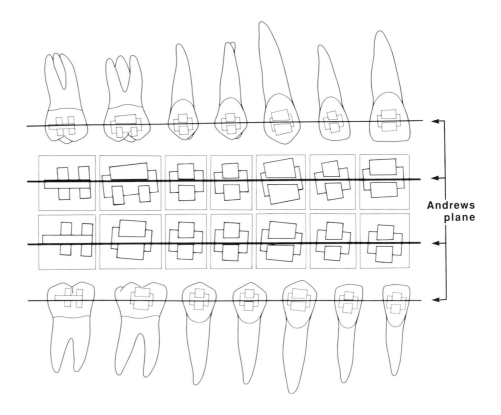

Fig. 11.7. Partly programmed slot siting. Even when partly programmed brackets with correct amounts of slot angulation and inclination are correctly sited as shown in Fig. 11.3, the slot points are directed above or below the Andrews plane. Enlarged bracket positions (*center*) are identical to those shown on teeth.

Andrews plane

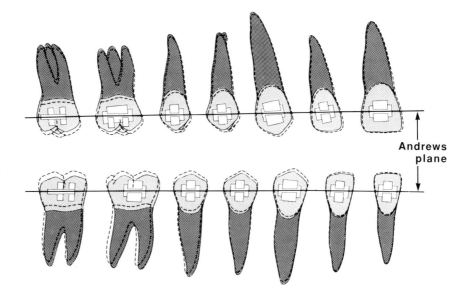

Fig. 11.8. The effects on crown angulation and occlusogingival position when the slots of brackets sited as shown in Figs. 11.3 and 11.7 are made passive to full-size unbent archwires. Dashed lines represent optimal positions.

Andrews plane

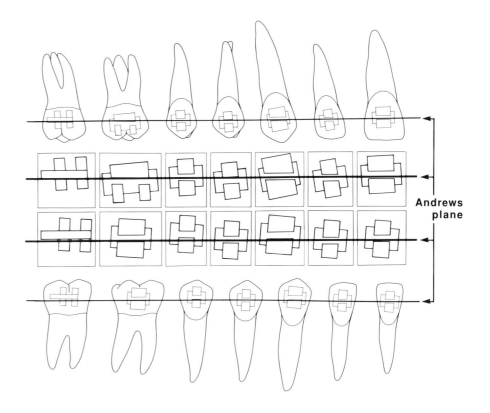

Fig. 11.9. Partly programmed slot siting. When partly programmed brackets are sited as shown in Fig. 11.5 they may be correctly angulated, but the slot points are above or below the Andrews plane even more than shown in Fig. 11.7. Enlarged bracket positions (*center*) are identical to those shown on teeth.

Andrews plane

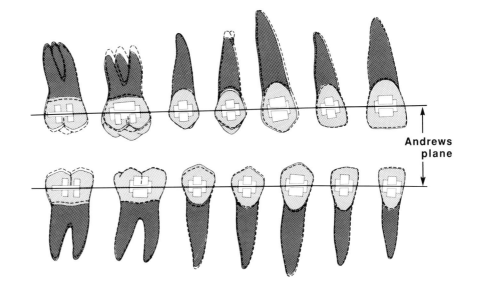

Fig. 11.10. The effects on crown angulation and occlusogingival position when the slots of brackets sited as shown in Figs. 11.5 and 11.9 are made passive to full-size unbent archwires. Dashed lines indicate optimal positions.

Andrews plane

219

the manufacturers; they may or may not be the same as for the Straight-Wire Appliance. If they are not, an appliance will not reliably locate the midsagittal plane of the bracket stem and slot on the crown's midsagittal plane.

Patents restrict translation slot-siting features to the Straight-Wire Appliance (Chapter 10); therefore none of the partly programmed appliances offer fully programmed translation brackets. This means that unless treated with combinations of wire bending and wire forming, and possibly with auxiliary rotation devices, none of the teeth requiring translation will translate, nor will they be sufficiently overinclined, overangulated, or overrotated after translation. However, teeth that are moved mesially or distally tend to rebound whether translated and overcorrected or not. If not overcorrected they are likely to rebound to an undertreated condition (see "Methods and Results" in Chapter 5).

Bracket Siting

Manufacturers' literature for nonprogrammed and partly programmed brackets does not specify that they are to be exactly located on the bracket site that Andrews earlier identified, described, and labeled as the FACC and FA point. Yet that is the site from which the measurements for the Straight-Wire Appliance were taken. These measurements have been adopted by most manufacturers. However, even when an attempt is made to place those brackets properly, the quality and quantity of their slot-targeting features prevent dependable slot siting. The slot-siting error may, in fact, be greater than illustrated in this book if partly programmed brackets are not sited on the FACC and FA point. Bracket and slot-siting features and bracket siting determine whether the slot will be sited within 2° and 0.5 mm of the slot-target site.

Appliance Data

The categories nonprogrammed, partly programmed, and fully programmed should be used to indicate the fundamental design distinctions among edgewise appliances. Each category can then be supplemented to provide additional slot-siting information, i.e., data about landmarks, design, bracket siting, and sets. For the nonprogrammed appliance, only landmark and bracket-siting information is required, because the slot-siting features for all brackets for that appliance are alike. For the fully programmed appliance, only information about the anterior and posterior sets is required, because the appliance is fully programmed and the landmarks and bracket siting are prespecified. The partly programmed category, however, requires information about landmarks, design, and siting.

Nonprogrammed Appliances

For adequate records when a nonprogrammed appliance is used—and for transferring a patient, conferring, lecturing, and reporting—certain information must be available. The landmarks used for bracket siting, and the degrees of bracket angulation, if any, are essential in conveying knowledge of where the slot is targeted. A form like this may be employed:

Appliance classification: Nonprogrammed
Landmarks for: angulation _____ inclination _____
Bracket angulation: no_____ yes _____
  Degrees:
    maxillary teeth   1__ 2__ 3__ 4__ 5__ 6__ 7__ 8__
    mandibular teeth 1__ 2__ 3__ 4__ 5__ 6__ 7__ 8__

Partly Programmed Appliances

The following information about any partly programmed appliance is necessary to begin an analysis of how the slots may be targeted:

Appliance classification: Partly programmed
Name of appliance _____
Data source for appliance design_____
Landmarks for: angulation _____ inclination ____
Bracket angulation: slot _____ bracket _____
  Degrees:
    maxillary teeth   1_ 2_ 3_ 4_ 5_ 6_ 7_ 8_
    mandibular teeth 1_ 2_ 3_ 4_ 5_ 6_ 7_ 8_
Bracket inclination: face _____ base _____
  Degrees:
    maxillary teeth   1_ 2_ 3_ 4_ 5_ 6_ 7_ 8_
    mandibular teeth 1_ 2_ 3_ 4_ 5_ 6_ 7_ 8_
Bracket prominence: no _____ yes _____
Bracket-base contour: horizontal only _____
                horizontal and vertical _____

Fully Programmed Appliances

This information is essential to a reader, listener, or transferring orthodontist about a fully programmed appliance:

Appliance classification: Fully programmed
Name of appliance _____
Data source for appliance design _____
Anterior set _____
Posterior set_____

Discussion

An individualized and correctly sited fully programmed appliance provides optimal guidance with unbent wires when tooth morphology and optimal position vary no more than 0.5 mm and 2° from the averages found in the optimal sample. In an estimated 90 percent of our patients, differences are so minor that they fall within the 2° and 0.5-mm guidelines; such dentitions can be properly and efficiently treated to the positional goals described as the Six Keys to Optimal Occlusion with little wirebending or none. The remaining 10 percent will require wirebending to the extent of the variations.

Therefore, since inconsistences in tooth morphology do exist, it is counterproductive to compound that problem with slot-siting variables imposed by brackets with incorrect bracket-siting and slot-siting features, and by inadequate bracket-siting techniques. How many features are programmed into a bracket has limited relevance if the bracket is not sited correctly or if its features do not direct the slot to the slot-target site (Chapter 8).

Because brackets are small, it is difficult to see how they differ, much less how their slots are sited individually and collectively. Appliances that purportedly can be used with unbent archwires, but that in fact do not deliver their slots to the slot-target sites, will create occlusion disharmonies unless some wirebending is done. Some occlusion disharmonies are as visually imperceptible as are discordancies among incorrectly sited bracket slots; nevertheless, they can be stressful and debilitating to the patient. To avoid treatment detours, and as an imperative for planning treatment, transferring patients, and scientific reporting, orthodontists should be aware of each slot-siting feature of the appliance being used, and know its effect.

As orthodontics moves further into the gnathological era, accurate bracket siting and slot siting become even more essential. The amount of slot-siting error that can be imposed by partly programmed appliances is considered by some to be minor; but when casts are mounted on articulators, the occlusal errors are seen to be clinically significant by gnathological standards, unless those errors first have been compensated for with wire bending.

Chapter 12

Arch Lines and Treatment Strategies

The Six Keys are more readily attained with any appliance when the clinician understands that there are three arch lines, not one, and that each must be optimal for occlusion to be optimal. This chapter will (1) define each arch line, (2) identify the components of each arch line, (3) explain how each component can affect the length of an arch line, (4) specify which components can be controlled orthodontically, and (5) discuss strategies for controlling the components efficiently. Some new terminology is necessary.

Abnormal malocclusion. A condition in which the occlusion or the anterior limit of the dentition cannot be treated to optimal goals without jaw surgery.

Angulating. Changing the mesiodistal cant of a tooth when the axis of rotation is in the crown.

Angulation. The mesiodistal cant of the facial axis of the clinical crown (FACC) relative to a line perpendicular to the occlusal plane. Angulation is "positive" when the occlusal portion of the FACC is mesial to the gingival portion, "negative" when distal.

Contact area. The portion of the mesial or distal surface of a tooth that will touch an adjacent tooth when both teeth are optimally positioned.

Contact point. The centermost portion of a crown's contact area.

Inclination. The faciolingual cant of the FACC when measured from a line perpendicular to the occlusal plane. Inclination is "positive" when the occlusal portion of the FACC is facial to its gingival portion, "negative" when lingual.

Inclining. Changing the faciolingual cant of the FACC when the axis of rotation is in the crown or bracket.

Normal malocclusion. A condition in which the occlusion and the anterior limit of the dentition can be treated to optimal goals without surgery.

Tip. The mesiodistal or faciolingual angle of the long axis of a tooth when measured to a line perpendicular to the occlusal plane. Tip is "positive" when the occlusal portion of the tooth's long axis is either mesial or facial to its apical portion, "negative" when distal or lingual.

Tipping. Changing the mesiodistal or faciolingual angle of the long axis of a tooth when the axis of rotation is in the root.

Arch Lines

Several imaginary lines have been proposed for measuring the existing or proposed length of an arch [9,3,1,20]. The three proposed here are the core, midsagittal, and perimeter lines. These lines correlate the most closely with the Six Keys to Optimal Occlusion [4]. In fact, they too work like an interconnected system: when one or more of the lines is incorrect, then one or more of the Six Keys is incorrect.

Core Line

The arch core line is an imaginary line that best represents the length of the dental arch at its core. It passes mesiodistally through the center of each crown whose alignment conforms to the arch form. It extends to the distal surface of the last teeth in each arch to be included in treatment. It is short when its length is less than the sum of the mesiodistal diameters of normal crowns at their contact points (Fig. 12.1), optimal when it equals that sum (Fig. 12.2).

Midsagittal Line

The arch midsagittal line is an imaginary line that best represents the anteroposterior length of an arch. It is measured in the midsagittal plane of an arch from the anterior limit of the core line to a line connecting the most

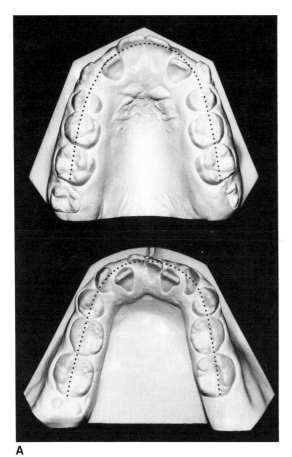

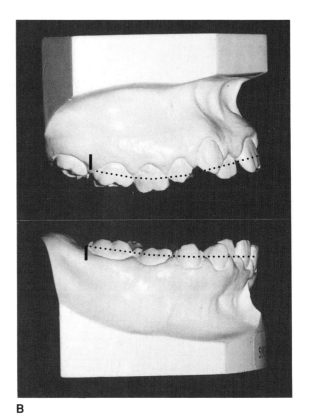

A
B

Fig. 12.1. Short arch core lines: *A*, occlusal view; *B*, buccal view.

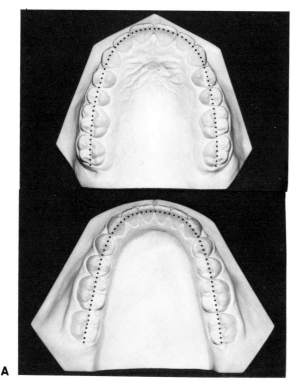

distal aspects of the core line. The midsagittal line is short when the core line is short (Fig. 12.3) or when the core line's occlusogingival form or buccolingual form are incorrect. The midsagittal line is optimal when the core line's length and form are optimal (Fig. 12.4).

Perimeter Line

The arch perimeter line is an imaginary line that best represents the length of the occlusofacial portion of the dental arch. It is measured along a line that connects the most facial points of the occlusal surfaces of the crowns that are on the core line, and extends as far distally as does the core line. A short perimeter

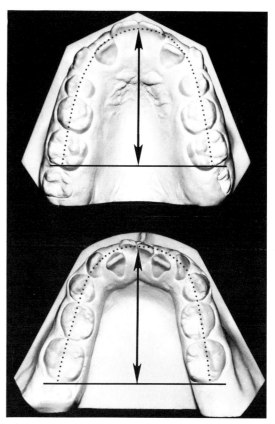

Fig. 12.2. Optimal arch core lines: *A*, occlusal view; *B*, buccal view.

Fig. 12.3. Short midsagittal lines.

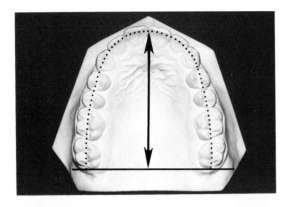

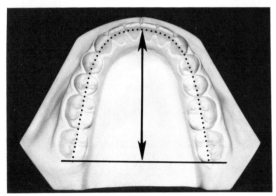

Fig. 12.4. Optimal midsagittal lines.

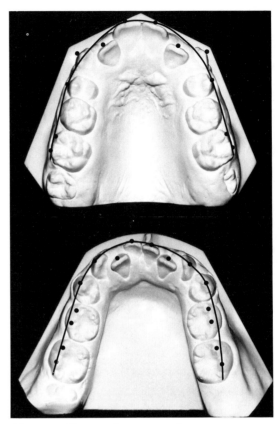

Fig. 12.5. Short arch perimeter lines.

line exists when the teeth on the core line are correctly inclined but the core line is short (Fig. 12.5), or when the core line is correct but the teeth on the core line are less than optimally inclined. The perimeter line is optimal when all the teeth are on the core line and the teeth are correctly inclined (Fig. 12.6).

Arch-Line Components

Normal teeth not optimally positioned, and normal jaws incorrectly related may produce incorrect arch lines. Incorrect inclination, angulation, or rotation can affect arch lines; so can faulty mesiodistal, faciolingual, or occlusogingival positions. Jaw conditions that affect arch lines include Class II or III interjaw relationships and incorrect jaw form. Some of these problems will instantly affect one or more of the

arch lines; some will later affect them; some will have no effect. For example, a rotated molar will instantly occupy more mesiodistal space, a rotated incisor will not. However, in time, a rotated incisor may affect one or more arch lines because of drift. A rotated canine or first premolar will have no effect on arch lines.

Table 3 indicates the immediate effect of each problem. This immediate effect may or may not adversely affect an arch line. (Problems that may later affect an arch line are not indicated.) The following discussion explains which arch lines are affected by each errant tooth position and how tooth position is affected by interjaw relationship. Most of the treatment results used as examples of the

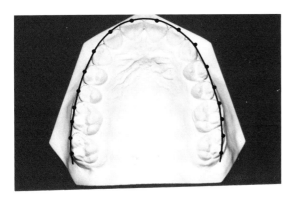

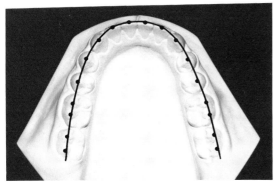

Fig. 12.6. Optimal arch perimeter lines.

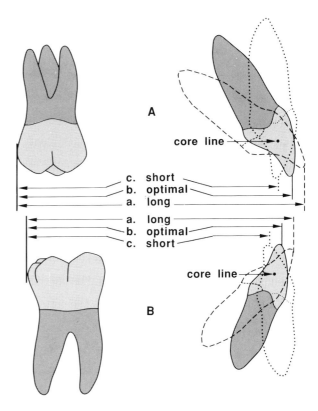

Fig. 12.7. In the maxillary arch (*A*), the perimeter line is: *a*, long when incisor inclination is excessively positive; *b*, optimal when inclination is moderately positive; *c*, short when inclination is negative. In the mandibular arch (*B*), the perimeter line is: *a*, long when the incisors are inclined positively; *b*, optimal when inclination is slightly negative; *c*, short when inclination is excessively negative.

arch-line conditions discussed in this chapter are from the 1960s or 1970s American Board samples (Chapter 5). When an appropriate example was not available from those sources an alternative source was used and the source identified.

Inclination

Maxillary and mandibular incisor inclination, when positive, can affect only the perimeter line; when negative, it can affect all three arch lines. Inclination of posterior teeth in either arch affects only the perimeter line.

Maxillary Incisors

Assuming an optimal core line, the maxillary perimeter line is long when the inclination of the maxillary incisors is excessively positive, optimal when the inclination is mod-

erately positive, and short when the inclination is negative (Fig. 12.7A).

If, assuming Class I molars and correct mandibular arch lines, the inclination of the maxillary incisors is negative or insufficiently positive, the maxillary perimeter line will be short, but the maxillary core and midsagittal lines will be long (Fig. 12.8). Under the same incisor conditions as shown in Figure 12.8, but with optimal maxillary core and midsagittal lines, the posterior teeth will, to some extent, have a Class II relationship (Fig. 12.9). Under these conditions the maxillary perimeter line will be even shorter.

Under the same incisor conditions as

227

Table 3
Components and Positions or Conditions That Affect Arch Lines

Components	Positions	Core	Midsagittal	Perimeter
Teeth	**Inclination**			
Maxillary incisors	Positive			x
	Negative	x	x	x
Mandibular incisors	Positive			x
	Negative	x	x	x
Canines, premolars, and molars	Positive			x
	Negative			x
	Angulation			
Maxillary incisors	Positive	x	x	x
	Negative	x	x	x
Mandibular incisors	Positive			
	Negative			
Canines, premolars, and molars	Positive			
	Negative			
	Rotation			
Incisors				
Canines				
First premolars				
Second premolars		x	x	x
Molars		x	x	x
	Mesiodistal			
The most posterior tooth		x	x	x
	Faciolingual			
Incisors (as a group)		x	x	x
Canines, premolars, and molars (as a group)		x		x
	Occlusogingival			
Maxillary arch				
Concave			x	
Convex			x	
Mandibular arch				
Concave			x	
Convex			x	
	Conditions			
Jaws	**Relationship**			
	Class II			
Maxilla		x	x	x
Mandible				x
	Class I			
Maxilla				
Mandible				
	Class III			
Maxilla				x
Mandible		x	x	x
	Width			
	Wide			
Maxilla		x		x
Mandible		x		x
	Narrow			
Maxilla		x		x
Mandible		x		x

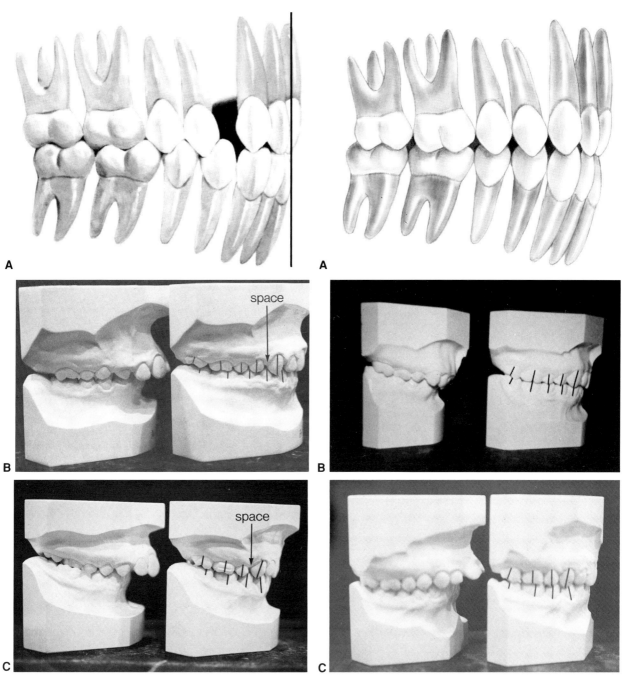

Fig. 12.8. When the molars are Class I but the maxillary incisor inclination is insufficiently positive, the perimeter line is short and the midsagittal and core lines are long, resulting in interdental space. *A*, The principle illustrated; *B*, nonextraction example; *C*, extraction example. Casts are from the mid-1960s American Board sample (Chapter 5). Lines on teeth indicate FACC.

Fig. 12.9. When maxillary incisor inclination is insufficiently positive and there is no interdental space, the core or midsagittal lines will be correct, but the perimeter line will be short and the molar relationship (assuming optimal mandibular arch lines and Class I incisor relationship) will tend to be Class II. *A*, The principle illustrated; *B*, nonextraction example; *C*, extraction example. Casts are from the mid-1960s American Board sample (Chapter 5). Lines on teeth indicate FACC.

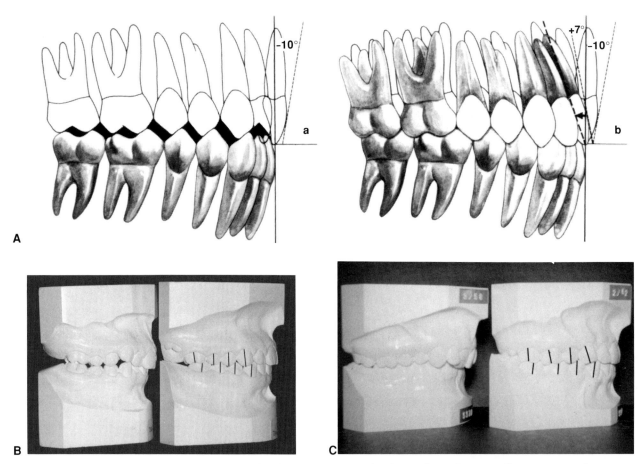

Fig. 12.10. The effects on the perimeter line and on posterior interarch relationship when maxillary incisor inclination is changed from negative (*Aa*) to positive (*Ab*). *B,* Nonextraction example (treatment by L. F. Andrews); *C,* extraction example (casts from the mid-1960s American Board sample). Lines on teeth indicate FACC.

shown in Figure 12.9, changing the incisors' inclination from negative to positive changes the length of the perimeter line from short to optimal without changing the already optimal midsagittal and core lines (Fig. 12.10). This act results in an incisor interarch discrepancy equal to that of the molars and allows the entire interarch relationship to be corrected. If the maxillary incisors shown in Figure 12.8 were to be inclined positively without changing the incisor or molar interarch relationship, the existing long maxillary core and midsagittal lines would become optimal, as would the short perimeter line.

Note: The interincisal crown angles are identical and *greater than* 180° in Figures 12.8A, 12.9A, and 12.10Aa. Under these conditions optimal occlusion cannot occur, regardless of the interarch or interjaw relationship.

Mandibular Incisors

The mandibular perimeter line is long when the inclination of the mandibular incisors is positive, optimal when the inclination is slightly negative, and short when the inclination is excessively negative (Fig. 12.7B).

A long mandibular perimeter line will result in long maxillary core, midsagittal, and

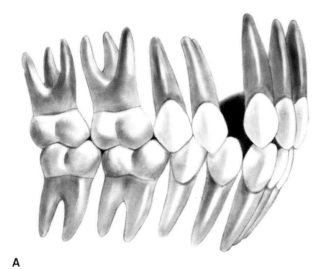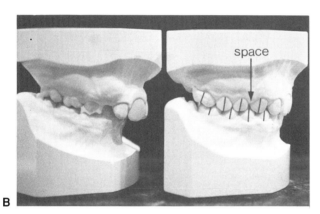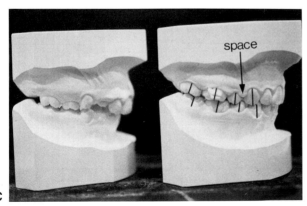

perimeter lines if the interarch relationship of the molars and incisors is correct (Fig. 12.11).

A long mandibular perimeter line will result in a Class II tendency of the posterior teeth if the incisor interarch relationship and the maxillary core and midsagittal lines are correct (Fig. 12.12).

The perimeter line in each arch is most likely to be optimal when inclination is moderately positive for the maxillary incisors (Fig. 12.7Ab) and slightly negative for the mandibular incisors (Fig. 12.7Bb). When the two perimeter lines are optimal the occlusion can be optimal (Fig. 12.13), though it may not be if one or more of the Six Keys is not attained or if the interjaw relationship is incorrect.

Excessive negative inclination of the mandibular incisors results in a short mandibular perimeter line (Fig. 12.7Bc). When this line is short the interarch relationships of the buccal segments will be Class III if the incisor interarch relationship is correct and if the core lines in each arch are comparable (Fig. 12.14).

Assuming correct incisor interarch relationship and comparable core lines, the interarch relationship of the posterior teeth can range from Class II to Class III, depending on the length of the perimeter line of each arch (Fig. 12.15).

Note: The dentitions illustrated in Figures 12.12A, 12.13A, and 12.14A are shown collectively in Figure 12.15. All of the interincisal crown angles are identical and *less than* 180°. An interincisal crown angle of less than 180°, a criterion of Key III [4], does not by itself ensure optimal occlusion; other factors, such as optimal arch lines and harmonious interjaw relationships, are also essential.

Posterior Teeth

Only the perimeter line is affected by inclination of posterior teeth.

Fig. 12.11. Positively inclined mandibular incisors lengthen the mandibular perimeter line, promoting maxillary interdental space when incisors and molars are Class I. *B,* Nonextraction example; *C,* extraction example. Casts are from the mid-1960s American Board sample (Chapter 5). Lines on teeth indicate FACC.

231

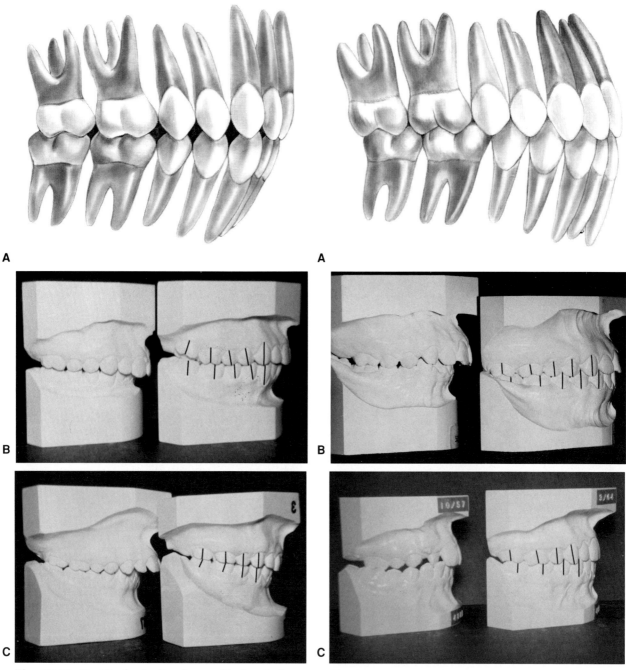

Fig. 12.12. Positively inclined mandibular incisors lengthen the mandibular perimeter line, causing the posterior teeth to have a Class II tendency if the incisor interarch relationship is Class I and there is no maxillary interdental space. *B*, Nonextraction example; *C*, extraction example. Casts are from the mid-1960s American Board sample (Chapter 5). Lines on teeth indicate FACC.

Fig. 12.13. Optimal perimeter lines occur when maxillary incisor inclination is moderately positive and mandibular incisor inclination is slightly negative. *B*, Nonextraction example (treatment by L. F. Andrews); *C*, extraction example (casts from the mid-1960s American Board sample). Lines on teeth indicate FACC.

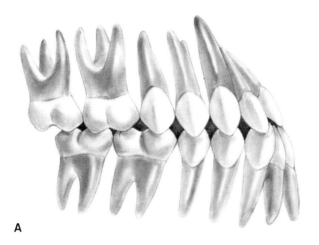

A

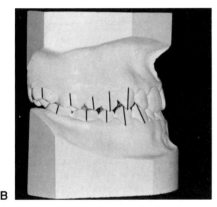

B

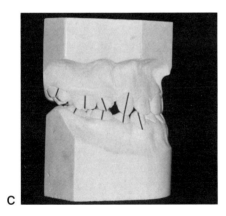

C

Fig. 12.14. Excessive negative inclination of mandibular incisors shortens the perimeter line. If the core lines in each arch are comparable and the incisors are Class I, the posterior teeth will have a Class III tendency. *B*, Nonextraction example (pretreatment casts, L. F. Andrews); *C*, extraction example (pretreatment serial extraction casts of a patient transferred to L. F. Andrews). Lines on teeth indicate FACC.

Angulation

The angulation of maxillary incisors can affect the core, midsagittal, and perimeter lines. Angulation of other teeth has little to no effect on the arch lines. The difference lies in the shapes of the mesiodistal crown surfaces in the contact areas when viewed from the facial perspective. In posterior crowns, these surfaces are, in effect, arcs of a circle; in mandibular incisors they resemble the sides of an isosceles triangle (Fig. 12.16). Teeth with such shapes, when angulated more or less than optimally, do not affect the mesiodistal space they occupy or the lengths of the three arch lines.

In contrast, the mesial and distal surfaces of maxillary incisor crowns are, in their areas of potential contact, like the sides of a trapezoid (Figs. 12.16, 12.17A). When the angulation of these teeth is zero, their contact points are at distinctively different distances from the occlusal plane of the arch; the distance between them when measured from vertical lines extending from the occlusal plane is less than the actual distance between them (Fig. 12.17B). Consequently, when these teeth are correctly angulated, the mesiodistal diameters are greater than when the teeth are upright (Fig. 12.17C).

The mesiodistal diameters of 120 maxillary incisors (30 of each type) were measured from positioner setups to determine how mesiodistal diameter was affected when angulation was changed from 0° to optimal (5° for centrals, 9° for laterals). The mesiodistal diameter of a maxillary central incisor is approximately 0.15 mm greater when it is angulated 5° than when 0°. For a maxillary lateral incisor, the mesiodistal diameter is about 0.25 mm more when angulated 9° than when 0°. The core line is 0.8 mm less when the maxillary incisors are upright than when they are optimally angulated (Fig. 12.18). (Unpublished study by Lawrence F. Andrews, 1986.)

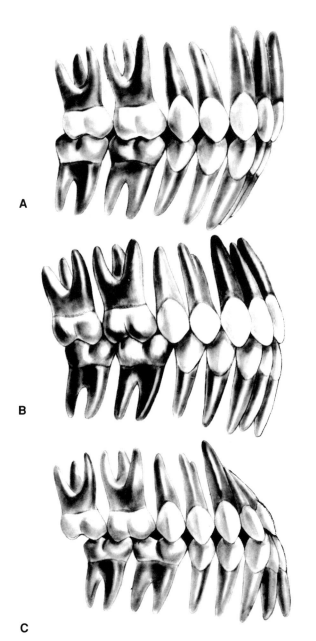

A

B

C

Fig. 12.15. Incompatible perimeter lines affect the inter-arch relationship of the posterior teeth if incisor relationships are Class I and the core and midsagittal line in each arch are comparable. Examples:
A, short maxillary perimeter line, long mandibular perimeter line—posterior Class II;
B, optimal maxillary and mandibular perimeter lines—posterior Class I;
C, long maxillary perimeter line, short mandibular—posterior Class III.

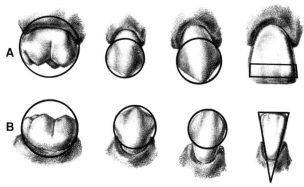

Fig. 12.16. The shape of the contact areas of crowns when viewed from the facial perspective. The mesiodistal surfaces of maxillary and mandibular posterior teeth are shaped like segments of a circle; mandibular incisors resemble the sides of a triangle; maxillary incisors resemble the sides of a trapezoid. *A,* Maxillary tooth types; *B,* mandibular tooth types.

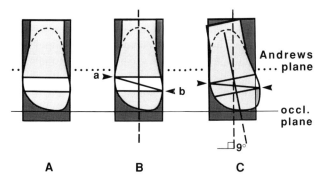

Fig. 12.17. *A,* From the facial aspect, the occlusal half of the middle third of a maxillary incisor crown resembles a trapezoid. *B,* When the FACC of a maxillary incisor is upright its distal contact point (*a*) is less occlusal than the mesial one (*b*). *C,* Unlike a circle or a triangle, a trapezoid occupies more mesiodistal space when angled.

Rotation

Rotating a first premolar, canine, or incisor will not immediately affect the arch core line, as will the rotation of second premolars and molars. But rotated incisors may cause broken contacts, allowing drift that can affect all three arch lines.

The mesiodistal diameters of maxillary and mandibular second premolars and first molars, in 20 positioner setups, were measured

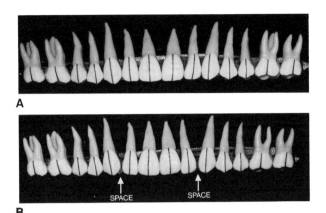

Fig. 12.18. Correctly angulated maxillary incisors occupy more mesiodistal space than upright incisors. In *A,* all maxillary crowns are correctly angulated; there is no interdental space. In *B,* the crowns are correctly angulated except for the upright incisors, which occupy less space (note interdental space between laterals and canines). Mesiodistal positions and angulations of the posterior teeth in both examples are identical. FACC of each crown is marked to highlight angulation.

to determine how much the core line would be increased by rotating the buccal surfaces of the teeth 20° mesially. The results were as follows: maxillary second premolars increased the core line by an average of .268 mm, and first molars by an average of .317 mm. (Unpublished study by Lawrence F. Andrews, 1987.)

Auxiliary rotation devices or built-in slot rotation features can correct or control tooth rotation and its effect on arch lines.

Mesiodistal Position

Long arch lines occur when there are interdental spaces (assuming no tooth size discrepancy or missing teeth). Correcting errant mesiodistal *crown* positions involves tooth tipping; correcting for errant mesiodistal *tooth* positions involves translation.

Faciolingual Position

Changing the faciolingual position of buccal segments will affect the core and perimeter lines. Palate splitting will increase those

lines in the maxillary arch. Facial tipping of buccal segments will increase those lines in either arch; lingual tipping will decrease them in either arch. Facial or lingual tipping of all four incisors will affect all three arch lines.

Occlusogingival Position

Changing the occlusogingival position of an isolated tooth will not immediately affect the arch lines. However, when the length of the arch core line is correct but its form is convex or concave, the midsagittal line will be short.

Under the same conditions, the midsagittal line will be correct if there is the right amount of interdental space for leveling the teeth without altering the anteroposterior positions of either the molars or the incisors. In that circumstance, the long core and perimeter lines will become optimal.

Table 4 shows how the core line is affected by leveling it within its *existing* anteroposterior and faciolingual borders (unpublished study by L.F. Andrews, 1976).

Interjaw Relationships

Inharmonious anteroposterior and buccolingual interjaw relationships can affect arch lines.

Table 4

**Effect of Leveling the Core Line
Within Its Existing Boundaries**

Depth of core line	Effect on length of core line
2 mm	1 mm
3 mm	2 mm
4 mm	3 mm
5 mm	5 mm
6 mm	7 mm

Anteroposterior

Class II jaws. Moderate-to-severe Class II jaws with Class I incisors result in negative maxillary incisor inclination and positive mandibular incisor inclination (Fig. 12.19A). The mandibular perimeter line is then long, and the maxillary perimeter line short (Fig. 12.12). If the molars are Class I and the inclination of the maxillary incisors is excessively negative, the maxillary core and midsagittal lines will be long (Fig. 12.11).

In Class II jaws, the cortical bone boundaries in each jaw prevent concurrently attaining optimal incisor interarch relationship and optimal incisor inclination (Fig. 12.19). Correction of jaw disharmony, therefore, is essential for correct incisor inclination and interarch relationship, and for optimal arch lines.

Class I jaws.* Class I jaws [16] present the best milieu for optimal arch lines and occlusion that conforms to the Six Key criteria [4] (Fig.12.20).

With Class I jaws, the orthodontist has the full range of alveolar bone to accommodate concurrent incisor inclination and interarch relationship. This condition yields optimal perimeter lines (Fig. 12.13).

Class III jaws. Class III jaws, with Class I incisors, cause excessively negative mandibular incisor inclination and excessively positive maxillary incisor inclination (Fig. 12.21). This condition results in a short mandibular perimeter line and a long maxillary perimeter line (Fig. 12.14).

In Class III jaws, the cortical plate boundaries in each jaw preclude concurrent optimal incisor inclination and interarch relationship.

---

*1 mm "Wits" for males, 0 mm "Wits" for females [16].

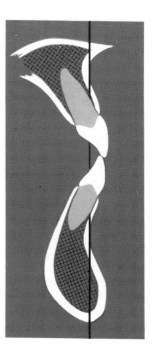

Fig. 12.19. A Class II jaw relationship restricts coincidentally attaining Class I incisors and optimal incisor inclination. Examples: *A*, Class I incisors with incorrect inclination; *B*, correct incisor inclination with Class II relationship. Vertical lines delimit jaw discrepancy.

Fig. 12.20. A Class I jaw presents the full range of alveolar bone for attaining optimal incisor inclination and Class I incisors.

Buccolingual

Widening a jaw may lengthen the core and perimeter lines; narrowing a jaw may shorten them. The midsagittal line will not be affected in either instance.

Note: Jaw surgery should be recommended when anteroposterior or buccolingual jaw position prevents treating the dentition to optimal arch lines, and to occlusal and anterior-limit goals. In this situation, when jaw disharmony is not correctible orthopedically, and when the patient refuses surgery, a less-than-optimal result is inevitable. Such treatment will lack the Six Keys, optimal arch lines, and facial harmony. Under these conditions the treatment result should be considered successful to the extent that lesser goals are attained, so long as the patient is better off as a result of such treatment.

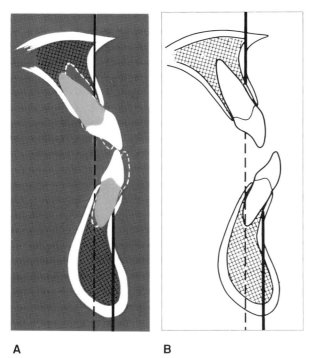

A   **B**

Fig. 12.21. A Class III jaw precludes coincidental Class I incisors and optimal inclination. *A*, Class I incisors with incorrect inclination; *B*, optimal incisor inclination with Class II relationship. Vertical lines delimit jaw discrepancy.

Etiology of Incorrect Arch Lines

Incorrect arch lines arise from varied sources, such as incorrect position or morphology of arch-line components, and missing or extra components. Such defects stem both from heredity and from environmental factors: some of each may be congenital (e.g., some teeth may be missing or malformed). Hereditary problems include some jaw abnormalities (e.g., morphology, size, and interjaw relationships) and some tooth abnormalities (e.g., teeth-to-jaw size, tooth-to-teeth size, and some malformed teeth). Environmental factors include the effects on jaw morphology and position, and on tooth position from thumb-sucking, tongue thrusting, missing teeth, and sometimes orthodontic treatment itself (iatrogenic disorders).

Treatment Strategies

Regardless of the etiology, part of our job as orthodontists is to correct the arch lines by correcting tooth positions and interarch relationships. Attaining optimal arch lines efficiently depends greatly on treatment strategies, which include goals, appliance selection and prescription, bracket and slot siting, and certain treatment procedures.

Goals

Treatment goals that do not include the Six Keys and optimal arch lines will not yield optimal occlusion.

Appliance Selection and Prescription

The category of edgewise appliance selected for treatment affects the efficiency of correcting tooth positions and arch lines. Three categories of edgewise brackets are available: nonprogrammed, partly programmed, and fully programmed (Fig. 11.1). Design differences cause the brackets of each category to site their slots differently, even when the brackets are matched to the same landmarks on optimally positioned teeth (Fig. 11.2).

When the base points of brackets in each appliance category are sited on the FACC and FA points of optimally positioned teeth, only the fully programmed appliance's slots (Fig. 9.3) will passively receive an unbent rectangular archwire (Figs. 7.3, 9.3, 11.3).

Another design contrast should be noted. Base-point-to-FA-point bracket siting is nearly impossible with a bracket whose base is not contoured vertically to match the tooth's curved surface (Fig. 7.7). Figures 7.8 and 11.5 show that when sited on optimally positioned teeth, flat-based nonprogrammed and partly programmed brackets are likely to site their slots with even greater irregularity than illustrated in Figures 7.3 and 11.3. Such variability requires a proportionally greater amount of trial-and-error wire bending. In contrast, the slots of fully programmed brackets line up when the teeth are optimally positioned (Fig. 9.3). Nonprogrammed and partly programmed brackets lack one or more of the eleven design features that are essential for siting their slots correctly. Eight features are needed for teeth not requiring translation (Chapter 9), up to eleven are needed for teeth requiring translation (Chapter 10). Each missing design feature can cause a slot to be sited beyond the clinically acceptable 2° or 0.5-mm allowable range.

Bracket Siting

Bracket siting is the first link in the chain of requirements for accurate slot siting. Accuracy in this matter means placing the vertical components of the bracket within 2° of the FACC, and the base point of the bracket within 0.5 mm of the FA point (Chapter 8).

Treatment Procedures

Archwire bending or forming can cause imperceptible yet clinically significant side effects that often result in unintended tooth movement.

A distinction must be made between wire bending and wire forming. *Wire bending* means to make one or more kinks in the archwire. Such bends sometimes are used to move one or more but never all of the teeth in an arch; examples are first-, second-, and third-order bends.

Wire forming is the shaping of an archwire to control the movement of all teeth within an arch in one or more planes. Wire forming is done to alter or maintain the existing core line, to alter or maintain the existing midsagittal line, or to alter or maintain the existing perimeter line.

Side effects from both wire bending and wire forming occur—as explained below—when a nonprogrammed or a partly programmed edgewise appliance is used.

To deliver the intended tooth movement with an archwire, the orthodontist must know (1) the goal position of each crown, relative to the site where the bracket is placed; (2) the extent to which each bracket slot reflects the position of the bracket site; and (3) the side effects of bending and forming archwires during treatment.

Wire Bending

Installing third-order archwire bends with the intent to positively incline the maxillary incisors will, as a side effect, change crown angulation. This change is important because aesthetics and the lengths of the core, midsagittal, and perimeter lines are all affected. As the maxillary incisors respond to the positive inclination installed in the anterior portion of a rectangular archwire, their angulation becomes either less positive, negative, or (if already negative) more negative. The ratio of the inclination-to-angulation side effect is approximately 4:1 (Fig. 12.22).

Wire bending and its side effects are, for the most part, eliminated with a correctly prescribed and sited fully programmed appliance. For example, the problem illustrated in Figure 12.22 is resolved when the correct inclination

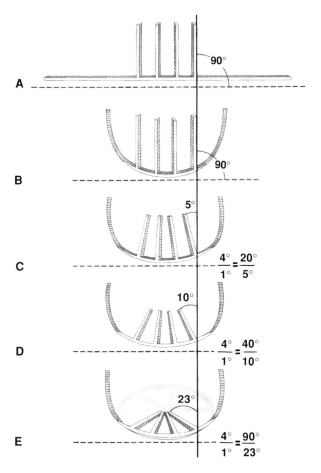

Fig. 12.22. Archwire inclination changes maxillary incisor angulation in a ratio of 4° to 1°. *A,* Four wires representing maxillary incisors connected to a flat, straight, rectangular wire. *B,* The wire is arched. *C,* 20° of positive inclination installed in the incisor portion of the wire. The angulation of the wires representing the incisors has changed from 90° to 85°, illustrating the ratio of 1° of crown angulation for every 4° of wire inclination. *D,* 40° of positive wire inclination results in 10° of negative crown angulation. *E,* If the anterior portion of the archwire is inclined 90°, the wires will resemble the spokes of a wagon wheel.

and angulation are built into maxillary incisor brackets to eliminate a need for wire bending.

Wire Forming

An arch with a deep curve of Spee and a concave core line is shown in Figure 12.23A. An archwire with a convex curve can be expected to level the core line. In addition, assuming an absence of interdental space, the arch's midsagittal length will increase. If a round wire with a convex curve is used to level the core line, the perimeter length will also increase in response to labial tipping of the mandibular incisors and as a result of intrusive force vectors (Fig. 12.23B). This wire-forming side effect will cause incisor inclination to become either less negative, positive, or (if already positive) more positive. Whether this side effect is desirable depends on the anterior limit and inclination goals for the incisors.

If a full-size rectangular wire is used to level the core line, additional incisor inclination can result from a side effect caused by installing a convex curve with the fingers and thumb. A 5-mm convex curve installed that way into a previously flat rectangular wire will change the inclination of the wire surfaces from zero to approximately 15° (Fig. 12.24). The ratio is approximately 3:1. Three degrees of inclination will accompany every millimeter of convexity. This side effect may cause the inclination of the incisor crowns to be more positive than if a similarly formed round wire is used (Fig. 12.23C). Such increased inclination results in a proportionally longer perimeter line (Fig. 12.7). Another probably unwanted consequence is the positive inclination of the posterior portion of the wire (Figs. 12.23C and 12.24).

Theoretically, the need to form the wire for leveling the core line could be eliminated or reduced with a fully programmed appliance, if bracket siting for the anterior teeth were to be altered from patient to patient in conformance with the depth of the curvatures of the core lines. Such an approach would be contradictory to the parallel-and-midpoint siting system and would introduce unwanted and unpredictable slot-siting variables. Efficient treatment requires that incisor brackets always be sited at the FA points even though that approach ensures a need for wire forming to level core lines. However, wire-forming side effects are predictable and quantifiable; therefore they can be neutralized or controlled, and often put to good use.

An example of a predictable and quantifiable wire-forming side effect is the inclina-

tion that occurs when a convex curve is installed, as discussed earlier and illustrated in Figures 12.23C and 12.24. It can be neutralized by first installing 15° of negative wire inclination throughout an otherwise flat archwire—using pliers, fingers, and thumb (Fig.

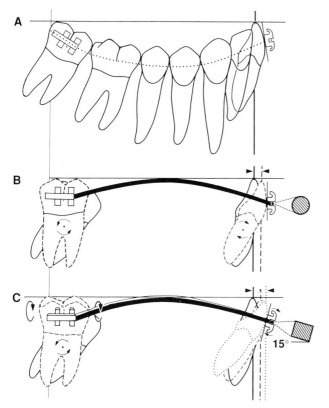

Fig. 12.23. Side effects from installing convex curves in archwires for leveling the core line. *A,* Concave core line (*dotted line*). *B,* Effect on incisors and molars from leveling the core line as seen in *A* with a round wire. An installed convex curve in the archwire tips the incisors labially and, to some extent, the molars distally (*dashed lines*) around their centers of rotation (*dots in roots*). *C,* Leveling a core line as seen in *A* with a full-size rectangular wire will, when a convex curve is installed, have the same effect on the teeth as a round wire (*dashed lines*), plus any difference between the slot inclination and wire inclination (*dotted lines*).

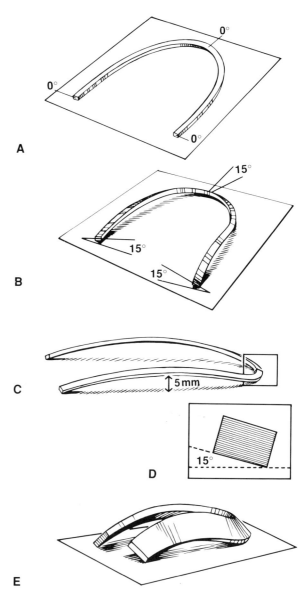

Fig. 12.24. Quantifying the inclination side effect from installing a convex curve. *A,* A flat rectangular archwire without inclination. *B, C, D,* A 15° inclination side effect resulting from installing a 5-mm convex curve. *E,* Exaggerated example.

12.25A–C). Installing a convex curve of approximately 5 mm then automatically erases the previously installed negative inclination (Fig. 12.25D,E).

When installing a concave curve into a rectangular wire to level the maxillary teeth (Fig. 12.26), one encounters side effects directly opposite to those discussed earlier for the mandibular arch (Fig. 12.23C and 12.24). The resulting positive-inclination side effect is often favored for the maxillary incisors, but is seldom wanted in the maxillary posterior teeth.

The positive wire inclination for the posterior teeth should be changed progressively from positive to negative, starting from the lateral incisors. This side effect can be controlled by holding the wire with one pair of pliers at a site immediately distal to the lateral incisor, and twisting with another pair at the end of the wire until there is 15° of negative inclination at the molar end (Fig. 12.27). The result will be 15° of positive incisor inclination and 15° of negative molar inclination, with the transition occurring gradually from the laterals through the molars. This approach will prevent the lingual cusps of the molars from obtruding.

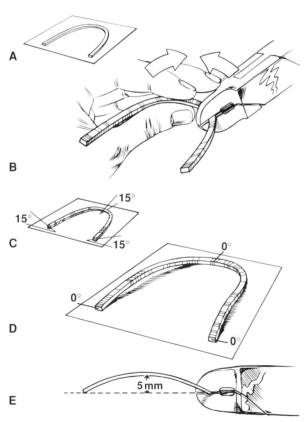

Fig. 12.25. Neutralizing a wire-forming side effect: preparing a rectangular wire with 5-mm convex curve and no inclination. *A*, A flat archwire without inclination. *B*, 15° of negative inclination is installed with fingers and pliers throughout the archwire while maintaining the flat vertical form (*C*). *D*, A 5-mm convex curve is then installed, automatically erasing the previously installed 15° of inclination. *E*, Final rectangular wire has a convex curve but no inclination.

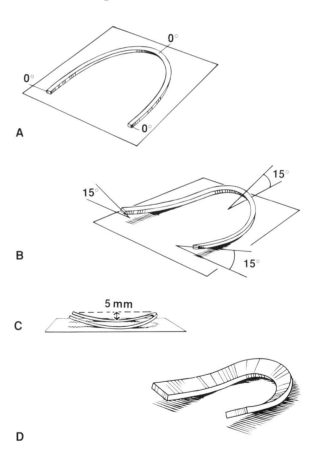

Fig. 12.26. A useful wire-forming side effect. *A*, A flat archwire blank without inclination. *B*, 15° of inclination results from installing a 5-mm concave curve into the wire. A side view (*C*) and an exaggerated example (*D*) of *B*.

241

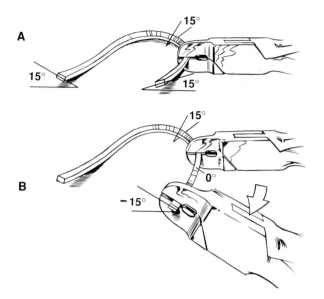

Fig. 12.27. Installing progressive negative inclination from the laterals through molars. *A,* A maxillary archwire with 15° of inclination throughout is grasped with pliers at a site between the lateral and canine. *B,* A second pliers, grasping the rear of the wire, is twisted to install −15° of inclination at the end of the wire.

Summary

Tooth positions and interjaw relationships determine the arch lines. Attaining optimal occlusion efficiently requires treatment strategies that include optimal arch lines, the Six Key goals, a fully programmed appliance, the FACC and FA point as landmarks for bracket siting, and understanding of wire-forming side effects.

Chapter 13

Fully Programmed
Appliance Prescription

Selecting the most suitable straight-wire brackets for each tooth in an arch begins with deciding which teeth must be moved mesio-distally, and how far they must be moved. The next step is to determine whether those teeth should be tipped or translated. Teeth to be translated will need translation brackets—minimum, medium, or maximum, depending on the distance to be moved. The other teeth need only standard brackets.

To make these distinctions, first measure the discrepancy between the size of the teeth and the space available for them within the existing arch. Then add or subtract the amount of space that would result from any proposed changes in the arch, such as its lateral anteroposterior limits, or its occlusogingival form. (For this exercise the existing posterior limit of the dentition is to be used.) These changes represent the portions of the treatment plan that can be achieved without mesial or distal movement of teeth. Any remaining discrepancy must be dealt with by mesial or distal movement. This discrepancy greatly in-

fluences whether extractions are required, not needed, or optional. Once a decision is made, it can be learned whether the mesial or distal movement still required must be tipping or translation, and what distance is involved for each tooth type.

For the portion of treatment involving mesial and distal movement there are only twelve possibilities for the maxillary arch, and eleven for the mandibular arch, each requiring a specific set of brackets if treatment is to be without wire bending and within 2° and 0.5 mm of optimal for each tooth. However, the possibilities for treatment other than mesio-distal movement would nearly equal the number of patients. Fortunately, the problems that do not involve mesial or distal movement do not require special built-in features or wire bending. They can all be resolved by wire forming with either standard or translation brackets because the translation features are not needed or used to correct those problems.

For convenient prescription, the portion

of the total plan that involves mesial or distal movement is identified and labeled, and its appropriate bracket set is given a matching or obvious label.

The following terminology is required for this prescription approach. Some of the terminology was defined earlier, but is also important in this chapter.

Alternate treatment plan. The less conservative of two treatment possibilities for a specified amount of interim core discrepancy (ICD).

Arch core discrepancy (core discrepancy). The difference between the length of the core line and the sum of the mesiodistal diameters of the crowns, measured at their contact points (after allowing for any planned correction of tooth size abnormality).

Another and quicker method of determining core discrepancy is to compute the difference between the sum of the mesiodistal diameters of only the malaligned teeth and the space on the core line available for them (Fig. 13.4).

Arch core line (core line). An imaginary line that best represents the form and length of the arch.* It passes mesiodistally through the center of each crown that is in line with the arch form (Figs. 12.1, 12.2). It can be indirectly represented from the occlusal perspective with a brass wire that is centered over the occlusal surface of each such crown (Fig. 13.3).

Basic treatment plan. Either the only or the most conservative treatment plan for an arch within a specified range of interim core discrepancy (ICD).

Interim core discrepancy (ICD). The difference between the sum of the mesiodistal diameters of the crowns at their contact points and the length of the interim core line.

Another and quicker method of determining ICD is to add to the core discrepancy the sum of the effects of changing the core line

in all ways proposed other than for its distal boundary.

This discrepancy is the portion of the problem that will be dealt with by mesial or distal movement of the posterior teeth, some or all of which may involve translation.

Interim core line. A proposed core line whose distal ends are those of the arch core line, but whose buccolingual and occlusogingival form and anterior boundary are treatment *goals.* Its length is the core-line length, plus the gain or loss from changing the core line in all ways intended except for distal boundary.

Normal arch. Any arch in which each tooth's existing position is within 7 mm of its proposed position. (This range allows a maximum core discrepancy of 14 mm through –14 mm.)

Subtypes. The eight ranges of interim core discrepancy within a normal arch, each representing where one basic treatment plan begins and ends: (positive discrepancy) 0–4 mm, 5–8 mm, 9–14 mm; (negative discrepancy) 0–6 mm, 7–8 mm, 9–10 mm, 11–13 mm, 14 mm.

Treatment core line. A line that conforms to all treatment goals for the arch core. Its length equals the sum of the mesiodistal diameters of the teeth when measured at their contact points (assuming no tooth size discrepancy).

Types. The three natural divisions of the range of core discrepancy or interim core discrepancy for a normal arch: Spaced (positive discrepancy), Classic (zero discrepancy), and Crowded (negative discrepancy).

Treatment Planning Components

Interim core discrepancy (ICD) is the portion of the treatment that must be dealt with by mesial or distal movement. The amount can be learned by comparing the mesiodistal space available for all crowns in an arch after the core-line length has been hypothetically corrected in all respects except

---

*Arch here refers to the portion of the arch that the clinician intends to include in treatment. Treatment of the entire arch is recommended.

distal boundary. The other aspects of the total treatment plan may include orthopedics, jaw surgery, and changes in position of individual teeth (other than by mesial or distal tipping or translation) such as buccolingual tipping, angulation, inclination, and rotation. All these other procedures are important in themselves, but they can be accomplished with equal efficiency with either standard or translation brackets. Only interim core discrepancy reveals whether there may be a need for translation brackets.

Just as no two individuals are identical, neither are any two malocclusions. Treatment plans, therefore, must be tailored for each person, except for the portion involving mesial or distal movement. For this portion there are only twelve treatment options for the maxillary arch and eleven for the mandibular arch. This is why it is practical to prearrange brackets into sets for prescription. Not all orthodontists will diagnose, for any one patient, the same amount of ICD; but all orthodontists will have the same treatment alternatives for all patients with matching amounts of ICD.

How to compute the ICD, decide the ICD portion of the treatment plan, and select the appropriate bracket set will be explained after a brief overview.

Overview

The core line can be efficiently corrected in all ways except for its distal boundaries with standard or translation brackets, because the tooth movements for these corrections do not require or use the translation features, even if they are present. Essential for appliance prescription is diagnosing the need, if any, for translation of any posterior teeth. For the most part that information is revealed by the ICD. If the ICD is positive, some posterior teeth must be translated mesially to occupy the excess space; if the ICD is zero, no mesial or distal movement is needed; if the ICD is negative, some posterior teeth must move mesially or distally. The direction and distance of movement, whether the movement will be tipping or translation, and which teeth, if any, need extracting will be discussed and illustrated.

This approach is feasible for the treatment of a normal arch, which—by definition—must fall within a range of 14 through –14 mm of ICD. To identify the nature (positive or negative) of the ICD, the full 28-mm spectrum is separated into three natural divisions called types: Spaced, Classic, and Crowded (Fig. 13.1A).

To show where one basic treatment plan ends and another begins, the Spaced and Crowded portions of the ICD spectrum are divided into a total of eight subtypes (Fig. 13.1B); Classic has no range, so it cannot be subdivided. Each boundary is based on need for a different set of brackets if treatment with unbent archwires is to meet the 2° and 0.5-mm tolerance guidelines for the position of each tooth. There is one basic treatment plan for each of the eight subtypes and one for type Classic. In addition there are three alternate plans: one for type Classic; one for type Crowded, subtype 0–6 mm; and one for type Crowded, subtype 14 mm that is for the maxillary arch only. These plans total twelve treatment possibilities for the maxillary arch and eleven for the mandibular arch for arches within the normal 28-mm ICD range.

Each treatment plan requires a different bracket set, except for the basic treatment plan for type Classic and for type Crowded, subtype 0–6 mm, which use the same set. Figure 13.1 lists the illustrations throughout this chapter that explain the treatment possibilities for each subtype range and for type Classic, as well as the suitable bracket for each tooth and the appropriate bracket set for each treatment plan. All of the brackets shown in these illustrations are from the inventory listed in Chapters 9 and 10.

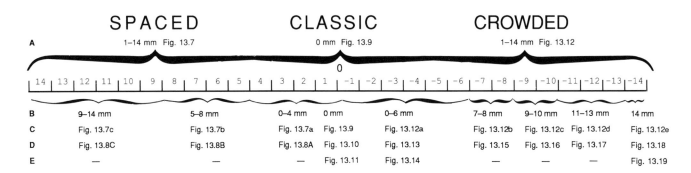

	SPACED		CLASSIC			CROWDED			

A — SPACED 1–14 mm Fig. 13.7 — CLASSIC 0 mm Fig. 13.9 — CROWDED 1–14 mm Fig. 13.12

B	9–14 mm	5–8 mm	0–4 mm	0 mm	0–6 mm	7–8 mm	9–10 mm	11–13 mm	14 mm
C	Fig. 13.7c	Fig. 13.7b	Fig. 13.7a	Fig. 13.9	Fig. 13.12a	Fig. 13.12b	Fig. 13.12c	Fig. 13.12d	Fig. 13.12e
D	Fig. 13.8C	Fig. 13.8B	Fig. 13.8A	Fig. 13.10	Fig. 13.13	Fig. 13.15	Fig. 13.16	Fig. 13.17	Fig. 13.18
E	—	—	—	Fig. 13.11	Fig. 13.14	—	—	—	Fig. 13.19

Fig. 13.1. The interim core discrepancy (ICD) for a normal arch may range from 14 to –14 mm. *A,* The ICD range includes types Spaced, Classic, and Crowded; the figure numbers illustrate examples of each. *B,* The ICD range for each subtype. *C,* Figure numbers that illustrate each subtype. *D,* Figure numbers that illustrate the basic treatment plan and bracket set for each subtype. *E,* Figure numbers that illustrate the alternate treatment plan and bracket set for each subtype that has an alternate treatment plan.

Fortunately, most arches can be assigned symmetrical bracket sets; i.e., mirror-image sets for the left and right quadrants. The crown positions of normal arches are not always bilaterally symmetrical, but the positions of the center of rotation of the teeth usually are (Fig. 13.2). In such arches, crowns that are mesial to a tooth's center of rotation can be uprighted by using teeth in the same quadrant whose crowns are distal to their centers of rotation, and, if needed, teeth on the other side of the arch or in the other arch if their positions would improve with the use of reciprocal force. This approach will convert most arches with asymmetrically positioned crowns to arches in which the crowns are as symmetrical as the centers of rotation of the teeth. If such an arch requires extractions, the energy and guidance required to translate the teeth on one side and to move only the roots on the other will be similar; and mirror-image translation brackets will be equally efficient for both sides.

The core line and interim core line for an arch are the same if the treatment plan calls for no change in either the form or the anterior

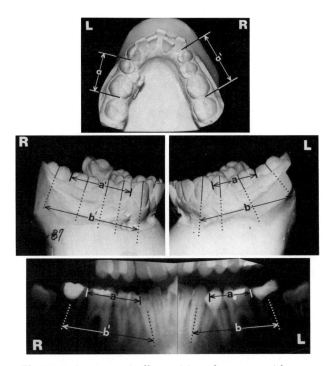

Fig. 13.2. Asymmetrically positioned crowns with symmetrically positioned roots (judged from centers of rotation). Distances between the left canine and second molar crowns (*a*), and the right canine and second molar crowns (*a'*) are unequal; distances between the canine and molar roots on left (*b*) and right (*b'*) sides are equal.

246

limit of the core line. When those lines are the same, all that is needed to determine the treatment plan and the appropriate bracket set for an arch is to (1) compute the discrepancy between the sum of the mesiodistal diameters of the teeth and the length of the interim core line (which, for the examples in this chapter, is the same as the core line); (2) match that number to the ICD range in Figure 13.1B; (3) refer to Figure 13.1C for an illustration of that condition; (4) refer to Figure 13.1D for the basic treatment plan, individual brackets, and the bracket set; and (5) refer to Figure 13.1E for an illustration of the alternate treatment plan, if there is one.

However, in most arches the interim core line differs from the core line, and that difference must be learned first (how will be explained later).

From this overview, we move on to the methods for computing core discrepancy and interim core discrepancy. Both measurements are essential for learning the treatment possibilities and matching bracket sets for any normal arch.

Core Discrepancy

As explained earlier, core discrepancy is the difference between the length of the core line and the sum of the mesiodistal diameters of the crowns measured at their contact points (after allowing for any planned correction of tooth size abnormality). A quicker method is to measure only the malaligned areas; both methods are explained below.

Measuring the Core Line and Teeth

The core line is an imaginary line that best represents the existing form and length of the arch. It passes mesiodistally through the center of each crown that is in line with the existing arch form. From the occlusal perspective it can be indirectly represented with a brass wire that is centered over the occlusal surface of each such crown (Fig. 13.3).

The mesiodistal diameter of a crown can be measured with dividers located as close to the contact points as possible.

Measuring Only the Malaligned Areas

Rather than measuring the length of the core line and all the crowns, a quicker method for determining core discrepancy is to compute the difference between the sum of the mesiodistal diameters of only the malaligned crowns and the sum of the space on the core line available for them (Fig. 13.4).

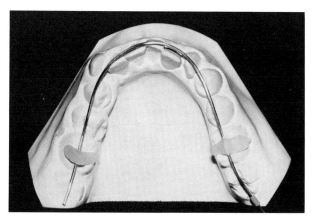
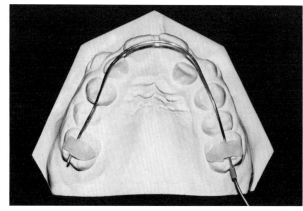

Fig. 13.3. Brass wire superimposed over contact points of teeth that are in line with the core form.

Interim Core Discrepancy

Orthodontic treatment alone will not provide all patients with optimal facial and occlusal results. Sometimes orthopedic treatment is needed; surgery may be indicated for those with abnormal jaws. The only difference in computing ICD for those who do require orthopedic treatment or surgery and those who do not is that, for those that do, the ICD is calculated with the jaws hypothetically located at their posttreatment positions.

As much latitude for professional judgment exists in planning treatment with this system as with any other. It is the orthodontist who decides the patient's proposed core form and its anterior limit. Any change in anterior limit or in buccolingual or occlusogingival form may change the length of the core line; if it does, it will also change the interim core discrepancy. Changed or not, the new line is called the interim core line. How to calculate the effects of changing the core line to the interim core line is explained below.

Buccolingual Effects

For every millimeter of proposed buccal movement of either side of the core line, add 1 mm to the core line and core discrepancy. Conversely, subtract 1 mm for every millimeter of lingual movement (Fig. 13.5).

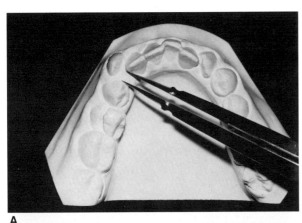

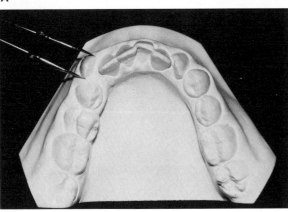

Fig. 13.4. Measuring core discrepancy for malaligned teeth: *A*, space; *B*, crown.

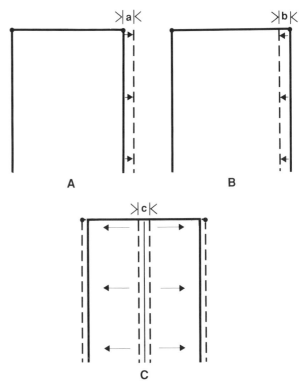

Fig. 13.5. Effects on the core-line length from arch expansion (*A*) and contraction (*B*) and from maxilla expansion (*C*). *Aa*, Add 1 mm to core line and to core discrepancy for every millimeter a buccal segment is moved laterally. *Bb*, Subtract 1 mm from the core line and core discrepancy for every millimeter a buccal segment is moved lingually. *Cc*, Add 1 mm to core line and core discrepancy for every millimeter of maxilla expansion. Solid line represents the occlusal view of an arch's core line. Dashed lines indicate proposed changes.

Anterior Limit Effects

For every millimeter of proposed advancement of the core line's anterior border, add 2 mm to the core line and core discrepancy; subtract 2 mm from each when it is to be retracted (Fig. 13.6).

Occlusogingival Effects

The occlusogingival form of the core line can be visualized as a line that nearly parallels the curve of Spee. Assuming a deep curve of Spee, no interdental space, and a fixed posterior boundary, a change in the occlusogingival form of the core line must be offset by a change in the buccolingual or anterior boundaries of the form. If the buccolingual boundary is also fixed, then the anterior boundary will have to move anteriorly when the concave form is leveled. If, under the same conditions, the anterior limit is also fixed, then the core line will have to be made shorter if it is to be level.

The effects on the length of a core line from leveling it within its existing borders have been computed for a range of depths, and recorded in Table 4 (p. 235). To use the table, measure the depth of the curve of Spee, which clinically is the same as the depth of the core line. Match that number with the same number found in the left column. Opposite that number, in the right column, is the amount of effect on core line length.

Treatment Possibilities and Bracket Sets

For each of the treatment plans illustrated in this chapter it is assumed that either (1) the core line and interim core line are coincidentally the same, or (2) the ICD illustrated is the amount remaining after the teeth have been hypothetically moved to the interim core line. It is also assumed that any interjaw treatment needed as a portion of the overall plan discussed earlier is to occur in conjunction with the orthodontic portion or has hypothetically been completed.

In each of the treatment plans illustrated, a letter S or number 1, 2, 3, or 4 on the surface of the crown indicates the category of bracket to be prescribed; arrows on the teeth indicate the direction of translation. S is the code for a standard bracket. The number 1 means minimum translation bracket; 2, medium; 3, maximum; and 4, Class II maxillary molar bracket. For certain teeth, some sets use some of the same brackets as other sets; this helps keep the inventory of brackets small, yet adequate.

It is not necessary to memorize the subtype ranges, treatment plans, labels, bracket sets, and other details for each ICD because Figure 13.1 will direct you to illustrations providing that information. The following discussion, however, explains all aspects for each of the basic and alternate treatment possibilities for each subtype.

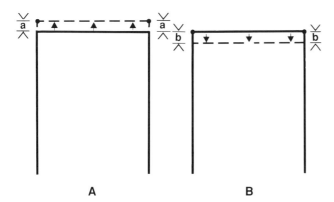

Fig. 13.6. Effects on the core-line length from changing the anteroposterior positions of incisor crowns. *Aa,* Add 2 mm to core line and core discrepancy for every millimeter that the incisor crowns are moved labially. *Bb,* Subtract 2 mm from core line and core discrepancy for every millimeter that the incisor crowns are moved lingually. Solid lines represent occlusal view of the arch core line. Dashed lines indicate proposed changes.

Type Spaced

The range of ICD for type Spaced is 0 through 14 mm. It is divided into three subtypes, each requiring a different set of brackets if treatment is to be without wire bends. The first subtype ranges from 0 to 4 mm (Fig. 13.7a); the next from 5 to 8 mm (Fig. 13.7b); and the final from 9 to 14 mm (Fig. 13.7c). The ICD for each quadrant is half that for the arch. The subtype ranges for each quadrant correspond with those for the three categories of translation brackets (minimum, medium, maximum). The treatment plans for the three subtypes differ only in how far the molars and second premolars must be mesially translated.

For each subtype range the appropriate brackets are matched to the distances the molars and second premolars must be translated mesially. Throughout type Spaced, the first premolars and canines will require only standard brackets (to review the explanation for this see Inventory in Chapter 10). The brackets that compose each set for the three Spaced subtypes are indicated in Figure 13.8. Each set is labeled for its type and treatment plan.

Subtype 0–4 mm (Fig. 13.7A)

Treatment plan, Spaced 0–4 mm. Advance molars and second premolars 0–2 mm per side (Fig. 13.8A).

Bracket set, Spaced 0–4 mm. Minimum translation brackets for molars and second premolars, and standard brackets for the first premolars and canines (Fig. 13.8A).

Subtype 5–8 mm (Fig. 13.7B)

Treatment plan, Spaced 5–8 mm. Advance molars and second premolars 2.5–4.0 mm per side (Fig. 13.8B).

Bracket set, Spaced 5–8 mm. Medium translation brackets for molars and second premolars, standard brackets for the first premolars and canines (Fig. 13.8B).

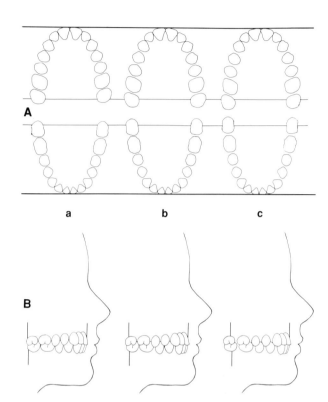

Fig. 13.7. Subtype examples for type Spaced: *A,* occlusal view; *B,* buccal view. Range of spacing for each: *a,* 0–4 mm; *b,* 5–8 mm; *c,* 9–14 mm. Lines indicate proposed A/P borders for arches.

Subtype 9–14 mm (Fig. 13.7C)

Treatment plan, Spaced 9–14 mm. Advance molars 4.5–7.0 mm per side (Fig. 13.8C).

Bracket set, Spaced 9–14 mm. Maximum translation brackets for molars and second premolars, standard brackets for first premolars and canines (Fig. 13.8C).

Type Classic

Type Classic indicates zero interim core discrepancy (Fig. 13.9). For this condition there is a basic and an alternate treatment plan (See Terminology on p. 244.)

Treatment plan, Classic. Type Classic indicates that even though the ICD is zero, some tooth repositioning is required, excluding any

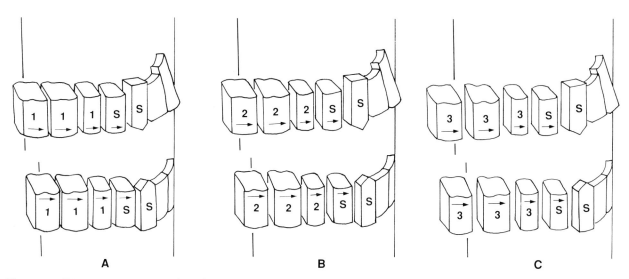

Fig. 13.8. Diagrammatic examples of spaced subtypes, with the direction of movement (*arrows*) and brackets (*numbers and letters*) most suitable for treating each: *A,* 0–4 mm; *B,* 5–8 mm; *C,* 9–14 mm. Lines indicate proposed A/P borders for arches.

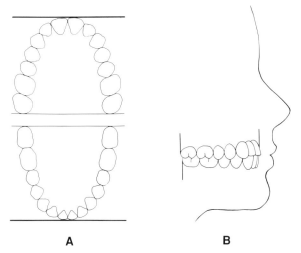

Fig. 13.9. Type Classic: *A,* occlusal view; *B,* buccal view. Lines indicate proposed A/P borders for arches.

mesial or distal movement. The needs may involve angulation, inclination, rotation, facial or lingual tipping, intrusion, or extrusion (Fig. 13.10).

Bracket set, Standard. The set for type Classic is composed entirely of standard brackets because the treatment plan does not call for translation of any teeth (Fig. 13.10).

When the anterior limit of the core line, the core form, and the positions of the teeth are all optimal, the condition is called Classic-Optimal. This label indicates that no treatment is needed.

Treatment plan, Classic-E4. The alternate treatment plan for type Classic calls for extraction of the first premolars (E4), and for the molars and second premolars to be translated mesially into the extraction sites (Fig. 13.11). This treatment plan is used for the mandibular arch when the mandibular posterior teeth are used to reciprocally retract protrusive maxillary anterior teeth after first premolar extraction in both arches. In this example the treatment plan for the maxillary arch is Crowded, 14 mm (explained later). For the maxillary arch the E4 plan would be used when the maxillary posterior teeth are used to reciprocally retract protrusive mandibular anterior teeth after first premolar extraction in both arches (usually when the mandible is to be surgically advanced). In this example the treatment plan for the mandibular arch is Crowded, 14 mm (explained later).

251

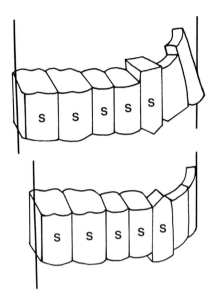

Fig. 13.10. Diagrammatic representation of type Classic and the brackets (*letters*) most suitable for the basic treatment plan. Lines indicate proposed A/P borders for arches.

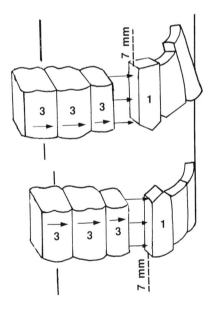

Fig. 13.11. Diagrammatic representation of type Classic, with the direction (*arrows*) and the amount (*mm*) of movement, and the brackets (*numbers*) most suitable for the alternate treatment plan. Lines indicate proposed A/P borders for arches.

Bracket set, Classic-E4. Maximum translation brackets are needed for molars and second premolars, and minimum brackets for canines (Fig. 13.11).

Type Crowded

Type Crowded spans a negative interim core discrepancy of from 0 through 14.0 mm. The range is divided into five subtypes (Fig. 13.12), each with its own basic treatment plan. The subtype boundaries, signaled by the need for a change in brackets to avoid wire bending, do not occur at conveniently equal spans of ICD as they do for type Spaced (Fig. 13.7). The ICD for the first crowded subtype is 0–6 mm (Fig. 13.12a); the second, 7–8 mm (Fig. 13.12b); the third, 9–10 mm (Fig. 13.12c); the fourth, 11–13 mm (Fig. 13.12d); and the fifth, 14.0 mm (Fig. 13.12e). These ranges, when halved, represent the ICD for each quadrant. In addition to its basic treatment plan, subtype 0–6 mm has an alternate plan, and subtype 14 mm has an alternate plan for only the maxillary arch. For type Crowded this makes a total of six treatment plans for the mandibular arch and seven for the maxillary arch.

Subtype 0–6 mm (Fig. 13.12a)

Treatment plan, Crowded 0–6 mm. The basic treatment plan for this range calls for the molars and possibly the premolars and canines to be tipped distally enough to neutralize the amount of the ICD (Fig. 13.13).

Bracket set, Standard. As explained in the Inventory section of Chapter 10, molars and second premolars do not need distal translation brackets; Chapter 9 explains that standard brackets are to be used for all tooth movements other than translation (Fig. 13.13).

Treatment plan, Crowded-E5. The alternate treatment plan is for precisely 6 mm of ICD. The plan is to extract the second premolars (E5) and translate the molars mesially 3 mm. Reciprocally, the first premolars and canines are translated distally 3 mm. The treatment plan is labeled Crowded-E5 (Fig. 13.14).

Bracket set, Crowded-E5. The set comprises medium translation brackets for all posterior teeth (Fig. 13.14).

* * *

First premolar extractions are required when the ICD is 7.0 mm or more, which is the condition for the treatment plans for the four remaining Crowded subtypes. Each calls for the canines to be moved distally one-half the total amount of ICD. Except when the canines are fully retracted, the posterior teeth are translated mesially into the remaining space.

Subtype 7–8 mm (Fig. 13.12b)

Treatment plan, Crowded 7–8 mm. Extract first premolars and retract canines 3.5–4 mm; advance molars and second premolars 3–3.5 mm (Fig. 13.15).

Bracket set, Crowded 7–8 mm. The set comprises medium translation brackets for all posterior teeth (Fig. 13.15).

Subtype 9–10 mm (Fig. 13.12c)

Treatment plan, Crowded 9–10 mm. Extract first premolars and retract canines 4.5–5 mm; advance molars and second premolars 2–2.5 mm (Fig. 13.16).

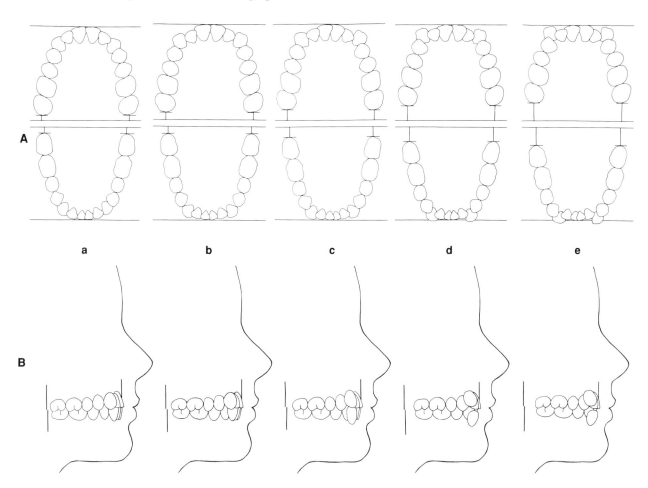

Fig. 13.12. Subtype examples for type Crowded: *A*, occlusal view; *B*, buccal view. Range of crowding for each: *a*, 0–6 mm; *b*, 7–8 mm; *c*, 9–10 mm; *d*, 11–13 mm; *e*, 14 mm. Long lines indicate optimal A/P core lines. Distance between posterior borders and posterior molars indicates core discrepancy.

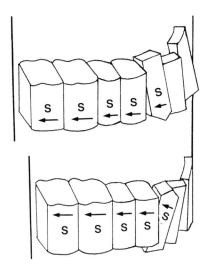

Fig. 13.13. Diagrammatic example for type Crowded 0–6 mm, with the direction of movement (*arrows*) and brackets (*letters*) most suitable for the basic treatment plan. Lines indicate proposed A/P borders for arches.

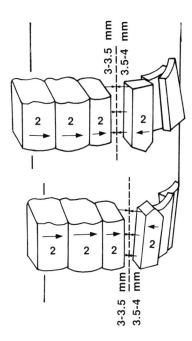

Fig. 13.15. Diagrammatic example for type Crowded 7–8 mm, with the direction (*arrows*) and the amount (*mm*) of movement, and the brackets (*numbers*) most suitable for the basic treatment plan. Lines indicate proposed A/P borders for arches.

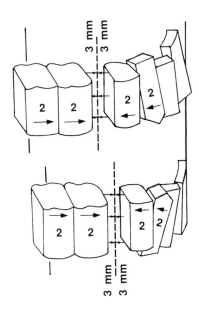

Fig. 13.14. Diagrammatic example for type Crowded 6 mm, with the direction (*arrows*) and the amount (*mm*) of movement, and the brackets (*numbers*) most suitable for the alternate treatment plan. Lines indicate proposed A/P borders for arches.

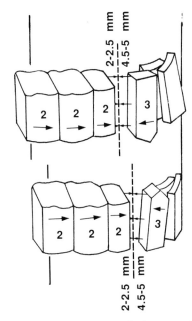

Fig. 13.16. Diagrammatic example for type Crowded 9–10 mm, with the direction (*arrows*) and the amount (*mm*) of movement, and the brackets (*numbers*) most suitable for the basic treatment plan. Lines indicate proposed A/P borders for arches.

Bracket set, Crowded 9–10 mm. The set comprises maximum translation brackets for canines, and medium for molars and second premolars (Fig. 13.16).

Subtype 11–13 mm (Fig. 13.12d)

Treatment plan, Crowded 11–13 mm. Extract first premolars and retract canines 5.5–6.5 mm; advance molars and second premolars 0.5–1.5 mm (Fig. 13.17).

Bracket set, Crowded 11–13 mm. The set comprises maximum translation brackets for the canines, and minimum for molars and second premolars (Fig. 13.17).

Subtype 14 mm (Fig. 13.12e)

Treatment plan, Crowded 14 mm. Extract first premolars and retract canines 7 mm (Fig. 13.18).

Bracket set, Crowded 14 mm. The set comprises maximum translation brackets for the canines, minimum for second premolars, and standard brackets for molars (Fig. 13.18).

Treatment plan, Crowded 14 mm Class II. The alternate treatment plan for subtype 14 mm is an alternative for the maxillary arch only. It is employed when a Class II molar relationship is left that way while treating the rest of the dentition to Class I (see Posterior Brackets in Chapter 9). The plan calls for first premolar extractions and for retracting the canines 7 mm (Fig. 13.19).

Bracket set, Crowded 14 mm Class II. The set is composed of maximum translation brackets for the canines, minimum for the second premolars, and Class II brackets for the molars (Fig. 13.19).

Set Inventory

When bands are used for posterior teeth it is economical for standard brackets to be

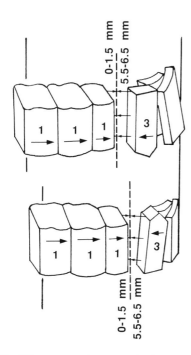

Fig. 13.17. Diagrammatic example for type Crowded 11–13 mm, with the direction (*arrows*) and the amount (*mm*) of movement, and the brackets (*numbers*) most suitable for the basic treatment plan. Lines indicate proposed A/P borders for arches.

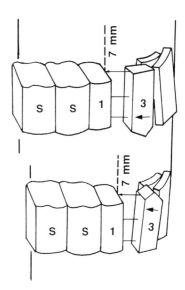

Fig. 13.18. Diagrammatic example for type Crowded 14 mm, with the direction (*arrows*) and the amount (*mm*) of movement, and the brackets (*numbers and letters*) most suitable for the basic treatment plan. Lines indicate proposed A/P borders for arches.

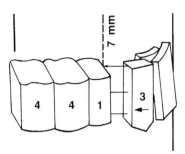

Fig. 13.19. Diagrammatic example for type Crowded 14 mm (maxillary arch), with the direction (*arrows*) and the amount (*mm*) of movement, and the brackets (*numbers*) most suitable for the alternate treatment plan. Lines indicate proposed A/P borders for arches.

prewelded to them, because such a high percentage of patients use standard brackets. However, this approach may not be economical for translation brackets. For the supply of translation bracket sets to be adequate and the cost minimal, the sets and blank bands should be purchased separately and welded only after the bands have been fitted. Inventory is not a problem when bonding is used.

For abnormal arches or teeth whose centers of rotation are not bilaterally symmetrical, sets can be broken and then prescribed by the quadrant, or brackets can be assigned individually. Given sufficient demand, manufacturers will surely provide sets for treatment plans not covered in this chapter.

Chapter 14

Implementing the Six Keys

Dental casts alone do not provide enough data for evaluating all aspects of orthodontic treatment. Other data, such as headfilms and photographs, are needed to judge such matters as interjaw relationship and how the jaws and teeth relate to the face. But the research leading to the Six Keys has upgraded orthodontists' ability to appraise occlusion either intraorally or with dental casts.

The measurement study (Chapter 4) yielded specific, quantitative data about crown positions and the depth of the curve of Spee, making it possible to assess results objectively. The Six Key approach uses facial grooves or ridges, and the gingiva and cusp tip (or incisal edge) as landmarks to locate the FACC and FA point. These landmarks hold several advantages—primarily tangibility—over traditional landmarks and referents. Finally, evaluation based on the Six Keys is more complete than other methods because it recognizes that premolars, canines, and lateral incisors are as important as molars and central incisors, and because it objectifies the positions and patterns required by teeth for optimal occlusion.

A clinician familiar with the Six Keys can immediately recognize whether optimal occlusion has been attained. But to implement the keys, an orthodontist must understand not only the definition of each key but also the role each tooth plays in static and functional occlusion, the effect of tooth and jaw position on arch lines, and the strategies most suitable for implementing the Six Keys and correcting arch lines. These matters are discussed key by key in the following sections.

Implementing Key I (Interarch Relationships)

Key I includes all the teeth. As it applies to the maxillary first molar, Key I has three parts (Fig. 3.15), not just the one advocated by Angle. This is evidenced by posttreatment dental casts that demonstrate suboptimal occlusion even though the alignment in each arch appears satisfactory and the mesiobuccal cusp of the maxillary first molar articulates in the mesiobuccal groove of the mandibular first molar (Fig. 5.1). Hundreds of other such examples can be observed in the treatment results from the mid-1960s and mid-1970s (Chapter 5), and to a slightly lesser extent in the mid-1980s treatment results shown in this chapter.

Concerning premolars, Key I requires that their maxillary buccal cusps occlude in the embrasures of their mandibular antagonists, and that the lingual cusps articulate with the distal fossae of the mandibular premolars (Fig. 3.15). It should be noted that the tips of the lingual cusps of maxillary premolars are mesial to the tips of their buccal cusps (Fig. 14.1). This relationship may not be generally known; in fact, some gnathologists perceive the lingual cusps to be directly lingual to the buccal cusps, and therefore advocate a slight Class II interarch relationship of the buccal segments to achieve the desired lingual cusp-fossa occlusion (Fig. 14.2) [25]. Such a relationship with natural teeth would require altering the occlusal anatomy of some posterior teeth and incisors for function and stability. The posterior teeth would require reshaping to avoid cusp collisions in lateral excursions, and the incisors would require greater faciolingual dimension to avoid excess overbite resulting from the excess overjet this interarch condition would cause.

The maxillary canine must occlude in the embrasure between the mandibular canine and first premolar, and its cusp tip must be slightly mesial to the embrasure (Fig. 3.15).

The maxillary incisors must overlap the mandibular incisors approximately 1–2 mm (Fig. 3.15) (clinically they appear to touch but shouldn't), and the midlines of both arches should match.

To set the stage for Key I premolar occlusion, the distal marginal ridge of the maxillary first molar must occlude with the mesial marginal ridge of the mandibular second molar (Fig. 3.15 and Fig. 14.3D). The absence of this condition can adversely affect occlusion elsewhere. As shown progressively in Figure 14.3A–D, the improvement in the Class II premolar interarch relationship is commensurate with the improvement in the proximation of the molar marginal ridges. Although the molar marginal-ridge condition pertains to occlusal surfaces, it can, like the other keys, be evaluated from the facial aspect of the crowns.

When the cusp-groove relationship of first molars is correct, but marginal-ridge contact with the mandibular second molar does not occur, the angulation of the maxillary first molar's crown is probably negative or insufficiently positive. This causes the mesiogingival

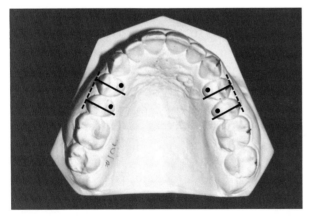

Fig. 14.1. Lingual cusps (*dots*) of correctly positioned maxillary premolars are mesial to the crown's midsagittal planes (*solid lines*).

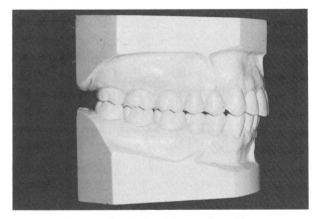

Fig. 14.2. Interarch relationships preferred by some noted gnathologists. Study casts courtesy of P. K. Thomas.

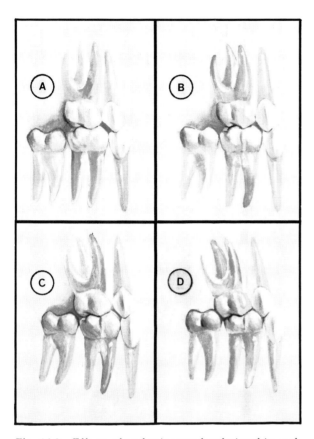

Fig. 14.3. Effects of molar interarch relationship and occlusion on premolar interarch relationship and occlusion: molars in *A, B,* and *C* satisfy the cusp-groove criterion for Key I, but only *D* also fulfills the marginal-ridge and premolar criteria.

portion of the maxillary first molar to occupy some of the space designated for the second premolar (Fig. 14.3A–C). Such a condition prohibits correct occlusion of some or all crowns that are mesial or distal to it. This condition may cause a chain reaction of errant teeth, poor aesthetics, and incorrect arch lines.

A deficient distal marginal-ridge occlusion of the maxillary first molar that is otherwise Class I can result from a variety of factors, such as the abandonment of the molars that have been tipped distally (Fig. 14.4B). Post-treatment settling cannot be relied on to correct this positional deficiency (Fig. 14.4C); the problem must be resolved by correcting the final molar angulation before completing treatment.

Headgear can promote tipping rather than translation of maxillary molars (Fig. 14.5). This problem can be reduced in part by prescribing brackets with the face-bow tube gingival to the archwire slot. In addition, the orthodontist can—with high-pull headgear, angulated slots, and wire bends—redirect the extraoral force closer to the tooth's center of resistance to encourage translation rather than tipping.

The third aspect of the molar portion of Key I involves seating the mesiolingual cusps of the maxillary molars in the central fossae of the mandibular molars (Fig. 3.15Bd, Ce). This requires the maxillary molars' mesiolingual

Fig. 14.4. Maxillary molars that are incorrectly angulated at the conclusion of active treatment do not always settle into the Key I position. *A,* Pretreatment casts; *B,* posttreatment casts with negative molar angulation; *C,* postretention casts, showing maxillary molars still with negative angulation. Lines indicate FACC.

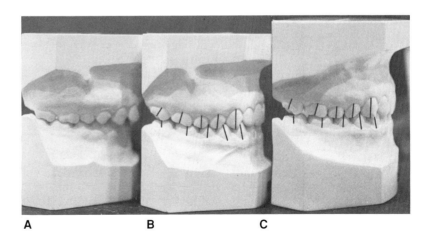

A   B   C

cusps to be more occlusally prominent than their buccal cusps. However, excessive prominence must be avoided to prevent bite opening, functional interferences (Fig. 14.6), bruxism, temporomandibular joint problems, and—over the long term—gingival deterioration (Fig. 14.7).

Cusps of teeth that encroach in the freeway space will generally not correct themselves, and must be dealt with by orthodontic treatment, equilibration, reconstruction, or surgery. Completing active treatment with molars

slightly intruded is preferable to extrusion, because self-correction usually will occur after natural settling if the molar position and interarch relationship are otherwise correct. A concave curve installed in a maxillary rectangular archwire, or a convex curve installed in a mandibular rectangular archwire will deal with occlusogingival tooth displacement, but such wire forming also alters the inclination of the wire's surfaces throughout (Figs. 12.24, 12.26). This side effect will positively incline all teeth. For molars it will cause excessive occlusal prominence of the lingual cusps. To deal with this side effect when unwanted, the curve in the wire should be maintained, but the inclination of the wire should be altered (Figs. 12.25, 12.27).

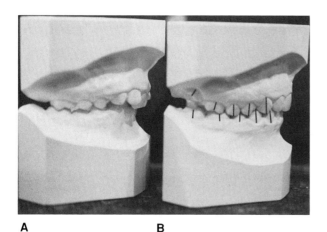

A   **B**

Fig. 14.5. Distally directed forces can cause molars to tip rather than translate distally: *A,* pretreatment casts with mesially tipped molars; *B,* posttreatment casts with distally tipped molars. Lines indicate FACC.

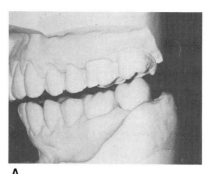

A

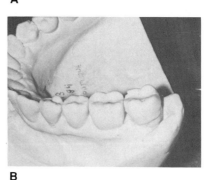

B

Fig. 14.7. Long-term effects of incorrect molar inclination: deterioration of the distal gingiva of mandibular second molar coincidental with working interferences resulting from excessive prominence of the mesiolingual cusp of the maxillary second molar. *A,* Molar cusps collide during working excursion. *B,* Periodontal deterioration around affected tooth.

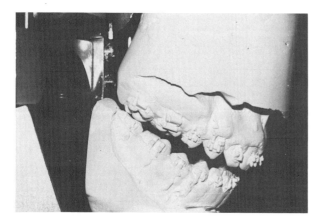

Fig. 14.6. Casts showing a maxillary second molar whose mesiolingual cusp is too occlusally prominent.

Incomplete correction of interarch relationship of the molars can result in incorrect interarch relationship of the premolars, canines, and incisors (Fig. 14.8).

As explained in Chapter 9, a limited exception to the molar portion of Key I is permissible when the treatment plan calls for the molars to be treated to a Class II relationship while treating the rest of the dentition to Class I, for example, after premolar extraction in the maxillary arch only.

The Key I standards for molars are not recommended for mixed dentitions, but they may be applied to all permanent dentitions, even in patients who are not physically mature. The Key I criteria are consistent with Björk's findings about how jaw growth affects interarch relationship of the permanent teeth:

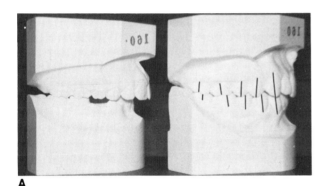

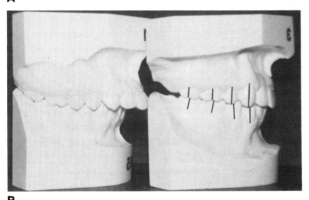

Fig. 14.8. Incomplete correction of molar interarch relationship may cause incorrect premolar, canine, and incisor interarch relationships. Pretreatment and posttreatment casts of nonextraction (A) and extraction (B) treatment. Lines indicate FACC.

"During the growth and development of the face, compensatory changes in the path of eruption of the teeth occur which tend to even out positional changes between the jaws" [10].

For some situations, Tweed advocated leaving molar crowns in excessive negative angulation and out of occlusion, relying on development and settling to establish full occlusal contact [27]. However, posttreatment dental casts demonstrate that development and settling do not always occur as hoped (Fig. 14.4).

Maxillary second molars normally emerge with negative crown angulation. As they further erupt, directed by the rounded distal surfaces of maxillary first molars, the second molars become partially upright and at the same time encourage the seating of the distal marginal ridges of the first molars. The same eruption pattern occurs later between the maxillary third and second molars. However, the effect of third-molar eruption on the second molars is lost once the maxillary first molars are moved mesially or distally, and when third molars are prematurely removed. Orthodontists are often criticized for failing to incorporate second molars into their treatment plans. These teeth, when routinely left unattended, can cause functional interferences that may induce bruxism, temporomandibular joint problems, and gingival recession (Figs. 14.6, 14.7).

Implementing Key II (Crown Angulation)

Key II states that the angulation of the facial axis of every clinical crown (FACC) should be positive. The extent of angulation varies according to tooth type. It is important to realize that the FACC is not parallel to the long axis of the crown or tooth, or to the mesial or distal surfaces of the crowns. For example, the average angulation of an optimally positioned maxillary molar, measured from the FACC to a line 90° to the occlusal plane, is 5°, but the long axis of the crown is more upright. For the same molar, the average FACC inclination is –9°, whereas the inclination of the long axis of the crown is positive [12,13,29] (Fig. 14.9).

The location of contact points, relative to other identifiable morphological features, is fairly consistent for each tooth type; therefore, from patient to patient, the optimal angulation of each tooth type must be equally consistent [29]. Landmarks traditionally used for judging tooth angulation and bracket angulation are inadequate for these purposes (Chapter 7). Contact points cannot be directly observed, nor can the long axis of the crown or tooth. Other landmarks, such as incisal edges, are tangible but have only limited value for banding, and less for bracketing. For bracketing, the incisal edge is simply too far from the bracket to serve as an effective guide for bracket placement for angulation. In the past we used to "band" rather than "bracket," and the band's edge was much closer to the incisal edge. Using the FACC is easier and more accurate because this landmark is visible, tangible, and close to the bracket.

An optimal maxillary core line is longer than its mandibular counterpart because the sum of the mesiodistal diameters of the maxillary crowns is greater. However, the crowns must be optimally angled. The sum of the average angulations of maxillary teeth for the optimal sample (excluding third molars) is 78° (Fig. 14.10). For the mandibular teeth, the combined angulations total 34° (Fig. 14.11).

Orthodontic treatment cannot cause teeth to be larger or smaller, but it can angulate them to occupy the space dictated by their mesiodistal diameters measured at the contact points (Figs. 12.17, 12.18).

In the study of optimal occlusions, the angulation pattern for maxillary crowns was found to differ from that for mandibular crowns. As discussed in Chapter 4, the angulation of the maxillary central incisors, lateral incisors, and canines is 5°, 9°, and 11°, respectively. The premolars are the most upright maxillary teeth, with an angulation of 2°.

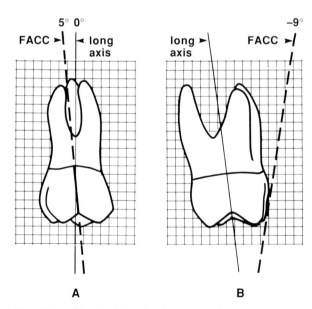

Fig. 14.9. The facial axis of a crown does not parallel the long axis of the crown or tooth. *A,* Facial view; *B,* distal view.

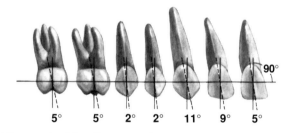

Fig. 14.10. Maxillary angulation patterns and average angulations in the optimal sample.

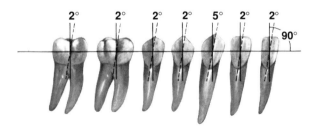

Fig. 14.11. Mandibular angulation patterns and average angulations in the optimal sample.

The maxillary molars are angulated 5° (Fig. 14.10).

In the mandibular crowns, the angulation pattern is a very subtle 2°, except for the canines, where it is 5° (Fig. 14.11).

To achieve optimal results, it may be necessary to overcorrect before completing treatment. For example, when translation is required, it is advisable to exaggerate angulation in anticipation of the rebound that will ultimately bring about the correct position.

Open extraction sites were frequently present in the sample of posttreatment dental casts (Chapters 1 and 5). This problem can perhaps be avoided by completely closing the space and overcorrecting the angulation of teeth requiring translation before completing treatment. Rebound then would be toward the space, rather than away from it. Such a procedure puts rebound to good use. Fortunately, overangulation of canines, premolars, and molars does not affect the space occupied by these teeth. The posterior teeth are different from maxillary incisors in this matter because of the oval shape of their mesial and distal surfaces. The posterior teeth are shaped like segments of a circle, whereas the maxillary incisors resemble the sides of a trapezoid (Fig. 12.16).

The study of posttreatment dental casts (Chapter 5) revealed that the maxillary lateral incisors and canines were, when compared to the optimal sample (Chapters 2 and 4), incorrectly angulated more often than any other teeth. In the case of the lateral incisors, one reason may be their unique shape. Furthermore, not all orthodontists agree on how much the crown should be angulated, or on the landmark from which angulation should be measured. In the past, brackets were precisely located on bands, then the band rims were oriented with tooth landmarks. This method used the band as a referent for locating the bracket. This proved a special problem for maxillary lateral incisors because of the comparative difficulty of accurately placing a band on these asymmetrical teeth. Other explanations for incorrect posttreatment angulation of the maxillary lateral incisors may include the side effects of wire bending and wire forming explained in Chapter 12 and illustrated in Figures 12.22–12.27. Figure 14.12 is an example of a posttreatment dentition in which the lateral incisor is negatively angulated, causing interdental space and compromised aesthetics.

Optimal canine and premolar angulation, especially when first premolars are extracted, is often not fully achieved (Fig. 14.13). Incorrect angulation does not affect the space that these crowns occupy, but it may affect stability, and will affect gingival health, occlusion, and aesthetics.

Most orthodontists do not angulate the maxillary canine as much as 11°. Doing so generally requires more effort than is required for leaving the crown upright, regardless of the appliance used. When the treatment goal includes functional occlusion, the merit of correct canine angulation becomes evident. The canine-rise concept of occlusion demands that only the incisors and canines on the working side meet in lateral excursions (Fig. 14.14).

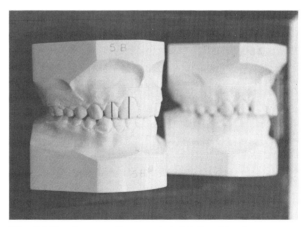

Fig. 14.12. Incorrectly angulated lateral incisor causes interdental space and compromised aesthetics. Lines indicate FACC.

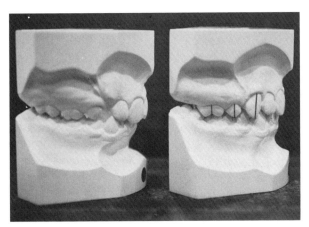

Fig. 14.13. Incorrect maxillary canine and premolar angulation. Lines indicate FACC.

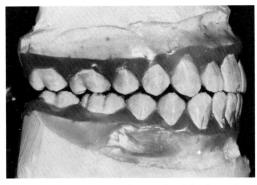

Fig. 14.14. Correct occlusion in right-lateral excursion: on the working side only canines and incisors should touch.

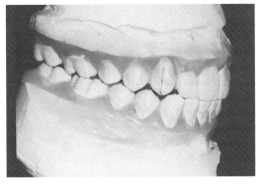

Fig. 14.15. Incorrect occlusion in right-lateral excursion: an upright maxillary canine fails to disclude the posterior teeth.

An upright maxillary canine, on the working side, will not disclude the premolars and molars in lateral excursions, because its cusp will pass through the embrasure between the mandibular canine and premolar (Fig. 14.15). Generally, this will put the burden of ripping and tearing on the incisors, which individually do not have enough root volume to handle this task as well as the canines.

In the protrusive excursion, the distal incline of the maxillary canine should ride on the mesial incline of the mandibular first premolar's buccal cusp, causing disclusion of the posterior teeth. It will do this in cooperation with the incisors if the canine is correctly angulated (Fig. 14.16). If the mandibular first premolar is extracted, the maxillary canine will articulate in the same way with the mandibular second premolar.

Maxillary and mandibular premolars require only 2° of angulation to allow the opposing teeth's buccal cusps to travel unscathed between their cusps during lateral working excursions (Fig. 14.17A). Premolars function best when their occlusion starts with a cusp-embrasure relationship of the buccal cusps (Fig. 3.15Ac), and a cusp-fossae relationship of the lingual cusps (Fig. 3.15Cf).

Maxillary first molars must be angulated 5° to position their distal marginal ridges for proper occlusion with the mesial marginal ridges of the mandibular second molars. This 5° angulation also positions the occlusal aspects of the maxillary molars' buccal cusps to parallel those of the mandibular molars, thus preventing interference during working excursions (Fig. 14.17B). Mandibular molar angulation is 2°.

Implementing Key III (Crown Inclination)

Crown inclination in the optimal sample followed a distinctive pattern for the maxillary arch. The incisors were generally positively inclined; the posterior crowns were always negatively inclined. As described in the measurement study in Chapter 4, the maxillary central incisors averaged 7° of inclination; the lateral incisors, 3°; the canines and premolars, –7°; and the molars, –9° (Fig. 14.18).

The inclination of the mandibular crowns also followed a consistent pattern. The incisors were generally negatively inclined, but not al-

ways. The canines and premolars were always negatively inclined, increasingly from the canines through the molars. The inclination portion of the measurement study in Chapter 4 provided the following averages for each tooth type: incisors –1°, canines –11°, first premolars –17°, second premolars –22°, first molars –30°, second molars –35° (Fig. 14.19).

Inclination of the posterior crowns has, in the past, been given less consideration than inclination of the incisors. This situation prevailed partly because the posterior crowns' in-

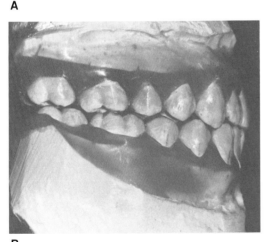

Fig. 14.16. Correct occlusion in protrusive excursion. The maxillary incisors should touch the mandibular incisors; the maxillary canine should touch the mandibular premolar. *A*, Disocclusion of maxillary premolars and mandibular second premolar when viewed facial to the canine and mandibular first premolar; *B*, molar disocclusion when viewed directly facial to the molars.

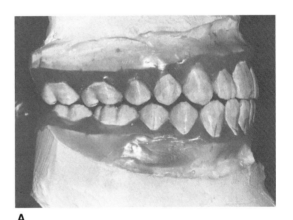

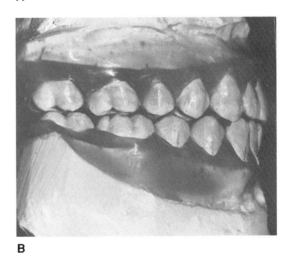

Fig. 14.17. Right-lateral excursion showing that correct crown angulations promote optimal disocclusion: *A*, premolar crown angulation of 2° prevents collision of cusps on the working side; *B*, maxillary molars' angulation must be 5°, and mandibular molars', 2°.

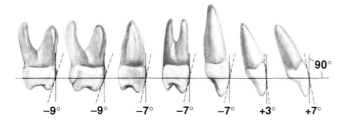

Fig. 14.18. Maxillary inclination patterns and average inclinations found in the optimal sample.

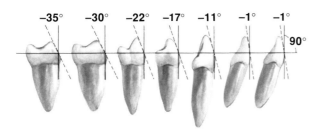

Fig. 14.19. Mandibular crown inclination patterns and average inclinations found in the optimal sample.

clination cannot be as readily measured cephalometrically. If mounting casts on articulators had been routine, perhaps the importance of posterior crown inclination would have been apparent sooner. Additionally, the literature contained no information about inclination that could be translated to the bracket slot until the measurement study described in Chapter 4 was first reported [2,5]. Earlier studies had dealt with the long axis of the crown or tooth [12,13]; however, these axes do not indicate how much a wire should be inclined for a nonprogrammed bracket, because the slot of that bracket represents the inclination of the face of the crown, not the inclination of the long axis of the tooth.

Optimal occlusion, both static and functional, requires that all crowns, not just incisors, be properly inclined. Maxillary molars must be inclined so that their lingual cusps will be more occlusally prominent than their buccal cusps. The objective is to position the tooth so that these lingual cusps are occlusally prominent enough to seat in the central fossae of the mandibular molars, but not so prominent as to encroach on the freeway space, where they would open the bite or interfere during function. Conversely, mandibular molars are to be positioned so their lingual cusps are less prominent occlusally than the buccal cusps. The occlusal prominence of molar cusps will be correct when the FACC of each crown is properly inclined.

One clinical advantage of using the FACC for planning and implementing treatment is that it is tangible; therefore crown inclination and intercrown angles can be seen and directly related to the occlusal plane. The long axis of a tooth, however, is intangible and—except for central incisors—it cannot be determined accurately, even with radiographs. Figure 14.20 illustrates the interincisal crown angle and the interincisal tooth angle. The average interincisal crown angle, in the optimal sample, was 174° (6° shy of a straight line); the

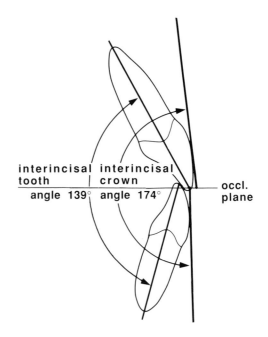

Fig. 14.20. Interincisal crown angle and interincisal tooth angle.

average interincisal tooth angle was 139°. In cephalometric analysis the long axes of the central incisors are generally used for measuring their inclination; however, for bracket selection the inclination of the incisors' facial axes, relative to the occlusal plane, is the more important measurement (Chapter 9).

Cephalometrically, the inclination of the FACC of a central incisor is not as discernible as the incisor's long axis. Therefore the average angular difference between the FACC and the long axis of an incisor is helpful information for wire bending and wire forming or bracket selection. An unpublished study (L. F. Andrews, 1968) of 100 cephalograms indicated an average difference of 18° between the inclination of the FACC and the long axis of the maxillary central incisor; for the mandibular central incisor the average difference was 16° (Fig. 9.14).

An interincisal tooth angle of 139° requires an interincisal crown angle of 174° (Fig. 14.20). The combined inclination of the crowns for the maxillary and mandibular centrals must be 6° from a line 90° to the occlusal plane. For example, for harmonious interjaw relationships, the maxillary central incisor should be at 7°, the mandibular incisor at –1° (Fig. 14.21).

As explained in Chapter 12, incisor inclination can affect perimeter length. Perimeter length has a direct correlation with interarch relationship (Fig. 12.15). Assuming optimal angulation of all maxillary teeth, the maxillary perimeter length will be short if the maxillary incisors are negatively inclined (Fig. 12.7Ac). This will lead to a Class II tendency in the interarch relationship (Fig. 12.10Aa). If the maxillary incisors are optimally inclined at 7° (Fig. 12.7Ab) the maxillary perimeter length and interarch relationship can be optimal (Fig. 12.10Ab).

Implementing Key IV (Rotations)

One way of saying that rotations do not exist in a given arch is to say that the crowns

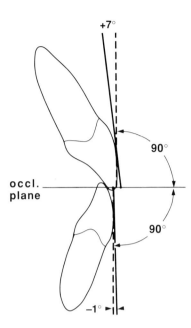

Fig. 14.21. Optimal maxillary and mandibular incisor crown inclination.

meet at their contact points. If they do not meet there, and their angulation is correct, they are rotated. As reported in Chapter 12, molars and premolars occupy more space when they are rotated. Figure 14.22 illustrates a rotated maxillary molar and its adverse affect not only on its own occlusion but also on the occlusion and position of all the other teeth.

Moderately rotated canines do not always occupy more (or less) space, because they are conical; however, aesthetics and occlusion can be affected. Rotated incisors generally occupy less space than those correctly aligned. With rotated mandibular incisors, a collapse of both arches can result from a breakdown of the gothic arch system. Rotated mandibular incisors usually stray from the core line, overlap, tip lingually, and extrude. Rotated teeth usually cause a chain reaction that affects the arch lines and one or more other keys.

Routinely including permanent second molars in treatment ensures that their optimal

267

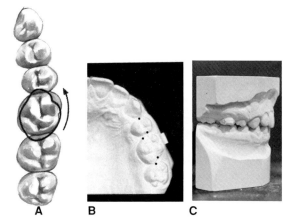

Fig. 14.22. Maxillary molars occupy excessive space when rotated: *A,* illustrated example; *B,* clinical example; *C,* effect on occlusion.

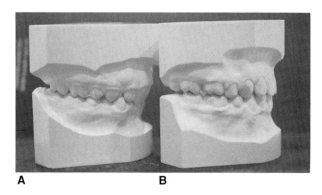

Fig. 14.23. Posttreatment rotations: molars that are not rotated at the beginning of treatment (*A*) often are rotated after treatment (*B*).

positioning is not left to chance. At the same time, second molars provide the needed buttress from which to control the permanent first molars. If the Six Keys and canine-rise functional occlusion are treatment goals, then it is almost always necessary to treat all teeth.

Naturally rotated teeth are usually dealt with early in treatment. Small-diameter wires are deflected, when engaged in the bracket, to the extent of the rotation for each individual tooth. Rotation springs and other devices are used when the wire is too stiff to flex.

Often, teeth requiring translation are found to be rotated at the conclusion of treatment, even though they may not have been rotated when treatment began (Fig. 14.23). It took years of inspecting examples of extraction treatment (Chapter 5) to find one posttreatment dental cast without one or more of the translated teeth rotated. Because a force cannot be applied directly to a tooth's center of resistance, tooth translation requires force to be applied there indirectly. Without a fully programmed appliance, such force is difficult to regulate. To ensure an ultimately correct position for a translated tooth, treatment must include overrotation to compensate for posttreatment rebound. The amount of overrotation should be proportional to the distance the

tooth is translated. Overcorrecting translated teeth without a fully programmed appliance requires springs or wire bends.

Implementing Key V (Tight Contacts)

Except for teeth with mesiodistal size discrepancy, adjacent teeth should touch at their contact points. Posttreatment spaces signify incomplete treatment, crown-size discrepancy, or treatment limitation. In most instances, the teeth in each dental arch can be positioned to satisfy Key V.

Orthodontists differ in the ways they handle discrepancies in mesiodistal crown diameter. Crowns that are abnormally large are no problem: they can be made narrower. The question is, What should be done with space from an occasional crown that is abnormally small? Some clinicians elect to close such spaces even though the occlusion will be compromised; other clinicians consider interdental spacing healthier than an occlusion that has been compromised just to achieve tight contacts. Generally, enlarging small crowns (with composites, or jacketing) is the best solution to the problem.

268

It was estimated that most interdental space in the treated sample resulted not from tooth size discrepancy, but from incomplete treatment—for example, insufficient maxillary incisor angulation (Fig. 5.8A); incorrect incisor inclination (Fig. 5.8B); or incorrect mesiodistal tooth position (Fig. 5.8C).

Implementing Key VI (Curve of Spee)

The occlusogingival form of the arch is one determinant of length of the midsagittal line. Leveling the curve of Spee will increase its length unless, for example, it is leveled within its existing boundaries. As explained in Chapter 12 and illustrated in Figure 12.23, leveling the curve of Spee may increase the midsagittal and perimeter lines, but not the core line. Treating to a level core line and curve of Spee is a form of overcorrection. Such treatment bares a slightly excessive amount of the occlusal surface of every mandibular crown, allowing ample room for the maxillary teeth to fully interface (Fig. 14.24B). A concave core line bares a less-than-optimal amount of the mandibular occlusal surfaces to the maxillary teeth (Fig. 14.24A). A mandibular core line that is slightly more concave than optimal may be an appropriate treatment goal if the maxillary core line is slightly short because the mesiodistal diameters of several teeth are slightly to moderately small. A convex mandibular core line bares excessive amounts of the occlusal surfaces (Fig. 14.24C). For individuals with normal teeth, however, a core line deeper than a 2.5-mm concave curve precludes attaining the Six Keys (Fig. 14.25).

In casts with optimal occlusion, the core line was never deeper than 2.5 mm (Chapter 4); but it was often deeper than that in the posttreatment sample (Chapter 5 and Fig. 14.25). If deep core lines are resolved with archwires, the side effects of wire forming can sometimes be put to good use. In other instances, they must be compensated for (Figs. 12.22–12.27).

Summary and Treatment Sample

Figures 14.26–14.235 are photographs of 210 pretreatment and posttreatment casts with grading forms. They constitute the 15 sets of casts used by 14 orthodontists to attain their diplomate status sometime in the mid-1980s. The orthodontists photographed their own

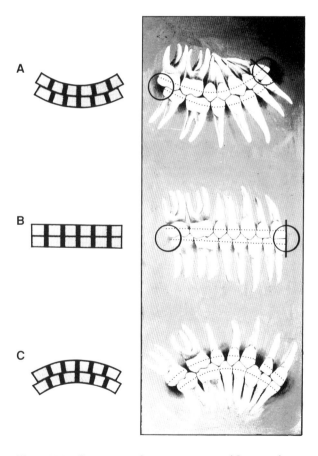

Fig. 14.24. Concave and convex curves of Spee and core lines. *A,* An excessively concave curve of Spee and mandibular core line restrict the occlusal surfaces available for maxillary teeth. *B,* A flat to slightly concave curve of Spee and mandibular core line bare the proper occlusal surfaces for optimal occlusion. *C,* A convex curve of Spee and mandibular core line bare excessive portions of the occlusal surfaces.

269

casts and agreed to have them shown anonymously in this book for whatever can be learned from them—as a benefit to other orthodontists.

By the mid-1980s the Six Key goals had been around long enough to be adopted, and the treatment results indicate that they had been adopted by some. Which results were appliance-aided cannot be surmised visually. Most patients were treated with a nonprogrammed appliance, some with a partly programmed appliance, and a few with a fully programmed appliance.

Earlier, readers were encouraged to ob-serve the casts and critique the grading of posttreatment results from the mid-1960s and mid-1970s. At that point in the book (Chapter 5) only the Six Keys had been introduced. Now that additional guidelines and information about arch lines and treatment strategies have been presented, the student should be prepared not only to judge and grade the treatment results from the 1980s but also to understand what should and could have been done if the results are incomplete.

The chance for reader involvement in grading these 210 examples may be the best summary this chapter and this book can offer.

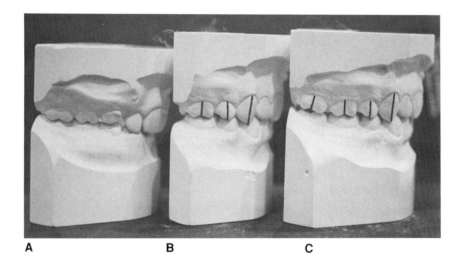

Fig. 14.25. Curves of Spee and core lines deeper than 2.5 mm generally preclude attaining Six Key occlusion: *A,* pretreatment casts; *B,* posttreatment casts; *C,* postretention casts. Lines on teeth indicate FACC.

A   B   C

ORTHODONTIST #1

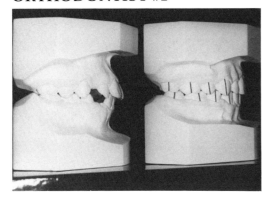
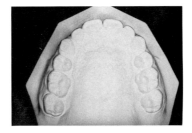
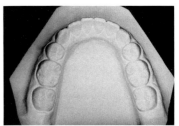

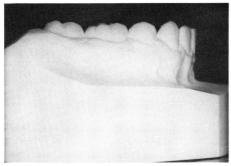

Fig. 14.26

Ortho 1   Patient 1   NE____   E____

Key	Grade	Key	Grade
I		IV	
II		V	
III		VI	

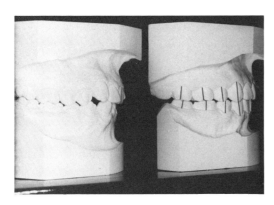
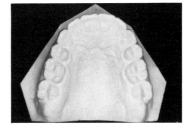
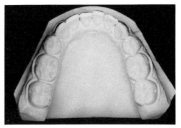

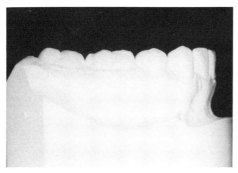

Fig. 14.27

Ortho 1   Patient 2   NE____   E____

Key	Grade	Key	Grade
I		IV	
II		V	
III		VI	

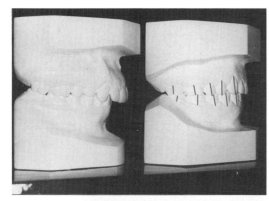
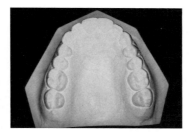
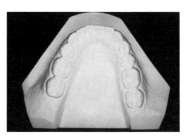
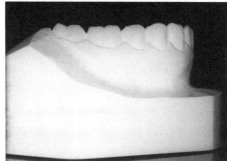

Fig. 14.28

Ortho___1___   Patient___3___   NE_____   E_____

Key		Grade	Key		Grade
I	_____	____	IV	_____|_____	_____
II	____|____	____	V	_____|_____	_____
III	___|____	____	VI	_____	_____

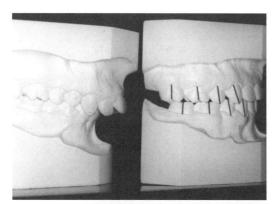
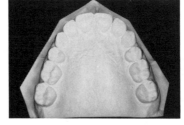
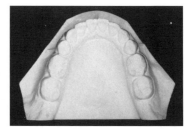
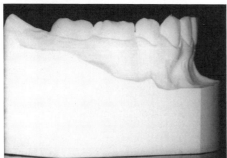

Fig. 14.29

Ortho___1___   Patient___4___   NE_____   E_____

Key		Grade	Key		Grade
I	_____	____	IV	_____|_____	_____
II	____|____	____	V	_____|_____	_____
III	___|____	____	VI	_____	_____

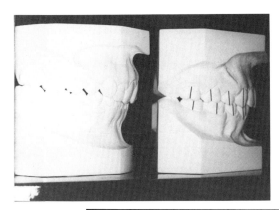
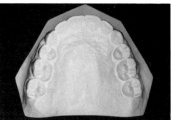
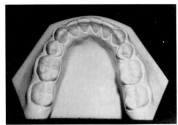

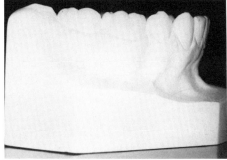

Ortho 1	Patient 5	NE	E
Key	Grade	Key	Grade
I		IV ─┼─	
II ─┼─		V ─┼─	
III ─┼─		VI	

Fig. 14.30

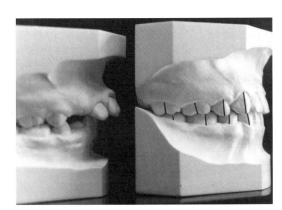
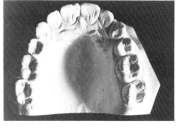
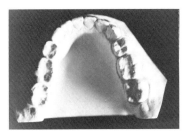

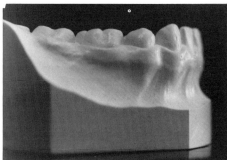

Ortho 1	Patient 6	NE	E
Key	Grade	Key	Grade
I		IV ─┼─	
II ─┼─		V ─┼─	
III ─┼─		VI	

Fig. 14.31

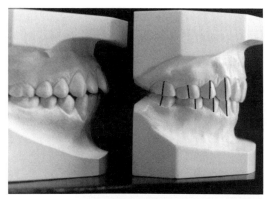
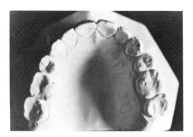
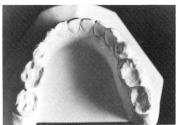

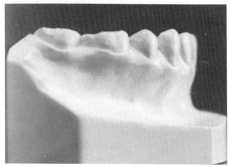

Fig. 14.32

Ortho___1___   Patient___7___   NE____   E____

Key		Grade	Key		Grade
I	_____	___	IV	___|___	___
II	___|___	___	V	___|___	___
III	___|___	___	VI	_____	___

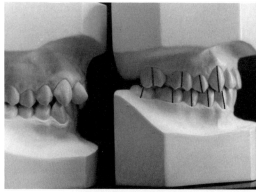
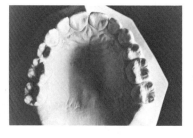
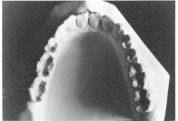

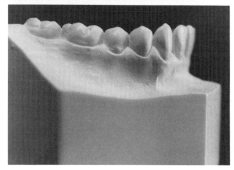

Fig. 14.33

Ortho___1___   Patient___8___   NE____   E____

Key		Grade	Key		Grade
I	_____	___	IV	___|___	___
II	___|___	___	V	___|___	___
III	___|___	___	VI	_____	___

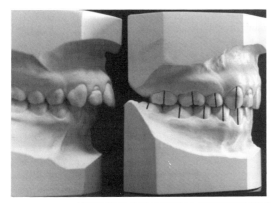
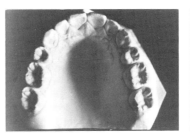
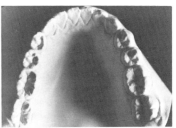

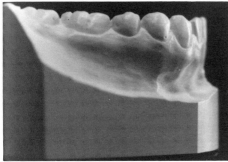

Fig. 14.34

Ortho __1__   Patient __9__   NE ____   E ____

Key	Grade	Key	Grade
I		IV	
II		V	
III		VI	

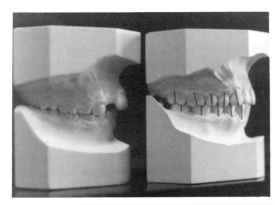
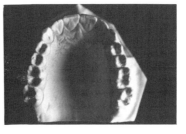
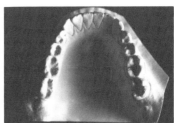

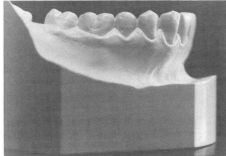

Fig. 14.35

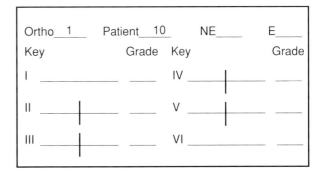

Ortho __1__   Patient __10__   NE ____   E ____

Key	Grade	Key	Grade
I		IV	
II		V	
III		VI	

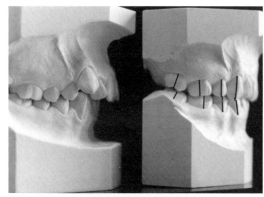
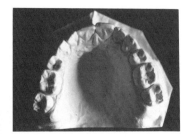
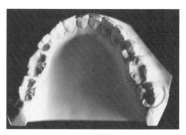
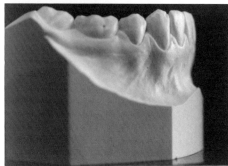

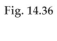
Fig. 14.36

Ortho __1__   Patient __11__   NE____   E____
Key   Grade   Key   Grade
I   _____   ___   IV   ___|_____   ___
II   _____|_____   ___   V   _____|_____ ___
III ____|_____   ___   VI   _____ ___

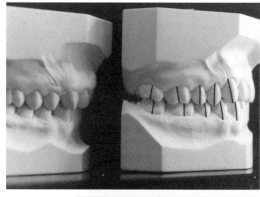
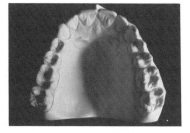
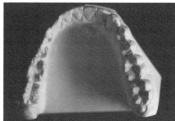
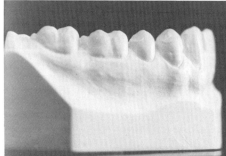

Fig. 14.37

Ortho __1__   Patient __12__   NE____   E____
Key   Grade   Key   Grade
I   _____   ___   IV   ___|_____   ___
II   ____|_____   ___   V   _____|_____ ___
III ____|_____   ___   VI   _____ ___

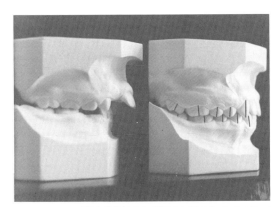
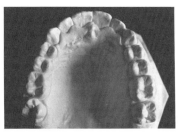
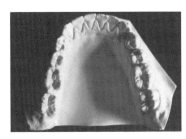

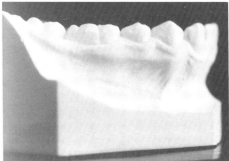

Fig. 14.38

Ortho ___1___   Patient ___13___   NE_____   E_____

Key	Grade	Key	Grade
I		IV	
II		V	
III		VI	

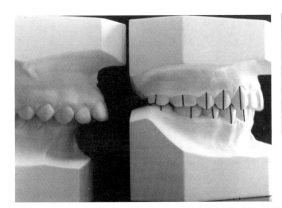
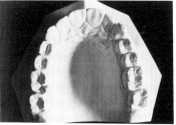
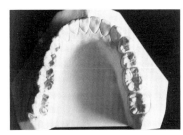

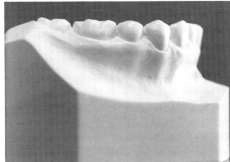

Fig. 14.39

Ortho ___1___   Patient ___14___   NE_____   E_____

Key	Grade	Key	Grade
I		IV	
II		V	
III		VI	

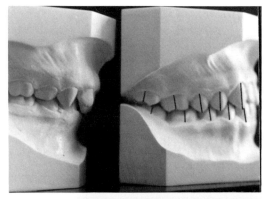
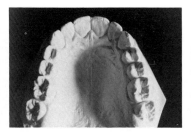
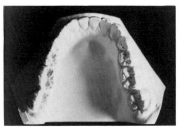
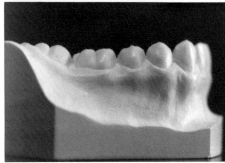

Fig. 14.40

Ortho __1__   Patient __15__   NE____   E____

Key		Grade	Key		Grade
I			IV		
II			V		
III			VI		

Summary for Orthodontist __1__

Patients __15__   NE____   E____

Keys	50% or more	Less than 50%, but significant	Grade
I			
II			
III			
IV			
V			
VI			

ORTHODONTIST #2

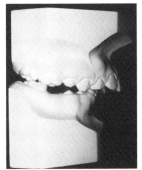
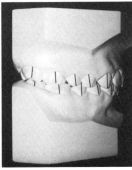
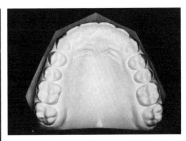
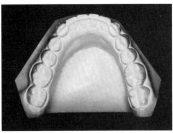

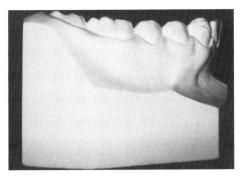

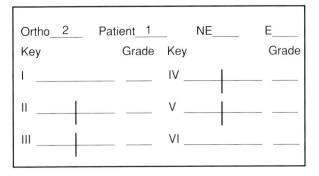

Ortho __2__   Patient __1__   NE____   E____

Key	Grade	Key	Grade
I _____	___	IV ___|___	___
II __|____	___	V __|____	___
III __|____	___	VI _____	___

Fig. 14.41

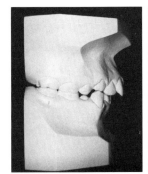
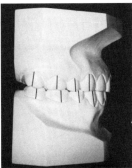
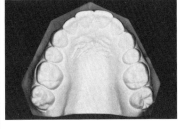
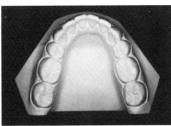

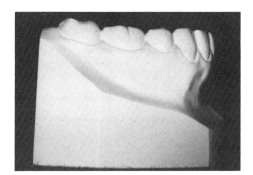

Ortho __2__   Patient __2__   NE____   E____

Key	Grade	Key	Grade
I _____	___	__|____	___
II __|____	___	V __|____	___
III __|____	___	VI _____	___

Fig. 14.42

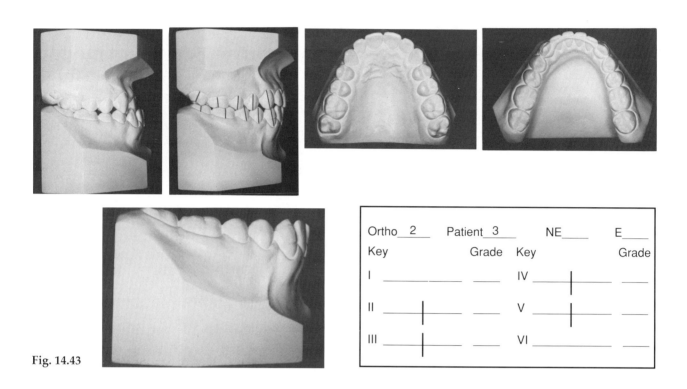

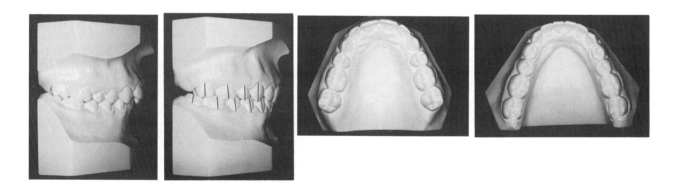

Fig. 14.43

Ortho 2	Patient 3	NE____	E____
Key	Grade	Key	Grade
I _____ ___		IV ___|___ ___	
II ___|___ ___		V ___|___ ___	
III ___|___ ___		VI _____ ___	

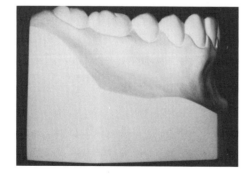

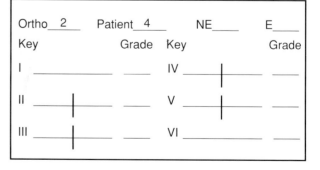

Fig. 14.44

Ortho 2	Patient 4	NE____	E____
Key	Grade	Key	Grade
I _____ ___		IV ___|___ ___	
II ___|___ ___		V ___|___ ___	
III ___|___ ___		VI _____ ___	

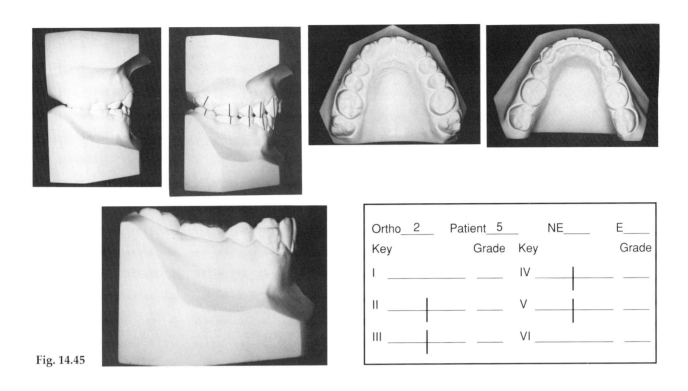

Fig. 14.45

Ortho __2__   Patient __5__   NE____   E____

Key		Grade	Key		Grade
I	_____	___	IV	__|__	___
II	__|__	___	V	__|__	___
III	__|__	___	VI	_____	___

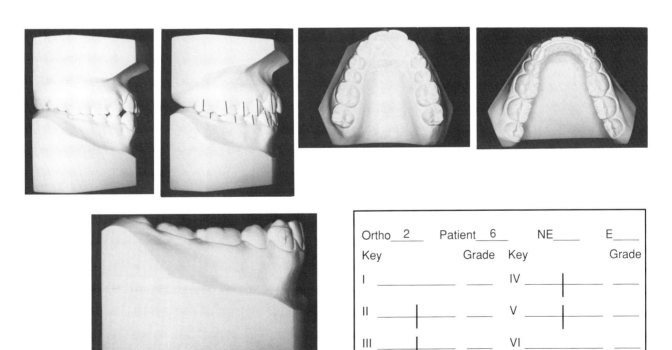

Fig. 14.46

Ortho __2__   Patient __6__   NE____   E____

Key		Grade	Key		Grade
I	_____	___	IV	__|__	___
II	__|__	___	V	__|__	___
III	__|__	___	VI	_____	___

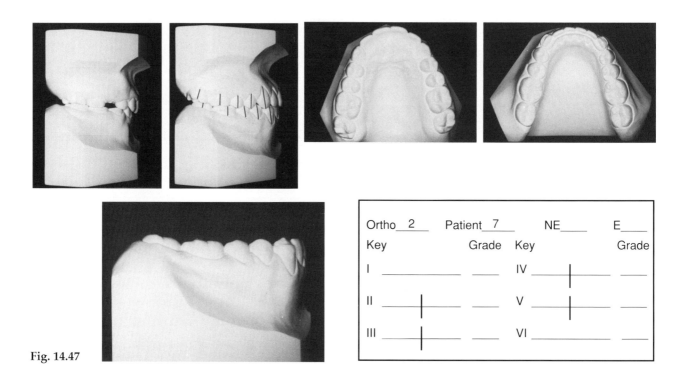

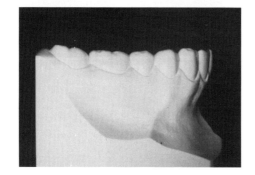

Fig. 14.47

Ortho 2	Patient 7	NE	E
Key	Grade	Key	Grade
I _____	___	IV __|___	___
II __|____	___	V __|___	___
III __|____	___	VI _____	___

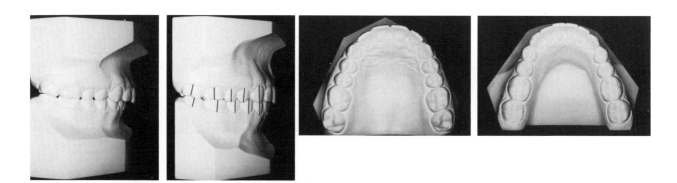

Fig. 14.48

Ortho 2	Patient 8	NE	E
Key	Grade	Key	Grade
I _____	___	IV __|___	___
II __|____	___	V __|___	___
III __|____	___	VI _____	___

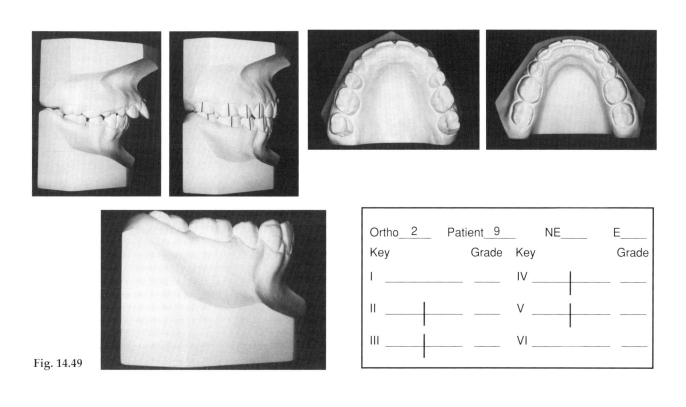

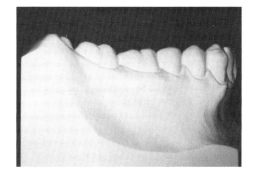

Fig. 14.49

Ortho 2   Patient 9   NE____ E____

Key	Grade	Key	Grade
I		IV	
II		V	
III		VI	

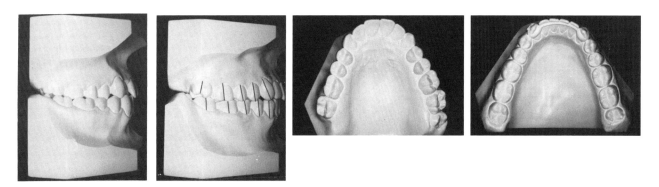

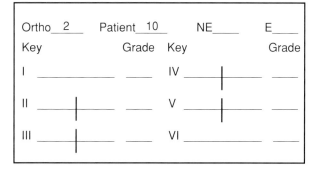

Fig. 14.50

Ortho 2   Patient 10   NE____ E____

Key	Grade	Key	Grade
I		IV	
II		V	
III		VI	

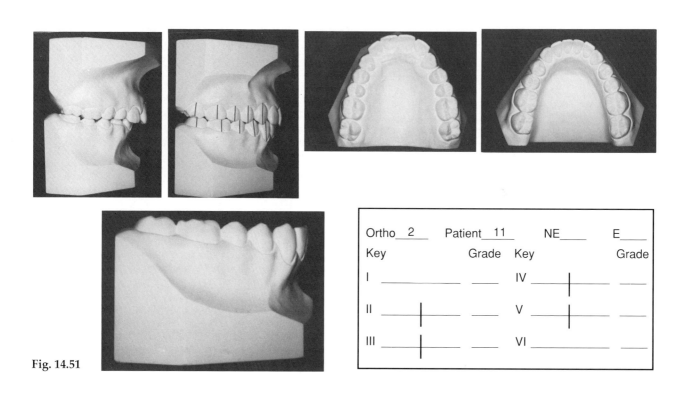

Fig. 14.51

Ortho __2__   Patient __11__   NE____   E____

Key		Grade	Key		Grade
I			IV		
II			V		
III			VI		

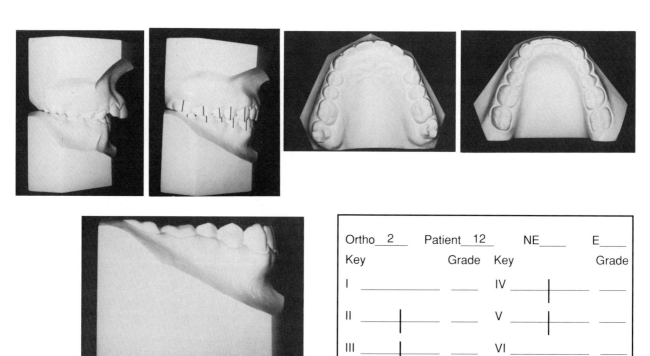

Fig. 14.52

Ortho __2__   Patient __12__   NE____   E____

Key		Grade	Key		Grade
I			IV		
II			V		
III			VI		

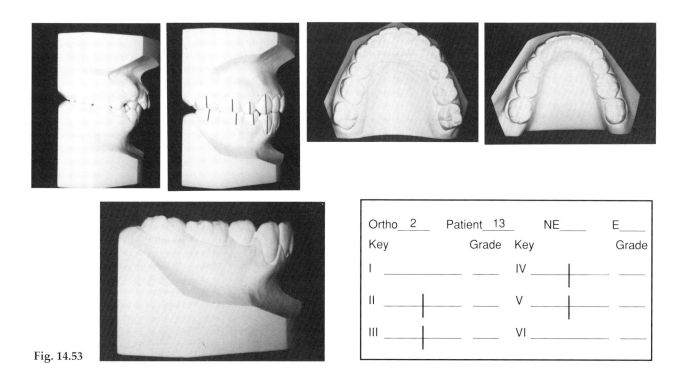

Fig. 14.53

Ortho __2__   Patient __13__   NE ____   E ____

Key	Grade	Key	Grade
I		IV	
II		V	
III		VI	

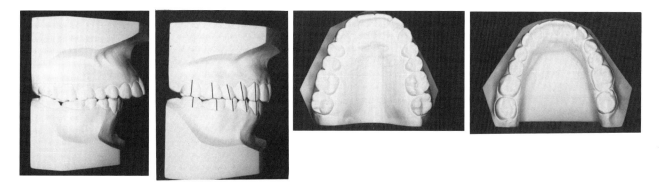

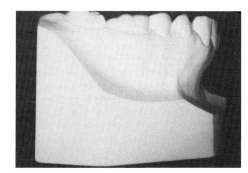

Fig. 14.54

Ortho __2__   Patient __14__   NE ____   E ____

Key	Grade	Key	Grade
I		IV	
II		V	
III		VI	

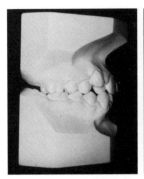
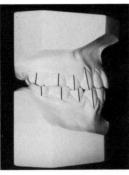
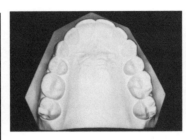
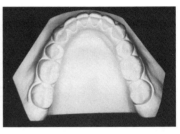

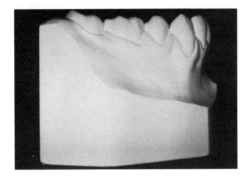

Fig. 14.55

Ortho __2__	Patient __15__	NE____	E____
Key	Grade	Key	Grade
I _____ ___		IV ___†___ ___	
II ___†___ ___		V ___†___ ___	
III ___†___ ___		VI _____ ___	

Summary for Orthodontist __2__			
Patients __15__	NE____	E____	
Keys	50% or more	Less than 50%, but significant	Grade
I	_____	_____	___
II	___†___	___†___	___
III	___†___	___†___	___
IV	___†___	___†___	___
V	_____	_____	___
VI	_____	_____	___

ORTHODONTIST #3

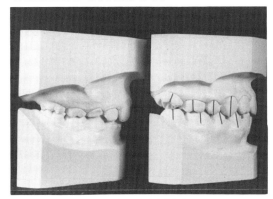
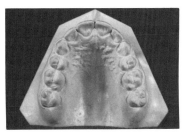
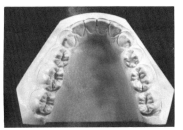

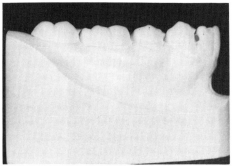

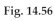

Fig. 14.56

```
Ortho  3      Patient  1        NE____      E____
Key                    Grade  Key                  Grade
I   _____   ___    IV _____|_____   ___
II  ____|_____   ___    V  _____|_____   ___
III ____|_____   ___    VI _____    ___
```

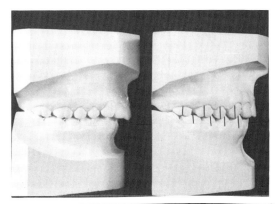
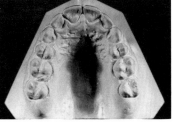
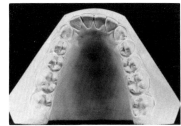

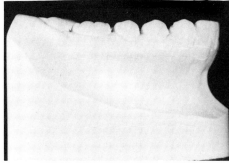

Fig. 14.57

```
Ortho  3      Patient  2        NE____      E____
Key                    Grade  Key                  Grade
I   _____   ___    IV _____|_____   ___
II  ____|_____   ___    V  _____|_____   ___
III ____|_____   ___    VI _____    ___
```

287

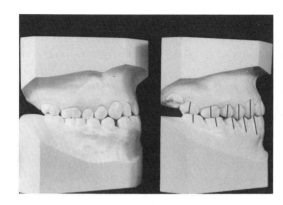
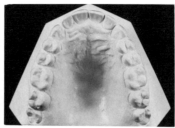
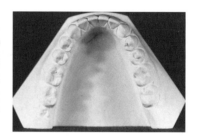

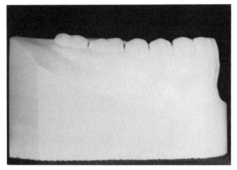

Fig. 14.58

Ortho __3__   Patient __3__   NE____   E____

Key	Grade	Key	Grade
I		IV	
II		V	
III		VI	

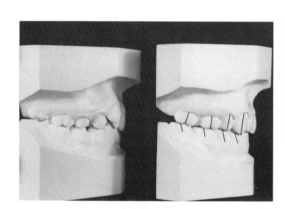
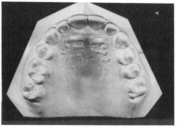
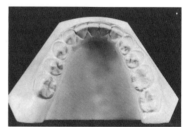

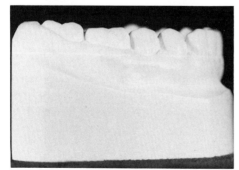

Fig. 14.59

Ortho __3__   Patient __4__   NE____   E____

Key	Grade	Key	Grade
I		IV	
II		V	
III		VI	

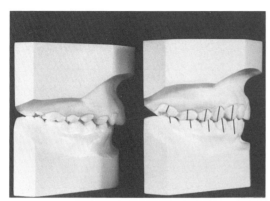
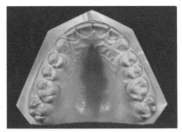
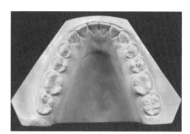

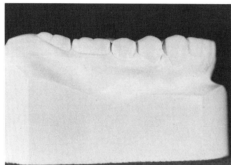

Fig. 14.60

Ortho __3__   Patient __5__   NE____   E____

Key	Grade	Key	Grade
I		IV	
II		V	
III		VI	

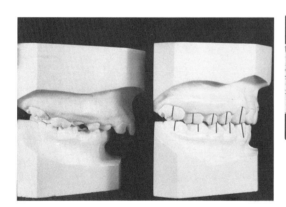
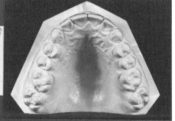
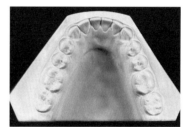

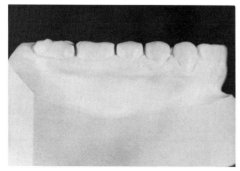

Fig. 14.61

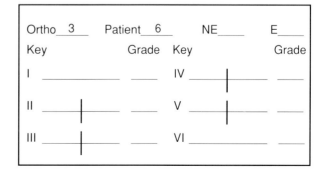

Ortho __3__   Patient __6__   NE____   E____

Key	Grade	Key	Grade
I		IV	
II		V	
III		VI	

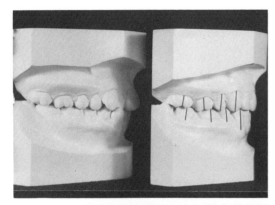
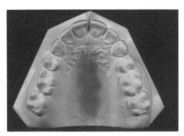
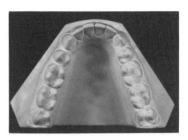

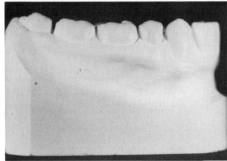

Fig. 14.62

Ortho ___3___   Patient ___7___   NE ____   E ____

Key		Grade	Key		Grade
I	_____	____	IV	___┼___	____
II	___┼___	____	V	___┼___	____
III	___┼___	____	VI	_____	____

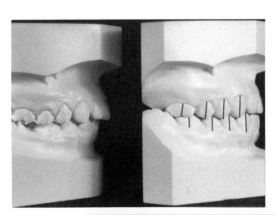
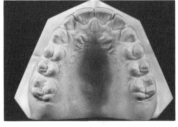
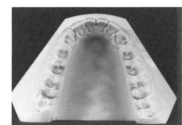

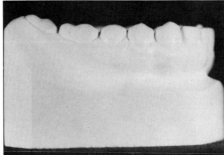

Fig. 14.63

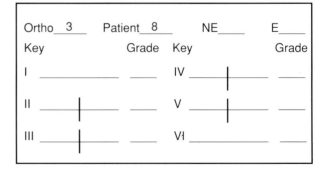

Ortho ___3___   Patient ___8___   NE ____   E ____

Key		Grade	Key		Grade
I	_____	____	IV	___┼___	____
II	___┼___	____	V	___┼___	____
III	___┼___	____	VI	_____	____

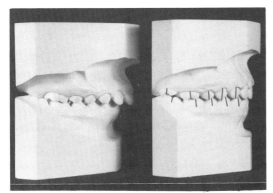
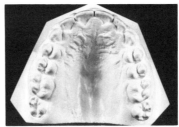
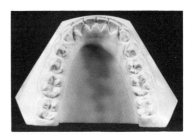

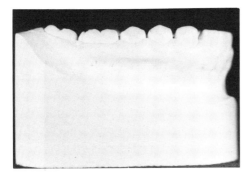

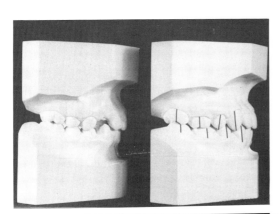

Ortho___3___   Patient___9___   NE_____   E_____

Key		Grade	Key		Grade
I	_____	____	IV	__|____	____
II	___|____	____	V	___|____	____
III	___|____	____	VI	_____	____

Fig. 14.64

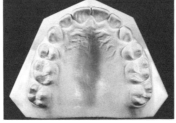
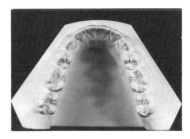

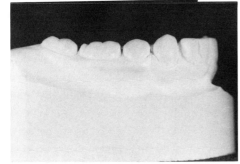

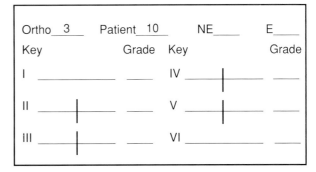

Ortho___3___   Patient___10___   NE_____   E_____

Key		Grade	Key		Grade
I	_____	____	IV	__|____	____
II	___|____	____	V	___|____	____
III	___|____	____	VI	_____	____

Fig. 14.65

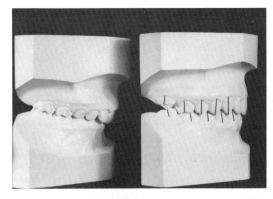
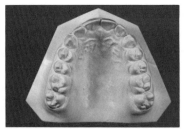
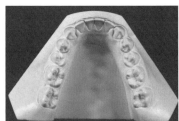

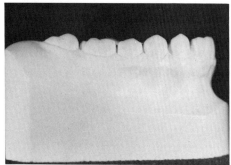

Fig. 14.66

Ortho 3	Patient 11	NE	E
Key	Grade	Key	Grade
I		IV	
II		V	
III		VI	

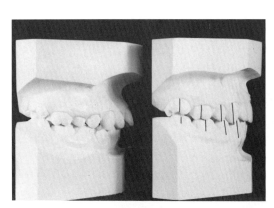
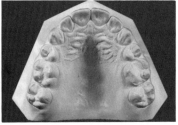
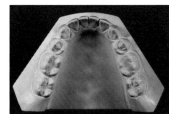

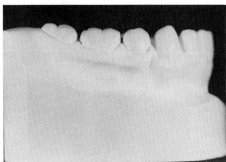

Fig. 14.67

Ortho 3	Patient 12	NE	E
Key	Grade	Key	Grade
I		IV	
II		V	
III		VI	

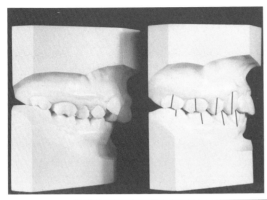
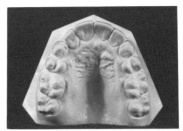
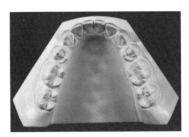

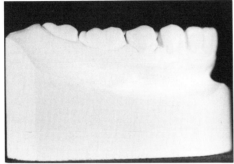

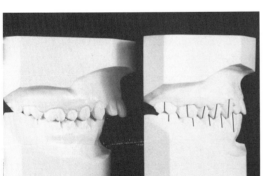

Fig. 14.68

Ortho 3	Patient 13	NE____	E____
Key	Grade	Key	Grade
I _____ ___		IV ___|___ ___	
II ___|___ ___		V ___|___ ___	
III ___|___ ___		VI _____ ___	

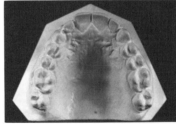
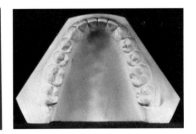

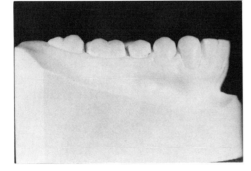

Fig. 14.69

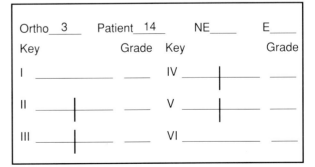

Ortho 3	Patient 14	NE____	E____
Key	Grade	Key	Grade
I _____ ___		IV ___|___ ___	
II ___|___ ___		V ___|___ ___	
III ___|___ ___		VI _____ ___	

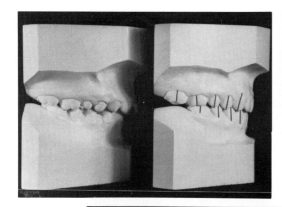
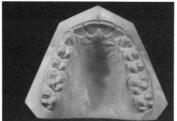
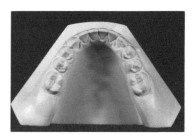

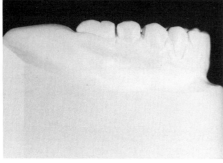

Fig. 14.70

Ortho __3__   Patient __15__   NE____   E____

Key		Grade	Key		Grade
I		____	IV	─┼─	____
II	─┼─	____	V	─┼─	____
III	─┼─	____	VI		

Summary for Orthodontist __3__

Patients __15__   NE____   E____

Keys	50% or more	Less than 50%, but significant	Grade
I			____
II	─┼─	─┼─	____
III	─┼─	─┼─	____
IV	─┼─	─┼─	____
V			
VI			

ORTHODONTIST #4

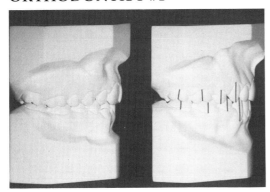
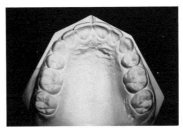
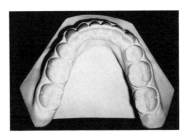

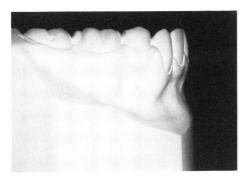

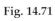

Ortho 4		Patient 1		NE___		E___
Key		Grade	Key			Grade
I	_____	___	IV	—┼—		___
II	—┼—	___	V	—┼—		___
III	—┼—	___	VI	_____		___

Fig. 14.71

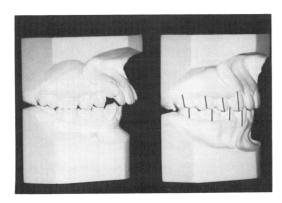
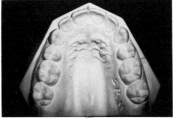
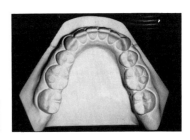

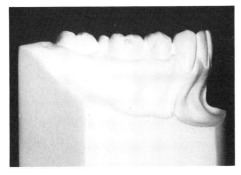

Ortho 4		Patient 2		NE___		E___
Key		Grade	Key			Grade
I	_____	___	IV	—┼—		___
II	—┼—	___	V	—┼—		___
III	—┼—	___	VI	_____		___

Fig. 14.72

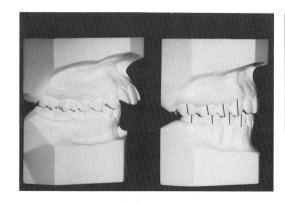
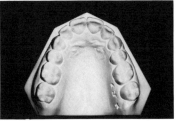
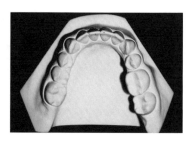

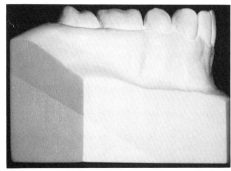

Fig. 14.73

Ortho __4__   Patient __3__   NE____   E____

Key		Grade	Key		Grade
I	_____	__	IV	—|—	__
II	—|—	__	V	—|—	__
III	—|—	__	VI	_____	__

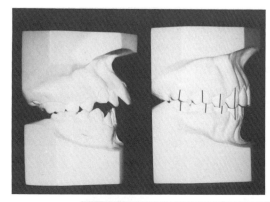
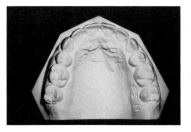
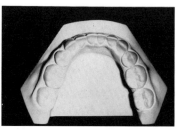

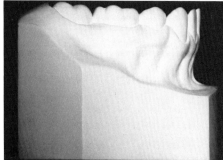

Fig. 14.74

Ortho __4__   Patient __4__   NE____   E____

Key		Grade	Key		Grade
I	_____	__	IV	—|—	__
II	—|—	__	V	—|—	__
III	—|—	__	VI	_____	__

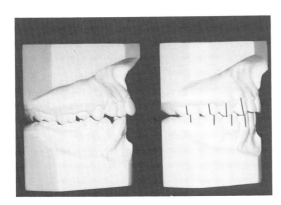
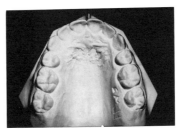
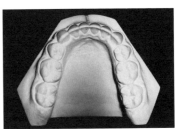

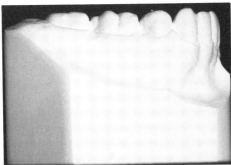
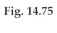

Ortho __4__   Patient __5__   NE ____   E ____

Key		Grade	Key		Grade
I	_____	___	IV	—┼—	___
II	—┼—	___	V	—┼—	___
III	—┼—	___	VI	_____	___

Fig. 14.75

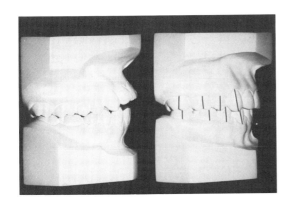
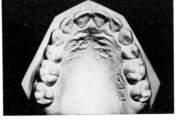
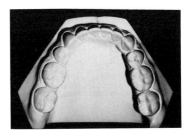

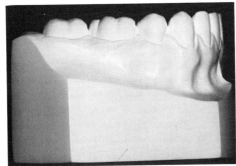

Ortho __4__   Patient __6__   NE ____   E ____

Key		Grade	Key		Grade
I	_____	___	IV	—┼—	___
II	—┼—	___	V	—┼—	___
III	—┼—	___	VI	_____	___

Fig. 14.76

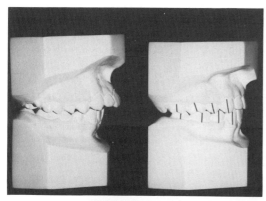
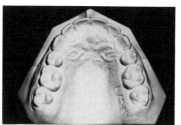
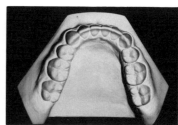

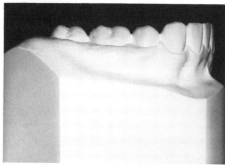

Fig. 14.77

Ortho 4		Patient 7		NE_____		E_____
Key		Grade	Key			Grade
I		___	IV			___
II		___	V			___
III		___	VI			___

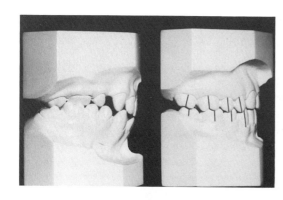
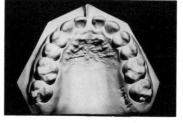
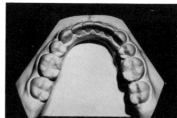

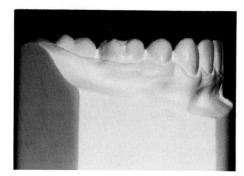

Fig. 14.78

Ortho 4		Patient 8		NE_____		E_____
Key		Grade	Key			Grade
I		___	IV			___
II		___	V			___
III		___	VI			___

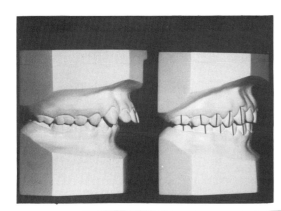

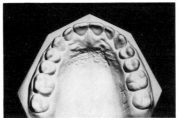

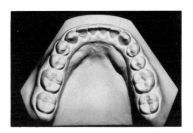

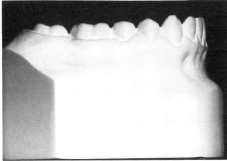

Ortho 4	Patient 9	NE___	E___
Key	Grade	Key	Grade
I _____	___	IV ___†___	___
II ___†___	___	V ___†___	___
III ___†___		VI _____	___

Fig. 14.79

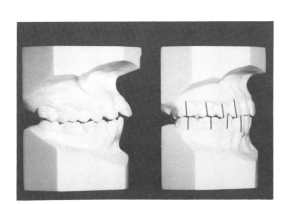

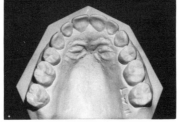

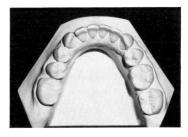

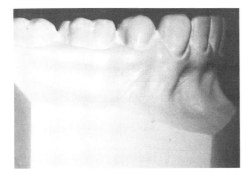

Ortho 4	Patient 10	NE___	E___
Key	Grade	Key	Grade
I _____	___	IV ___†___	___
II ___†___	___	V ___†___	___
III ___†___		VI _____	

Fig. 14.80

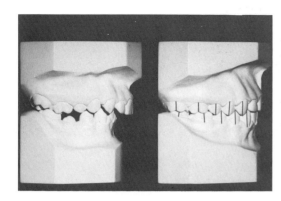
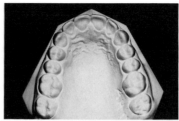
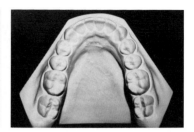

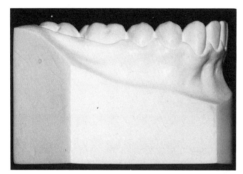

Fig. 14.81

Ortho 4	Patient 11	NE	E
Key	Grade	Key	Grade
I		IV	
II		V	
III		VI	

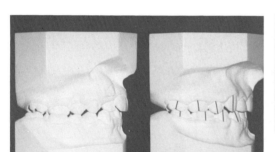
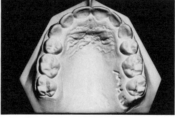
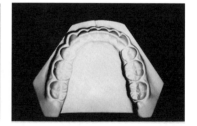

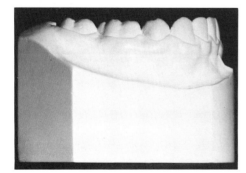

Fig. 14.82

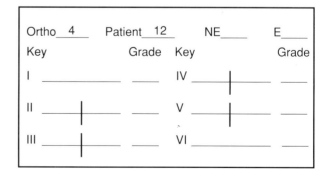

Ortho 4	Patient 12	NE	E
Key	Grade	Key	Grade
I		IV	
II		V	
III		VI	

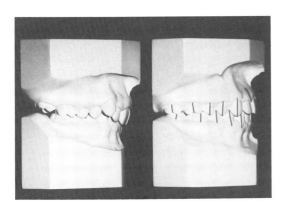
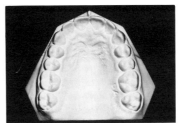
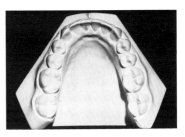

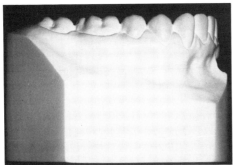

Fig. 14.83

Ortho __4__	Patient __13__	NE ____	E ____
Key	Grade	Key	Grade
I		IV	
II		V	
III		VI	

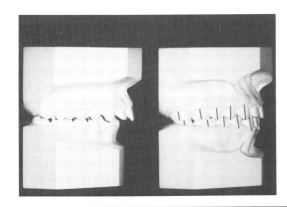
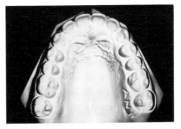
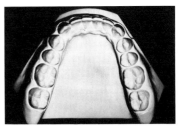

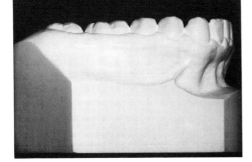

Fig. 14.84

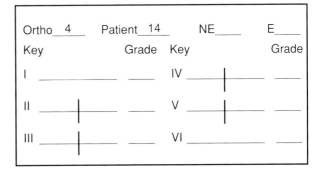

Ortho __4__	Patient __14__	NE ____	E ____
Key	Grade	Key	Grade
I		IV	
II		V	
III		VI	

301

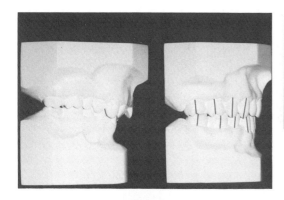

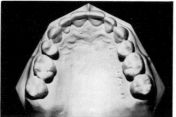

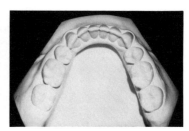

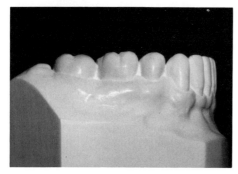

Fig. 14.85

Ortho 4	Patient 15	NE	E
Key	Grade	Key	Grade
I		IV	
II		V	
III		VI	

Summary for Orthodontist 4			
Patients 15	NE	E	
Keys	50% or more	Less than 50%, but significant	Grade
I			
II			
III			
IV			
V			
VI			

ORTHODONTIST #5

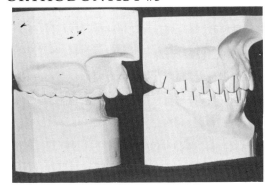 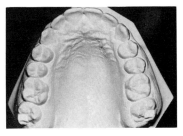 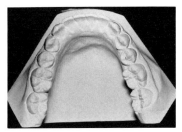

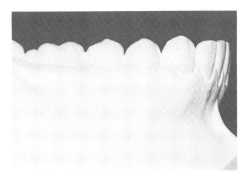
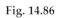

Ortho 5   Patient 1   NE____   E____

Key	Grade	Key	Grade
I		IV	
II		V	
III		VI	

Fig. 14.86

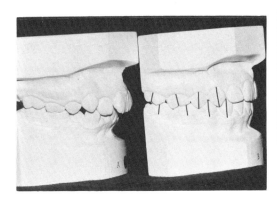 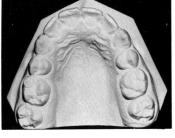 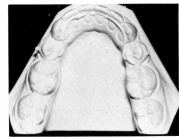

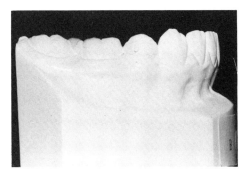

Ortho 5   Patient 2   NE____   E____

Key	Grade	Key	Grade
I		IV	
II		V	
III		VI	

Fig. 14.87

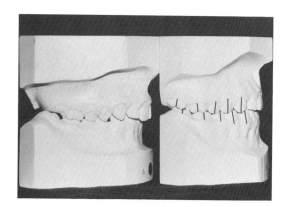
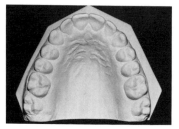
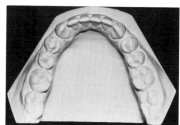

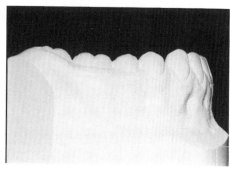

Fig. 14.88

Ortho 5	Patient 3		NE	E
Key		Grade	Key	Grade
I _____		____	IV ___|___	____
II ___|___		____	V ___|___	____
III ___|___		____	VI _____	

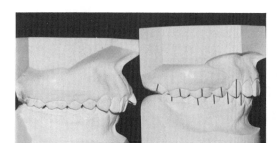
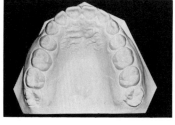
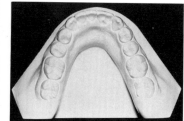

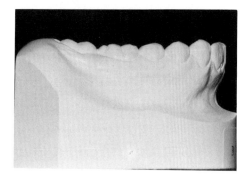

Fig. 14.89

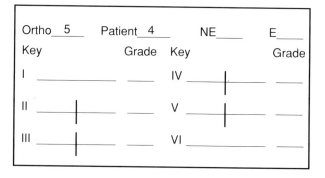

Ortho 5	Patient 4		NE	E
Key		Grade	Key	Grade
I _____		____	IV ___|___	____
II ___|___		____	V ___|___	____
III ___|___		____	VI _____	

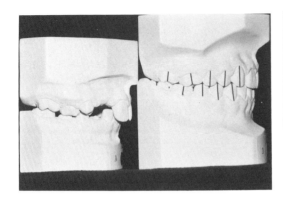
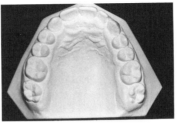
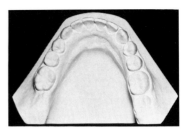

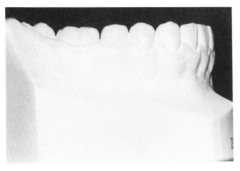

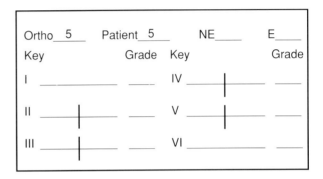

Ortho __5__   Patient __5__   NE____   E____

Key	Grade	Key	Grade
I		IV +	
II +		V +	
III +		VI	

Fig. 14.90

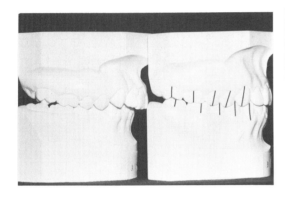
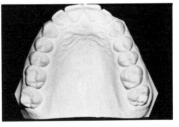
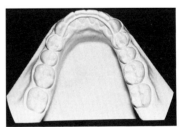

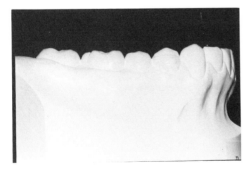

Ortho __5__   Patient __6__   NE____   E____

Key	Grade	Key	Grade
I		IV +	
II +		V +	
III +		VI	

Fig. 14.91

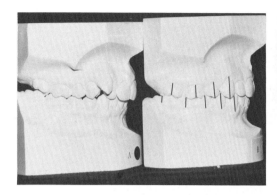
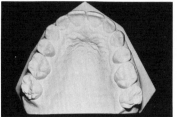
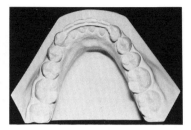

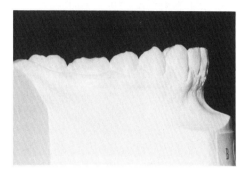

Fig. 14.92

Ortho __5__   Patient __7__   NE____   E____

Key	Grade	Key	Grade
I		IV	
II		V	
III		VI	

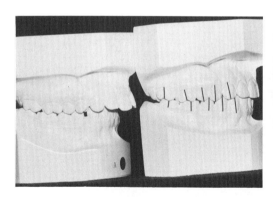
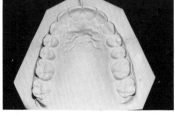
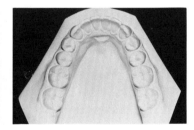

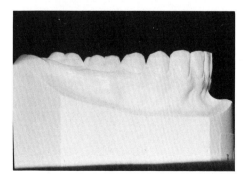

Fig. 14.93

Ortho __5__   Patient __8__   NE____   E____

Key	Grade	Key	Grade
I		IV	
II		V	
III		VI	

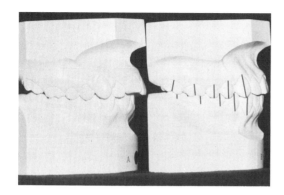
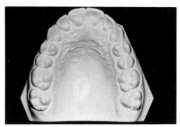
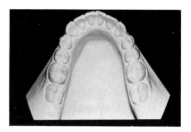

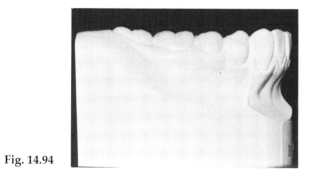

Fig. 14.94

Ortho __5__   Patient __9__   NE____   E____

Key	Grade	Key	Grade
I		IV	
II		V	
III		VI	

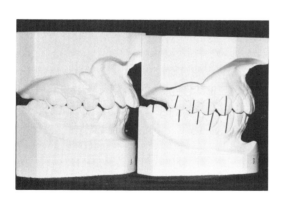
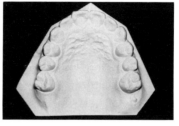
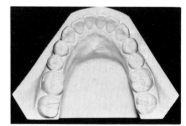

Fig. 14.95

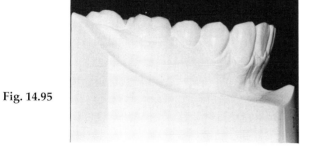

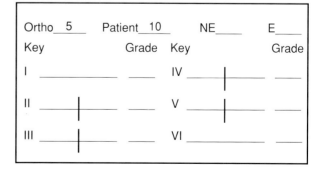

Ortho __5__   Patient __10__   NE____   E____

Key	Grade	Key	Grade
I		IV	
II		V	
III		VI	

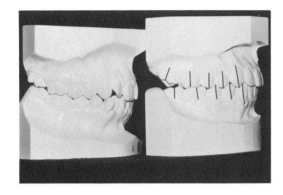
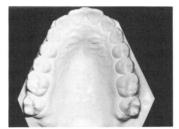
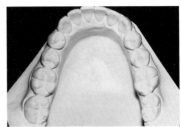

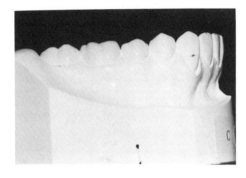

Fig. 14.96

Ortho __5__   Patient __11__   NE____   E____

Key	Grade	Key	Grade
I		IV	
II		V	
III		VI	

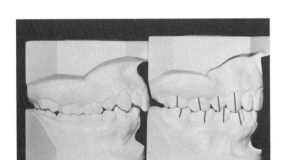
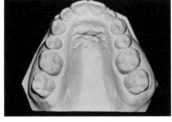
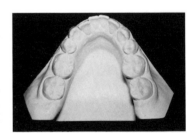

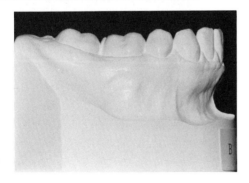

Fig. 14.97

Ortho __5__   Patient __12__   NE____   E____

Key	Grade	Key	Grade
I		IV	
II		V	
III		VI	

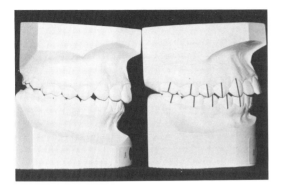
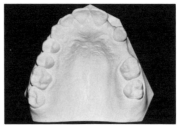
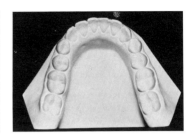

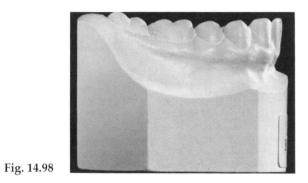

Ortho___5___ Patient___13___ NE_____ E_____

Key		Grade	Key		Grade
I			IV		
II			V		
III			VI		

Fig. 14.98

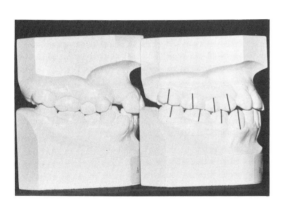
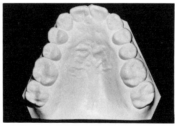
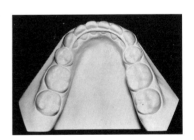

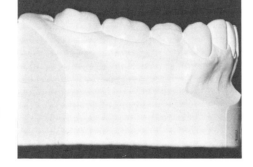

Ortho___5___ Patient___14___ NE_____ E_____

Key		Grade	Key		Grade
I			IV		
II			V		
III			VI		

Fig. 14.99

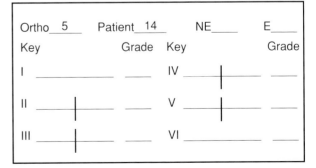

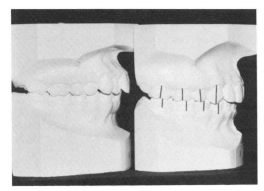

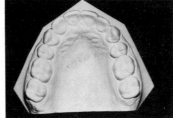

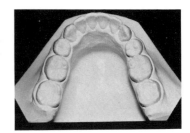

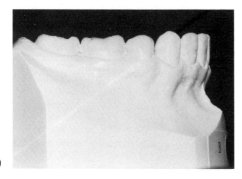

Fig. 14.100

Ortho __5__   Patient __15__   NE____   E____

Key		Grade	Key		Grade
I	_____	___	IV	—┼—	___
II	—┼—	___	V	—┼—	___
III	—┼—	___	VI	_____	___

Summary for Orthodontist __5__

Patients __15__   NE____   E____

Keys	50% or more	Less than 50%, but significant	Grade
I	_____	_____	___
II	—┼—	—┼—	___
III	—┼—	—┼—	___
IV	—┼—	—┼—	___
V	_____	_____	___
VI	_____	_____	___

310

ORTHODONTIST #6

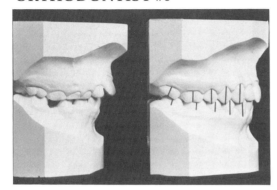
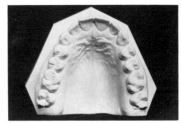
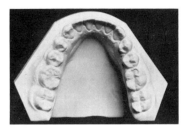

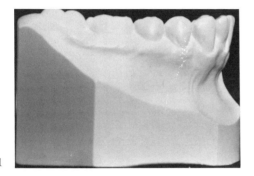

Fig. 14.101

Ortho 6	Patient 1	NE____	E____
Key	Grade	Key	Grade
I		IV	
II		V	
III		VI	

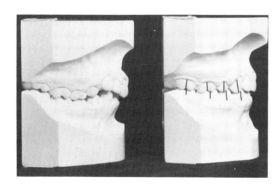
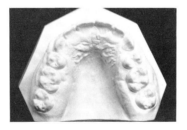
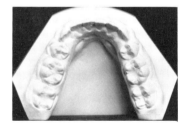

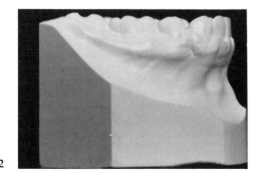

Fig. 14.102

Ortho 6	Patient 2	NE____	E____
Key	Grade	Key	Grade
I		IV	
II		V	
III		VI	

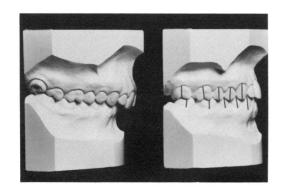
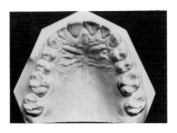
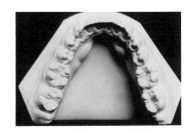

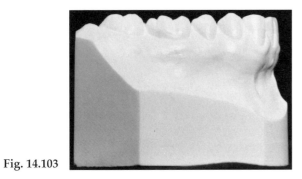

Fig. 14.103

Ortho 6	Patient 3	NE	E
Key	Grade	Key	Grade
I		IV ‖	
II ‖		V ‖	
III ‖		VI	

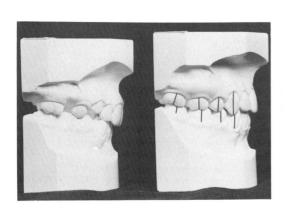
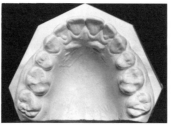
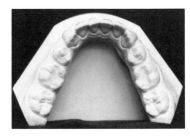

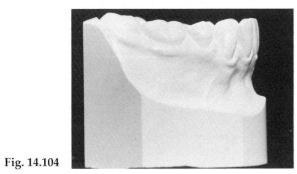

Fig. 14.104

Ortho 6	Patient 4	NE	E
Key	Grade	Key	Grade
I		IV ‖	
II ‖		V ‖	
III ‖		VI	

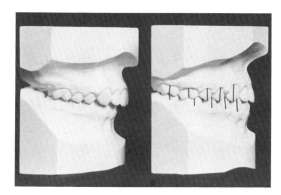
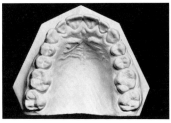
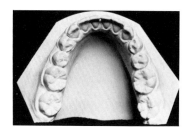

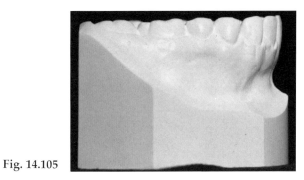

Fig. 14.105

Ortho___6___   Patient___5___   NE_____   E_____

Key		Grade	Key		Grade
I			IV		
II			V		
III			VI		

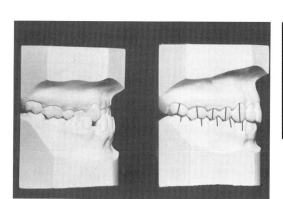
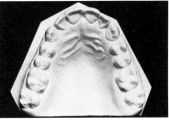
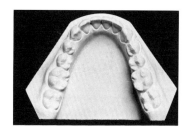

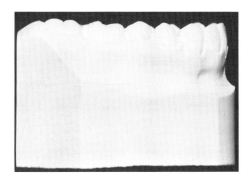

Fig. 14.106

Ortho___6___   Patient___6___   NE_____   E_____

Key		Grade	Key		Grade
I			IV		
II			V		
III			VI		

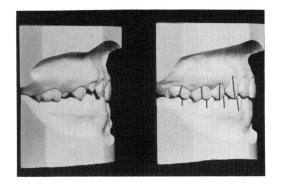
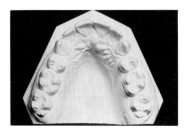
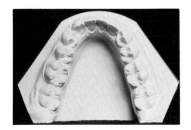

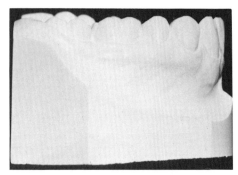

Fig. 14.107

Ortho 6	Patient 7	NE____	E____
Key	Grade	Key	Grade
I		IV	
II		V	
III		VI	

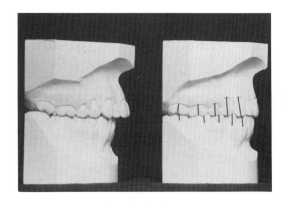
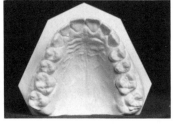
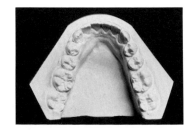

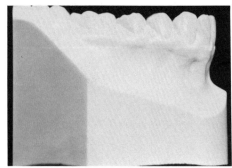

Fig. 14.108

Ortho 6	Patient 8	NE____	E____
Key	Grade	Key	Grade
I		IV	
II		V	
III		VI	

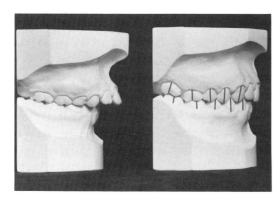
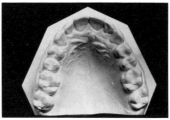
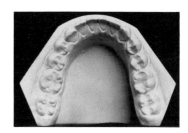

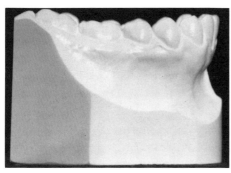

Fig. 14.109

Ortho __6__   Patient __9__   NE____   E____

Key		Grade	Key		Grade
I	_____	___	IV	__+__	___
II	__+__	___	V	__+__	___
III	__+__	___	VI	_____	___

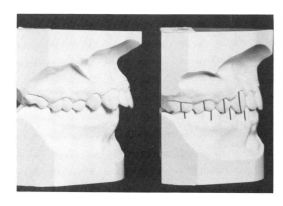
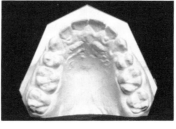
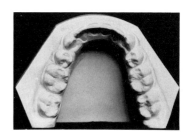

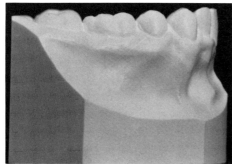

Fig. 14.110

Ortho __6__   Patient __10__   NE____   E____

Key		Grade	Key		Grade
I	_____	___	IV	__+__	___
II	__+__	___	V	__+__	___
III	__+__	___	VI	_____	___

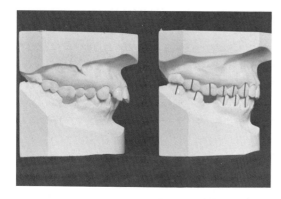
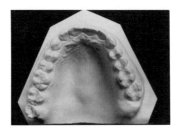
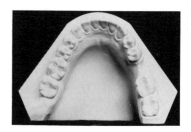

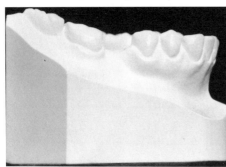

Fig. 14.111

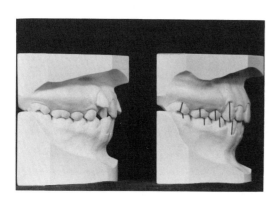
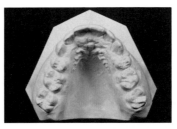
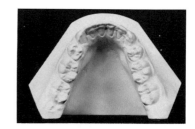

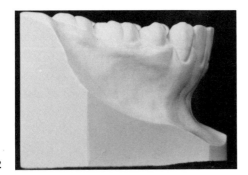

Fig. 14.112

Ortho 6	Patient 12	NE	E
Key	Grade	Key	Grade
I		IV ┼	
II ┼		V ┼	
III ┼		VI	

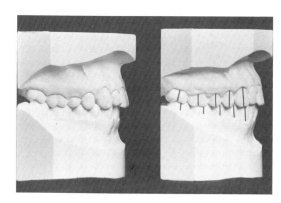
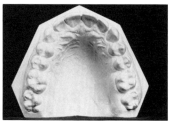
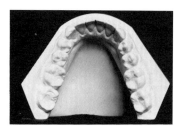

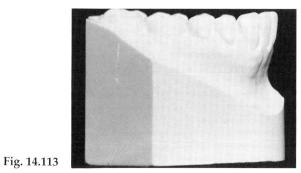

Fig. 14.113

Ortho 6	Patient 13	NE____	E____
Key	Grade	Key	Grade
I		IV	
II		V	
III		VI	

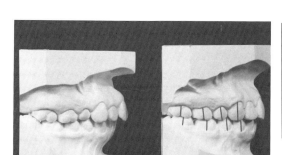
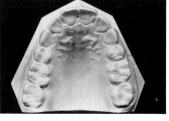
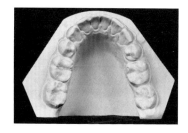

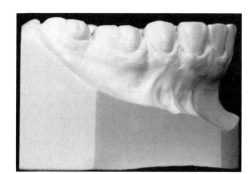

Fig. 14.114

Ortho 6	Patient 14	NE____	E____
Key	Grade	Key	Grade
I		IV	
II		V	
III		VI	

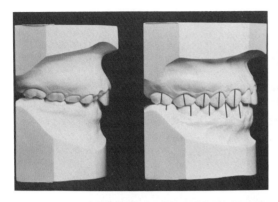
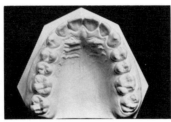
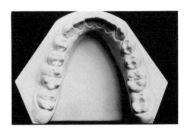

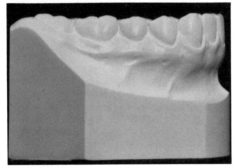

Fig. 14.115

Ortho ___6___ Patient ___15___ NE_____ E_____

Key		Grade	Key		Grade
I	_____	___	IV	__┼__	___
II	__┼__	___	V	__┼__	___
III	__┼__	___	VI	_____	___

Summary for Orthodontist ___6___

Patients ___15___ NE_____ E_____

Keys	50% or more	Less than 50%, but significant	Grade
I	_____	_____	___
II	__┼__	__┼__	___
III	__┼__	__┼__	___
IV	__┼__	__┼__	___
V	_____	_____	___
VI	_____	_____	___

ORTHODONTIST #7

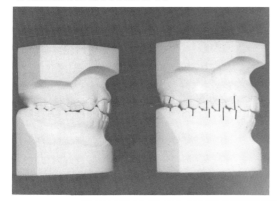
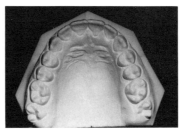
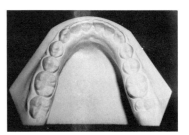

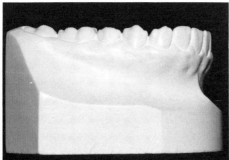

Fig. 14.116

Ortho 7 Patient 1 NE____ E____

Key	Grade	Key	Grade
I		IV	
II		V	
III		VI	

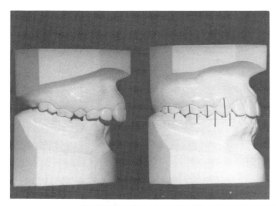
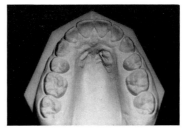
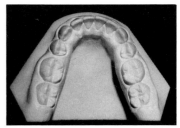

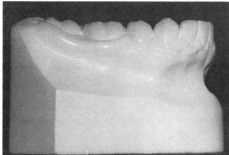

Fig. 14.117

Ortho 7 Patient 2 NE____ E____

Key	Grade	Key	Grade
I		IV	
II		V	
III		VI	

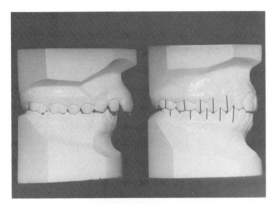
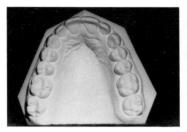
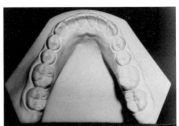
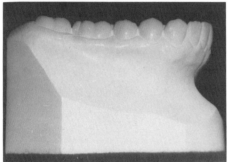

Fig. 14.118

Ortho __7__   Patient __3__   NE____   E____

Key	Grade	Key	Grade
I		IV	
II		V	
III		VI	

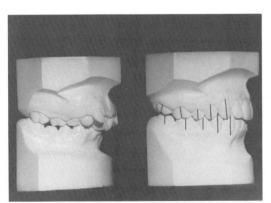
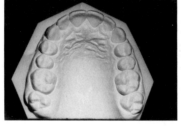
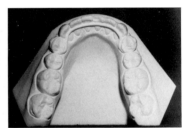
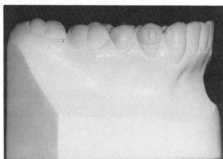

Fig. 14.119

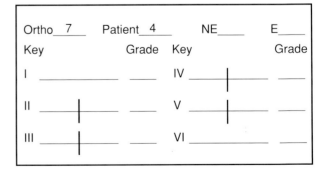

Ortho __7__   Patient __4__   NE____   E____

Key	Grade	Key	Grade
I		IV	
II		V	
III		VI	

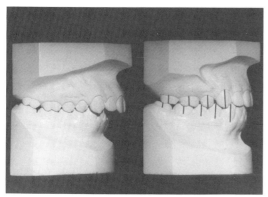
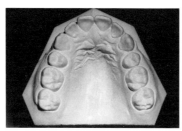
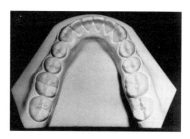

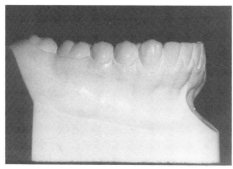

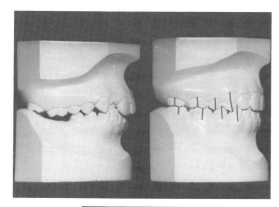

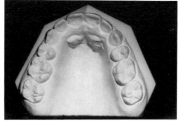
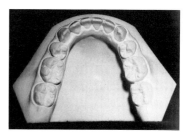

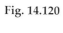
Fig. 14.120

Ortho __7__   Patient __5__   NE ____   E ____

Key	Grade	Key	Grade
I		IV	
II		V	
III		VI	

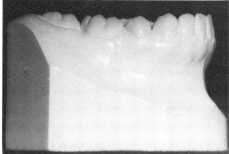
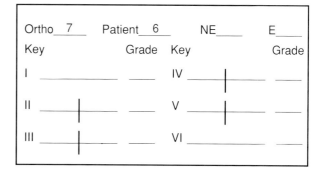

Fig. 14.121

Ortho __7__   Patient __6__   NE ____   E ____

Key	Grade	Key	Grade
I		IV	
II		V	
III		VI	

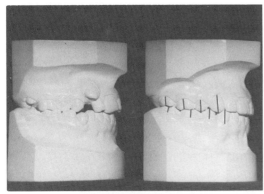
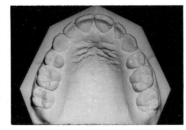
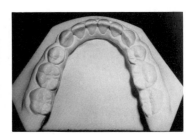
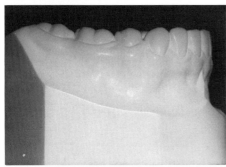

Fig. 14.122

Ortho 7	Patient 7	NE____	E____
Key	Grade	Key	Grade
I		IV	
II		V	
III		VI	

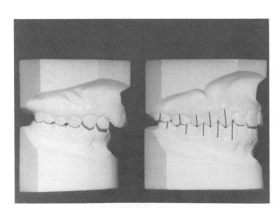
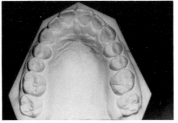
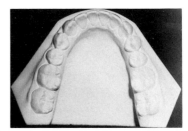
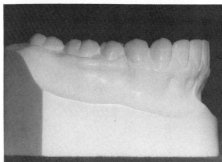

Fig. 14.123

Ortho 7	Patient 8	NE____	E____
Key	Grade	Key	Grade
I		IV	
II		V	
III		VI	

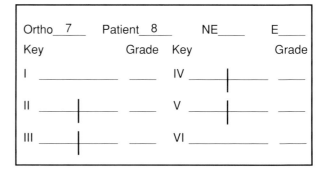

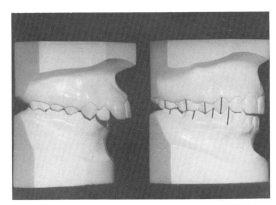
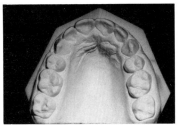
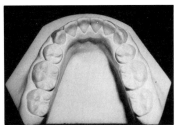
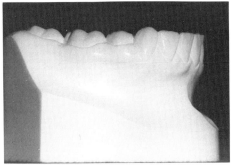

Fig. 14.124

Ortho __7__   Patient __9__   NE ____   E ____

Key	Grade	Key	Grade
I		IV	
II		V	
III		VI	

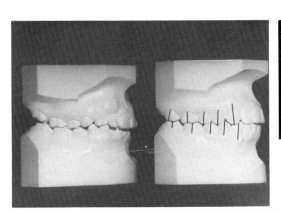
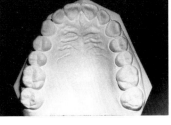
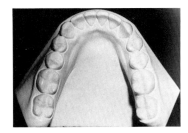
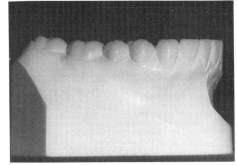

Fig. 14.125

Ortho __7__   Patient __10__   NE ____   E ____

Key	Grade	Key	Grade
I		IV	
II		V	
III		VI	

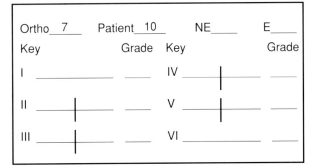

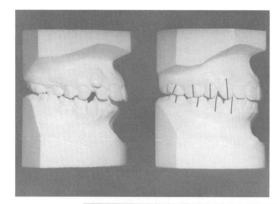

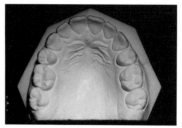

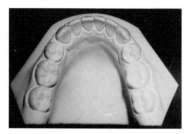

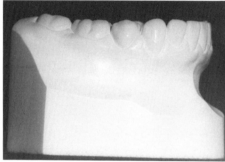

Fig. 14.126

Ortho __7__   Patient __11__   NE ____   E ____

Key		Grade	Key		Grade
I			IV		
II			V		
III			VI		

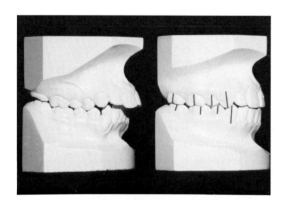

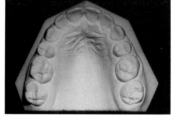

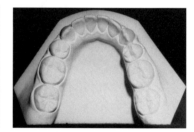

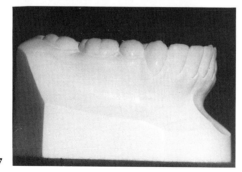

Fig. 14.127

Ortho __7__   Patient __12__   NE ____   E ____

Key		Grade	Key		Grade
I			IV		
II			V		
III			VI		

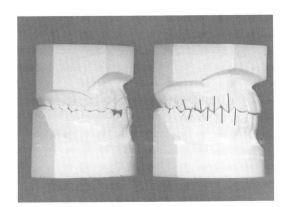

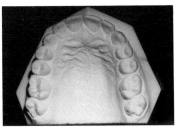

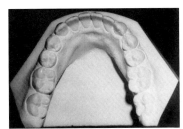

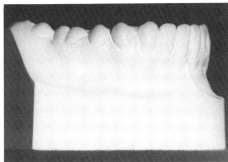

Ortho _7_	Patient _13_		NE____	E____
Key	Grade	Key		Grade
I _____	____	IV ___|___		____
II ___|___	____	V ___|___		____
III ___|___	____	VI _____		____

Fig. 14.128

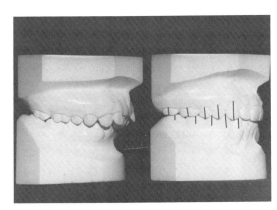

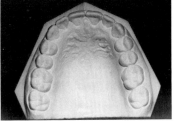

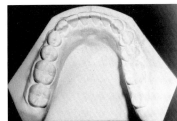

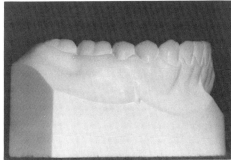

Ortho _7_	Patient _14_		NE____	E____
Key	Grade	Key		Grade
I _____	____	IV ___|___		____
II ___|___	____	V ___|___		____
III ___|___	____	VI _____		____

Fig. 14.129

325

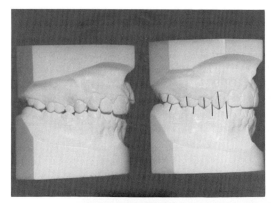

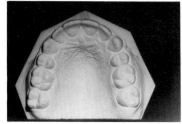

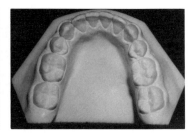

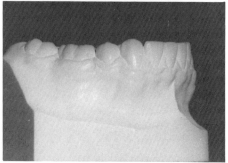

Fig. 14.130

Ortho __7__   Patient __15__   NE____   E____

Key		Grade	Key		Grade
I	_____	___	IV	___┼___	___
II	___┼___	___	V	___┼___	___
III	___┼___	___	VI	_____	___

Summary for Orthodontist __7__

Patients __15__   NE_____   E____

Keys	50% or more	Less than 50%, but significant	Grade
I	_____	_____	___
II	___┼___	___┼___	___
III	___┼___	___┼___	___
IV	___┼___	___┼___	___
V	_____	_____	___
VI	_____	_____	___

ORTHODONTIST #8

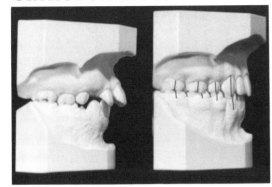
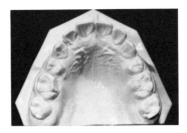
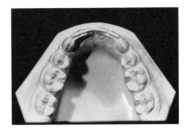

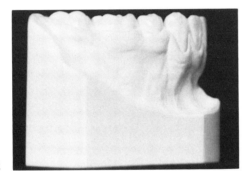

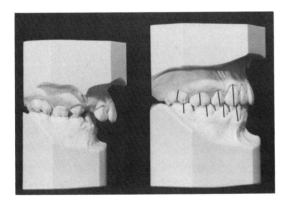

Fig. 14.131

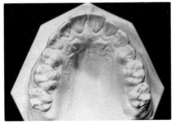
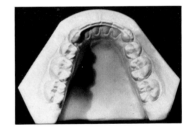

Ortho 8	Patient 1	NE____	E____
Key	Grade	Key	Grade
I _____ ___		IV ____|____ ___	
II ____|____ ___		V ____|____ ___	
III ____|____ ___		VI _____ ___	

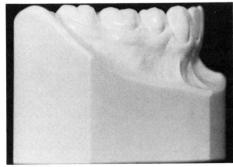

Fig. 14.132

Ortho 8	Patient 2	NE____	E____
Key	Grade	Key	Grade
I _____ ___		IV ____|____ ___	
II ____|____ ___		V ____|____ ___	
III ____|____ ___		VI _____ ___	

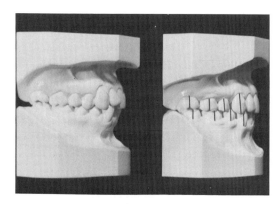
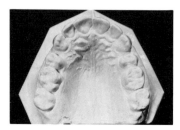
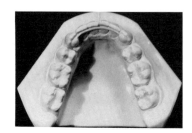

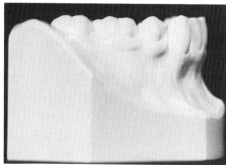

Fig. 14.133

Ortho __8__   Patient __3__   NE____   E____

Key		Grade	Key		Grade
I			IV		
II			V		
III			VI		

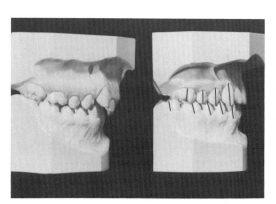
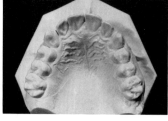
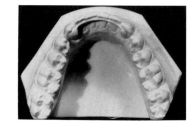

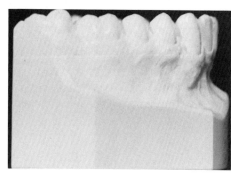

Fig. 14.134

Ortho __8__   Patient __4__   NE____   E____

Key		Grade	Key		Grade
I			IV		
II			V		
III			VI		

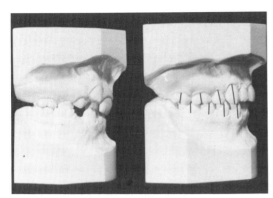
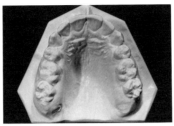
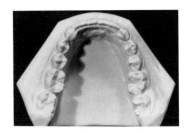

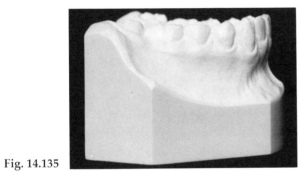

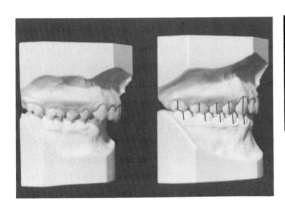

Fig. 14.135

Ortho __8__	Patient __5__	NE____	E____
Key	Grade	Key	Grade
I	___	IV ____┼____	___
II ____┼____	___	V ____┼____	___
III ____┼____		VI _____	

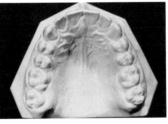
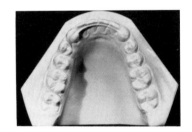

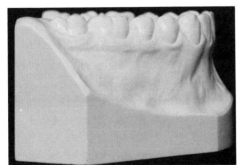

Fig. 14.136

Ortho __8__	Patient __6__	NE____	E____
Key	Grade	Key	Grade
I	___	IV ____┼____	___
II ____┼____	___	V ____┼____	___
III ____┼____		VI _____	

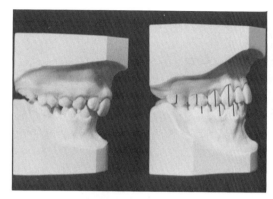
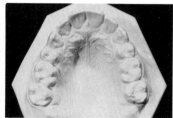
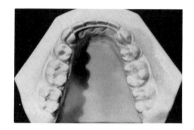

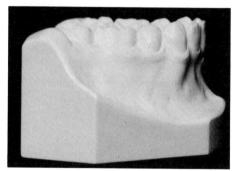

Fig. 14.137

Ortho 8   Patient 7   NE____   E____

Key	Grade	Key	Grade
I		IV	
II		V	
III		VI	

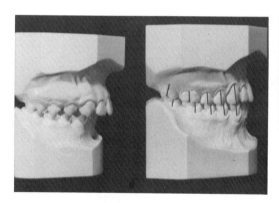
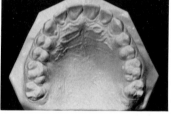
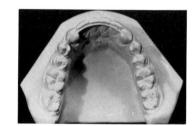

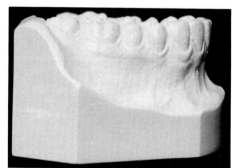

Fig. 14.138

Ortho 8   Patient 8   NE____   E____

Key	Grade	Key	Grade
I		IV	
II		V	
III		VI	

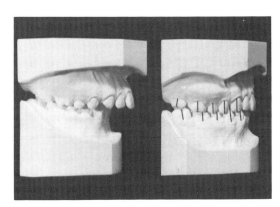
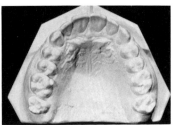
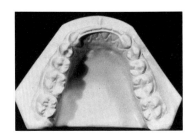

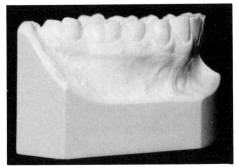

Ortho 8	Patient 9		NE____	E____
Key		Grade	Key	Grade
I	_____	___	IV ⊣	___
II ⊣		___	V ⊣	___
III ⊣		___	VI	___

Fig. 14.139

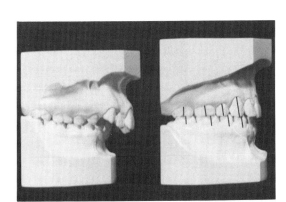
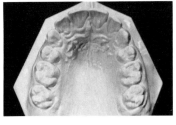
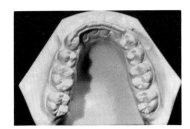

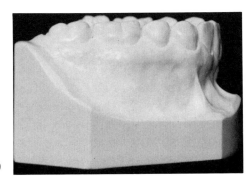

Ortho 8	Patient 10		NE____	E____
Key		Grade	Key	Grade
I	_____	___	IV ⊣	___
II ⊣		___	V ⊣	___
III ⊣		___	VI	___

Fig. 14.140

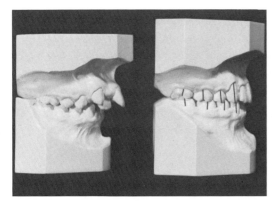
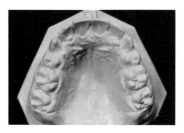
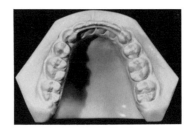
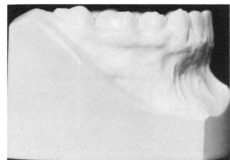

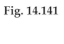
Fig. 14.141

Ortho __8__   Patient __11__   NE____   E____

Key	Grade	Key	Grade
I		IV	
II		V	
III		VI	

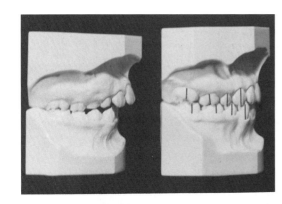
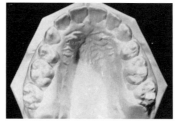
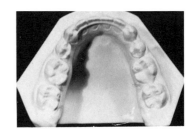

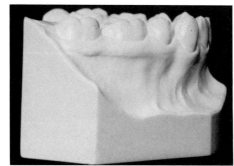
Fig. 14.142

Ortho __8__   Patient __12__   NE____   E____

Key	Grade	Key	Grade
I		IV	
II		V	
III		VI	

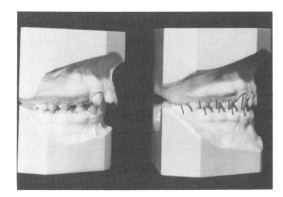
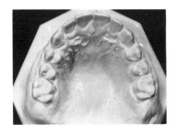
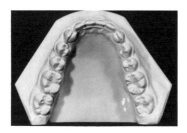

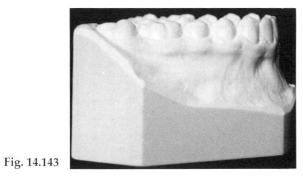

Fig. 14.143

Ortho 8	Patient 13	NE	E
Key	Grade	Key	Grade
I		IV ——+——	
II ——+——		V ——+——	
III ——+——		VI	

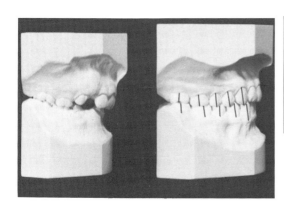
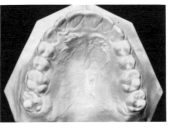
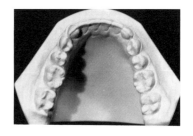

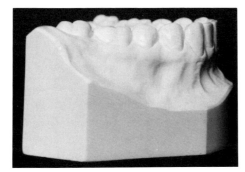

Fig. 14.144

Ortho 8	Patient 14	NE	E
Key	Grade	Key	Grade
I		IV ——+——	
II ——+——		V ——+——	
III ——+——		VI	

333

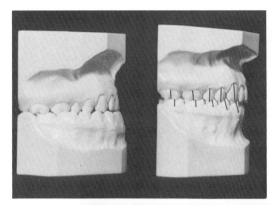
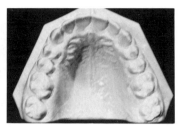
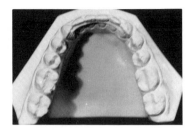

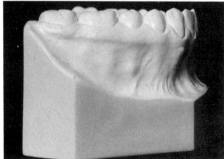

Fig. 14.145

Ortho 8	Patient 15	NE	E
Key	Grade	Key	Grade
I		IV ─┼─	
II ─┼─		V ─┼─	
III ─┼─		VI	

Summary for Orthodontist 8			
Patients 15	NE	E	
Keys	50% or more	Less than 50%, but significant	Grade
I			
II	─┼─	─┼─	
III	─┼─	─┼─	
IV	─┼─	─┼─	
V			
VI			

ORTHODONTIST #9

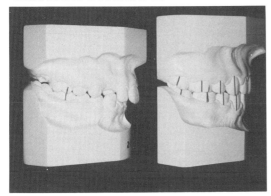
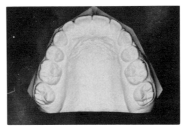
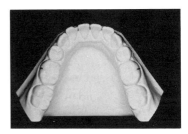

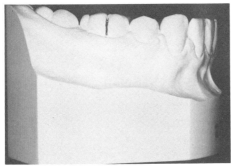

Ortho __9__   Patient __1__   NE____   E____

Key	Grade	Key	Grade
I		IV	
II		V	
III		VI	

Fig. 14.146

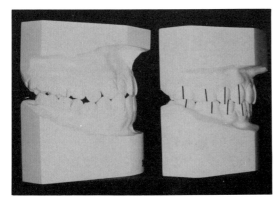
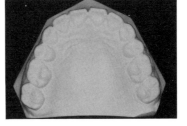
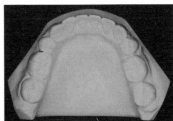

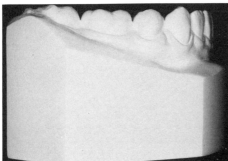

Ortho __9__   Patient __2__   NE____   E____

Key	Grade	Key	Grade
I		IV	
II		V	
III		VI	

Fig. 14.147

335

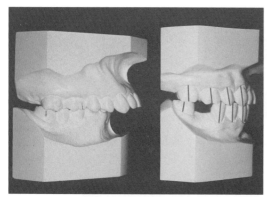

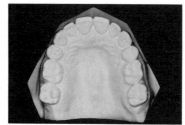

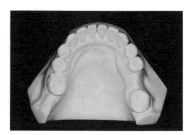

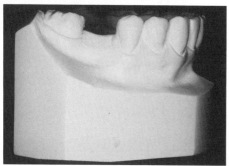

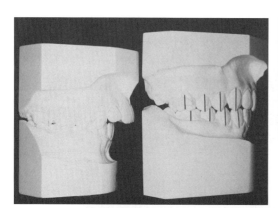

Fig. 14.148

Ortho __9__   Patient __3__   NE ____   E ____

Key		Grade	Key		Grade
I			IV	┼	
II	┼		V	┼	
III	┼		VI		

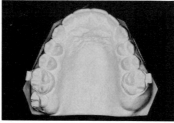

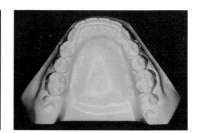

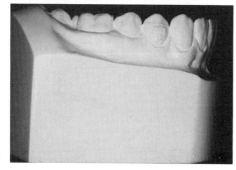

Fig. 14.149

Ortho __9__   Patient __4__   NE ____   E ____

Key		Grade	Key		Grade
I			IV	┼	
II	┼		V	┼	
III	┼		VI		

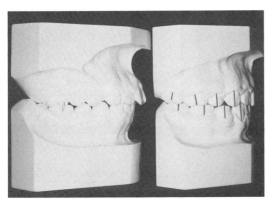
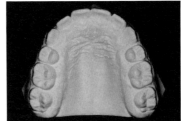
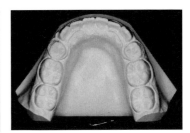
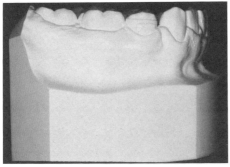

Ortho 9	Patient 5	NE	E
Key	Grade	Key	Grade
I		IV	
II		V	
III		VI	

Fig. 14.150

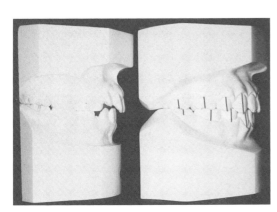
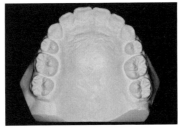
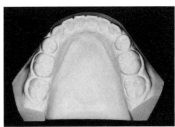
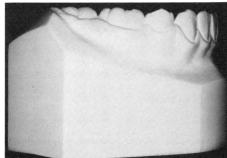

Ortho 9	Patient 6	NE	E
Key	Grade	Key	Grade
I		IV	
II		V	
III		VI	

Fig. 14.151

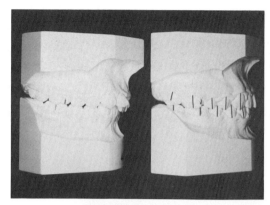

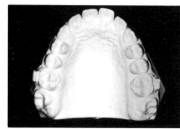

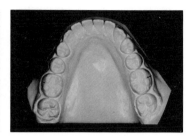

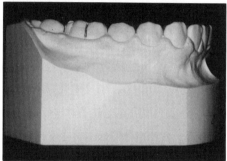

Fig. 14.152

Ortho __9__   Patient __7__   NE____   E____

Key	Grade	Key	Grade
I		IV	
II		V	
III		VI	

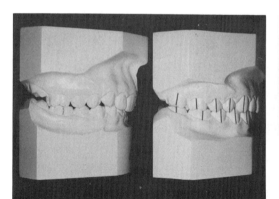

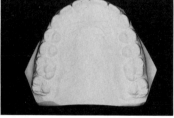

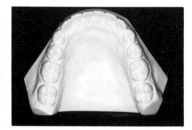

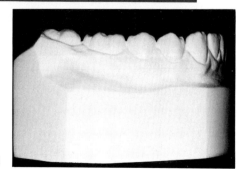

Fig. 14.153

Ortho __9__   Patient __8__   NE____   E____

Key	Grade	Key	Grade
I		IV	
II		V	
III		VI	

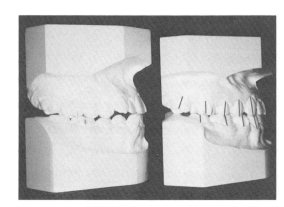
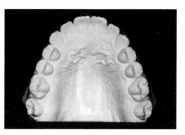
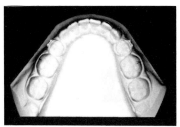

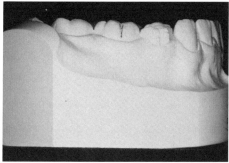

Fig. 14.154

Ortho __9__   Patient __9__   NE ____   E ____

Key		Grade	Key		Grade
I			IV		
II			V		
III			VI		

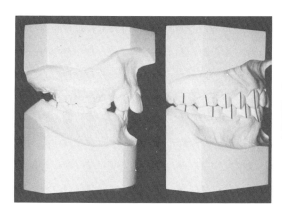
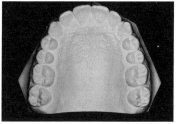
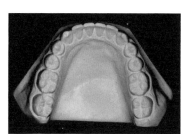

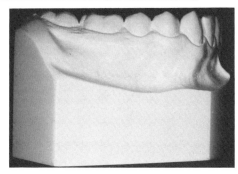

Fig. 14.155

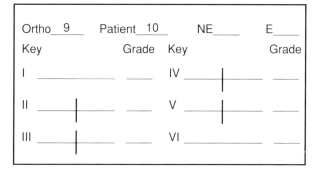

Ortho __9__   Patient __10__   NE ____   E ____

Key		Grade	Key		Grade
I			IV		
II			V		
III			VI		

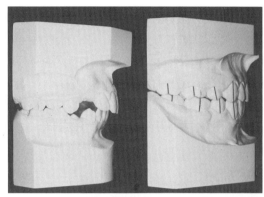
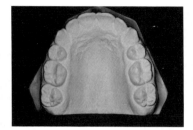
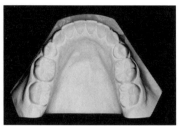
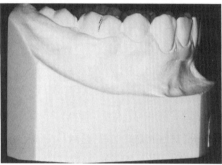
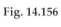

Fig. 14.156

Ortho __9__   Patient __11__   NE____   E____

Key		Grade	Key		Grade
I	_____	___	IV	─┼─	___
II	─┼─	___	V	─┼─	___
III	─┼─	___	VI	_____	___

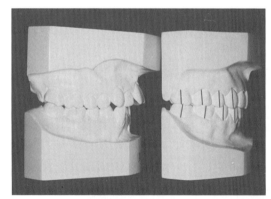
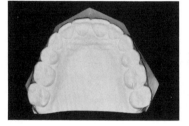
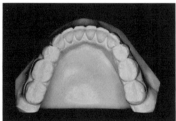
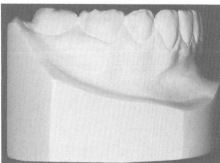

Fig. 14.157

Ortho __9__   Patient __12__   NE____   E____

Key		Grade	Key		Grade
I	_____	___	IV	─┼─	___
II	─┼─	___	V	─┼─	___
III	─┼─	___	VI	_____	___

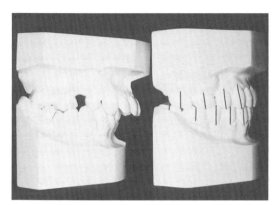
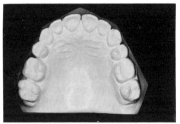
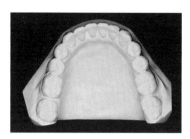

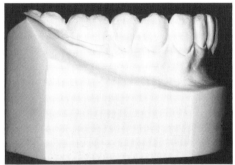

Fig. 14.158

```
Ortho   9      Patient   13        NE____       E____
Key                  Grade  Key                    Grade
I  _____  ___    IV _____|_____  ___
II _____|_____ ___   V  _____|_____  ___
III _____|_____ ___  VI _____  ___
```

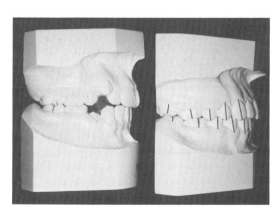
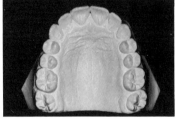
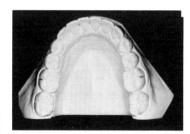

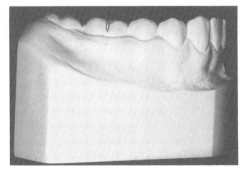

Fig. 14.159

```
Ortho   9      Patient   14        NE____       E____
Key                  Grade  Key                    Grade
I  _____  ___    IV _____|_____  ___
II _____|_____ ___   V  _____|_____  ___
III _____|_____ ___  VI _____  ___
```

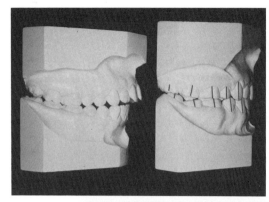

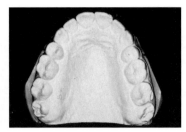

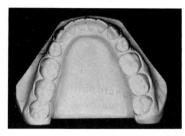

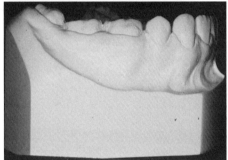

Fig. 14.160

Ortho 9	Patient 15	NE____	E____
Key	Grade	Key	Grade
I	____	IV ———|———	____
II ———|———	____	V ———|———	____
III ———|———	____	VI ————————	____

Summary for Orthodontist 9			
Patients 15	NE____	E____	
Keys	50% or more	Less than 50%, but significant	Grade
I	————————	————————	____
II	———|———	———|———	
III	———|———	———|———	
IV	———|———	———|———	
V	————————	————————	
VI	————————	————————	

ORTHODONTIST #10

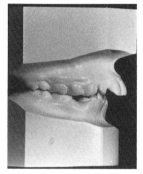
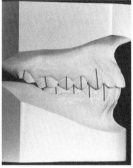
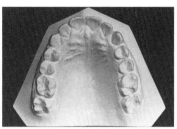
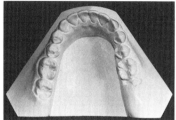

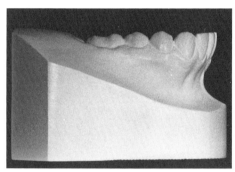

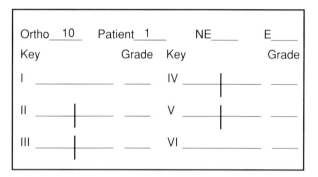

Fig. 14.161

Ortho 10	Patient 1	NE	E
Key	Grade	Key	Grade
I		IV	
II		V	
III		VI	

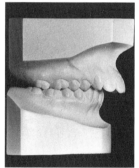
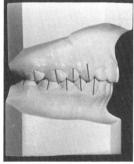
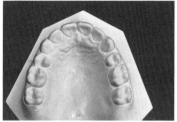
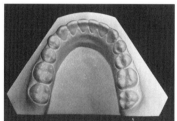

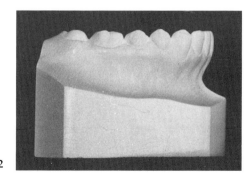

Fig. 14.162

Ortho 10	Patient 2	NE	E
Key	Grade	Key	Grade
I		IV	
II		V	
III		VI	

343

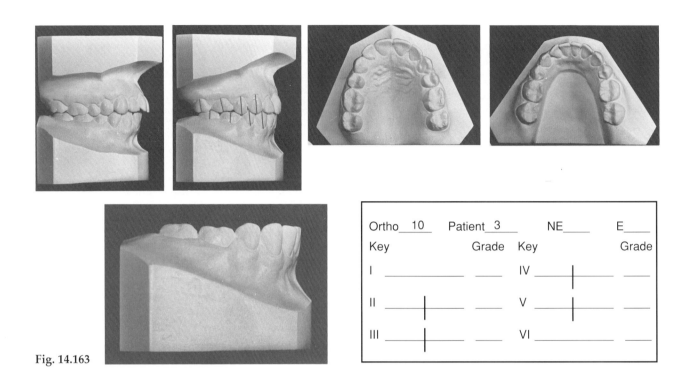

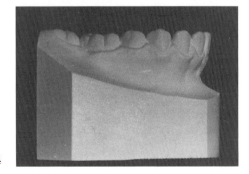

Fig. 14.163

Ortho __10__	Patient __3__		NE____		E____
Key		Grade	Key		Grade
I			IV	╪	
II	╪		V	╪	
III	╪		VI		

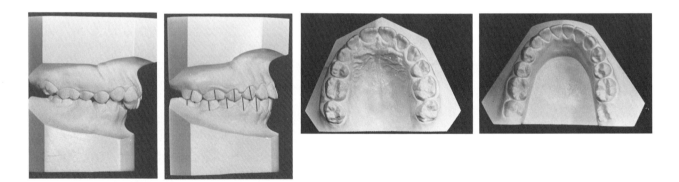

Fig. 14.164

Ortho __10__	Patient __4__		NE____		E____
Key		Grade	Key		Grade
I			IV	╪	
II	╪		V	╪	
III	╪		VI		

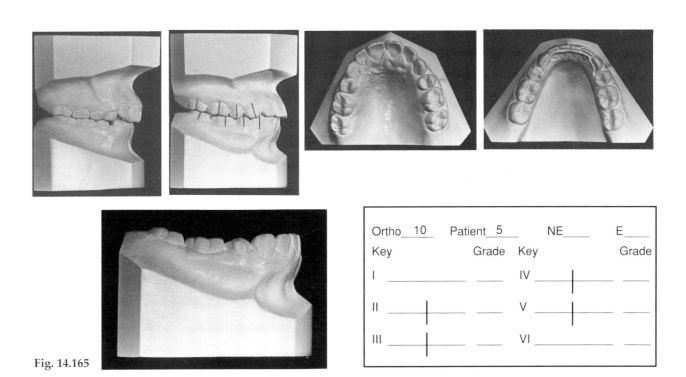

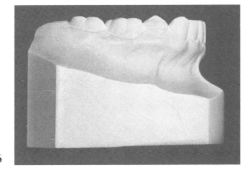

Fig. 14.165

Ortho___10___   Patient___5___   NE_____   E_____

Key		Grade	Key		Grade
I	_____	___	IV	_╪_	___
II	_╪_	___	V	_╪_	___
III	_╪_	___	VI	_____	___

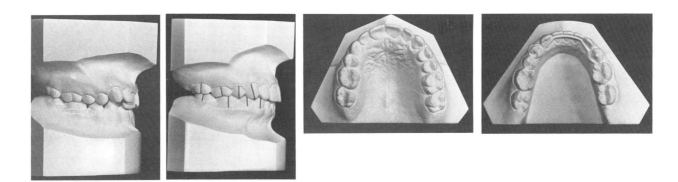

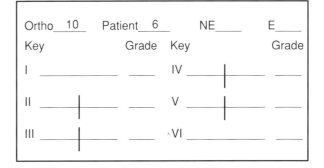

Fig. 14.166

Ortho___10___   Patient___6___   NE_____   E_____

Key		Grade	Key		Grade
I	_____	___	IV	_╪_	___
II	_╪_	___	V	_╪_	___
III	_╪_	___	VI	_____	___

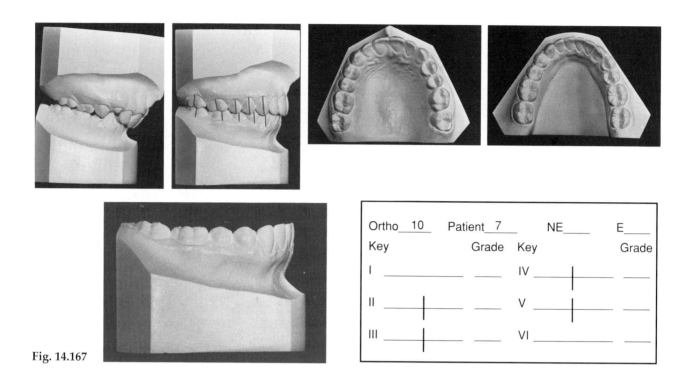

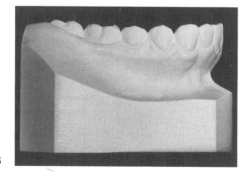

Fig. 14.167

Ortho 10	Patient 7		NE____	E____
Key		Grade	Key	Grade
I			IV	
II			V	
III			VI	

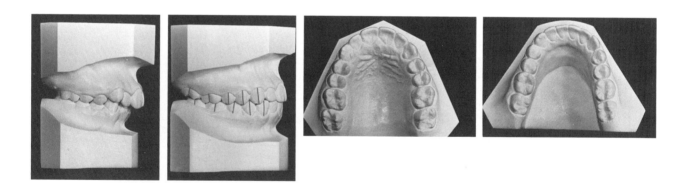

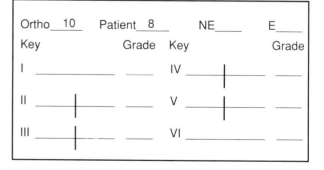

Fig. 14.168

Ortho 10	Patient 8		NE____	E____
Key		Grade	Key	Grade
I			IV	
II			V	
III			VI	

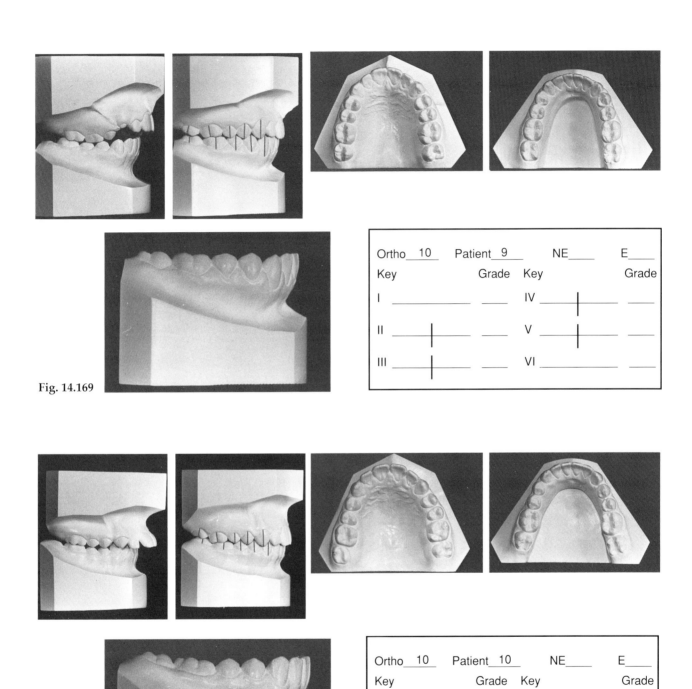

Fig. 14.169

Ortho __10__ Patient __9__ NE____ E____

Fig. 14.170

Ortho __10__ Patient __10__ NE____ E____

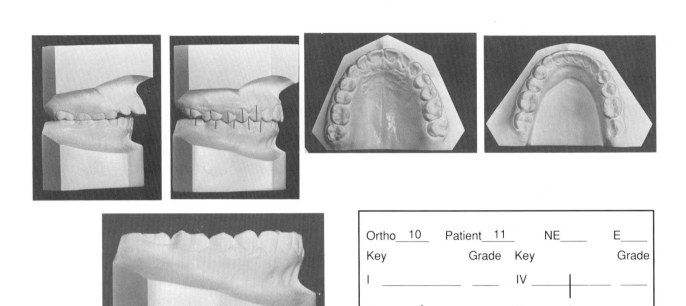

Fig. 14.171

Ortho __10__   Patient __11__   NE ____   E ____

Key	Grade	Key	Grade
I		IV ——┼——	
II ——┼——		V ——┼——	
III ——┼——		VI	

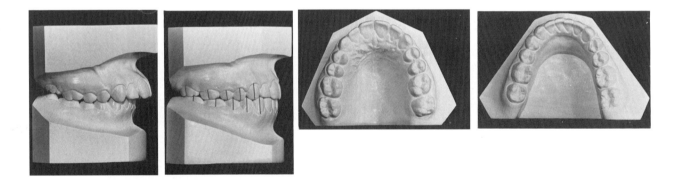

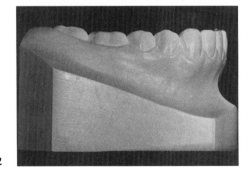

Fig. 14.172

Ortho __10__   Patient __12__   NE ____   E ____

Key	Grade	Key	Grade
I		IV ——┼——	
II ——┼——		V ——┼——	
III ——┼——		VI	

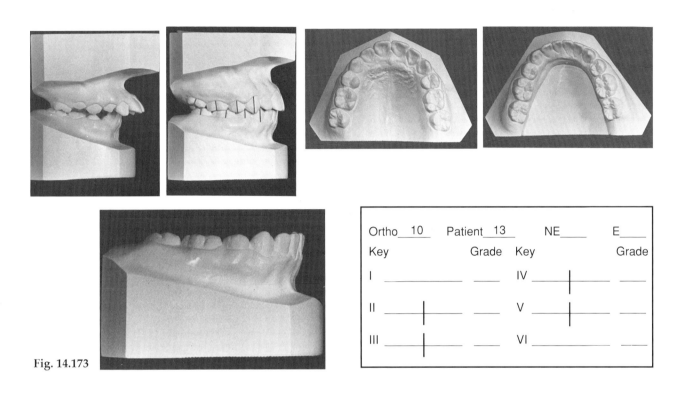

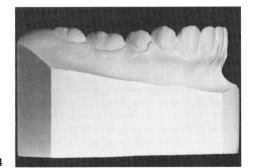

Fig. 14.173

Ortho 10   Patient 13   NE____   E____

Key		Grade	Key		Grade
I	_____	___	IV	___╫___	___
II	___╫___	___	V	___╫___	___
III	___╫___	___	VI	_____	___

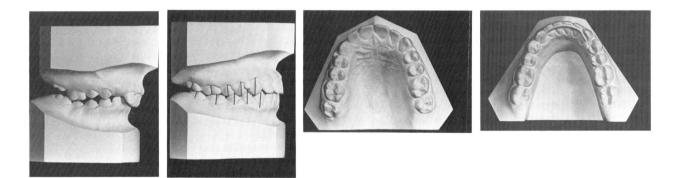

Fig. 14.174

Ortho 10   Patient 14   NE____   E____

Key		Grade	Key		Grade
I	_____	___	IV	___╫___	___
II	___╫___	___	V	___╫___	___
III	___╫___	___	VI	_____	___

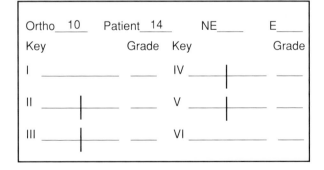

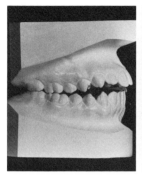 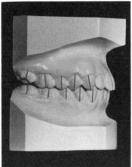 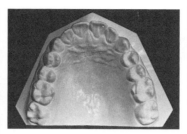 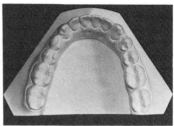

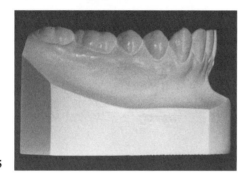

Fig. 14.175

Ortho___10___   Patient___15___   NE_____   E_____

Key		Grade	Key		Grade
I	_____	____	IV	_____+_____	____
II	_____+_____	____	V	_____+_____	____
III	_____+_____	____	VI	_____	____

Summary for Orthodontist ___10___

Patients ___15___   NE_____   E_____

Keys	50% or more	Less than 50%, but significant	Grade
I	_____	_____	____
II	_____+_____	_____+_____	____
III	_____+_____	_____+_____	____
IV	_____+_____	_____+_____	____
V	_____	_____	____
VI	_____	_____	____

ORTHODONTIST #11

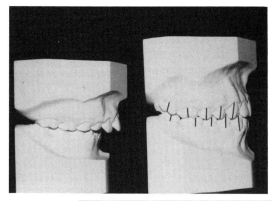
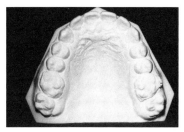
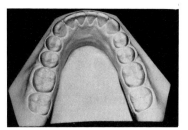

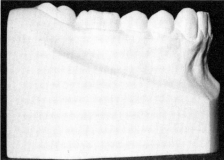

Ortho __11__ Patient __1__ NE____ E____

Key		Grade	Key		Grade
I	_____	___	IV	___|___	___
II	__|___	___	V	___|___	___
III	__|___	___	VI	_____	___

Fig. 14.176

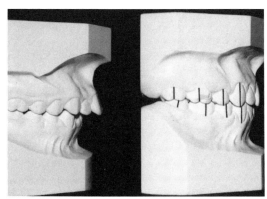
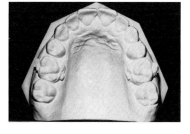
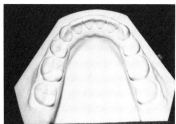

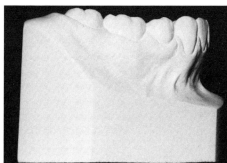

Ortho __11__ Patient __2__ NE____ E____

Key		Grade	Key		Grade
I	_____	___	IV	___|___	___
II	__|___	___	V	___|___	___
III	__|___	___	VI	_____	___

Fig. 14.177

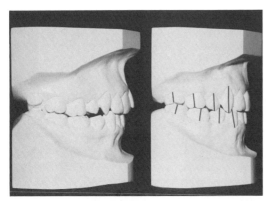
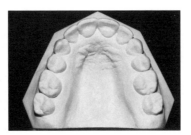
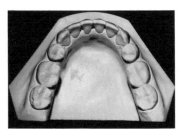

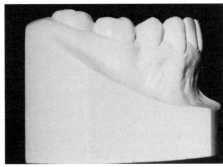

Fig. 14.178

Ortho __11__   Patient __3__   NE____   E____

Key		Grade	Key		Grade
I			IV	╪	
II	╪		V	╪	
III	╪		VI		

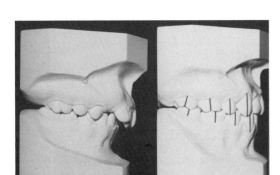
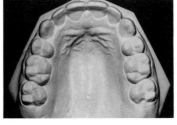
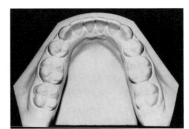

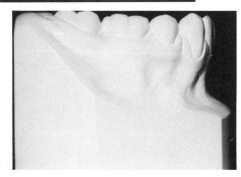

Fig. 14.179

Ortho __11__   Patient __4__   NE____   E____

Key		Grade	Key		Grade
I			IV	╪	
II	╪		V	╪	
III	╪		VI		

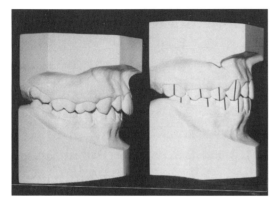
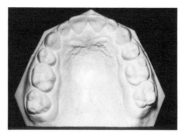
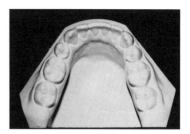

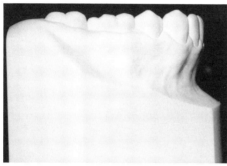

Fig. 14.180

Ortho 11	Patient 5	NE____	E____
Key	Grade	Key	Grade
I _____ ___		IV _____|___ ___	
II _____|___ ___		V _____|___ ___	
III _____|___ ___		VI _____ ___	

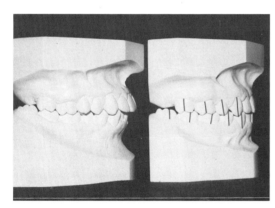
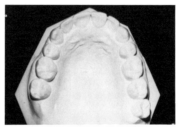
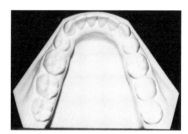

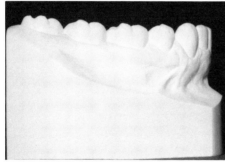

Fig. 14.181

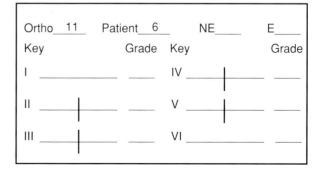

Ortho 11	Patient 6	NE____	E____
Key	Grade	Key	Grade
I _____ ___		IV _____|___ ___	
II _____|___ ___		V _____|___ ___	
III _____|___ ___		VI _____ ___	

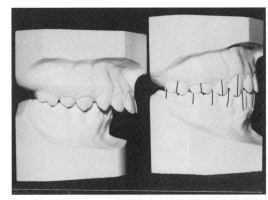
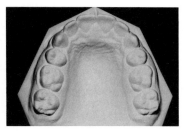
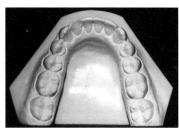

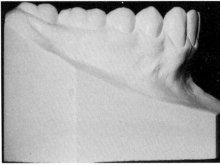

Fig. 14.182

Ortho __11__   Patient __7__   NE____   E____

Key		Grade	Key		Grade
I			IV		
II			V		
III			VI		

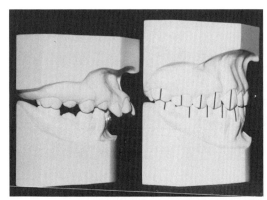
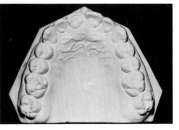
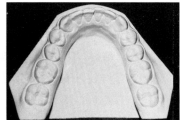

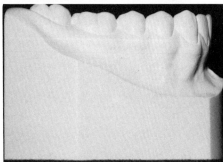

Fig. 14.183

Ortho __11__   Patient __8__   NE____   E____

Key		Grade	Key		Grade
I			IV		
II			V		
III			VI		

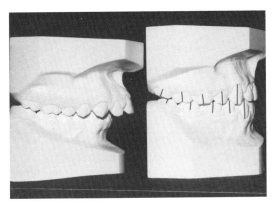
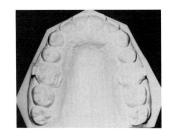
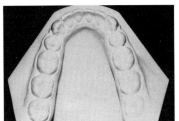

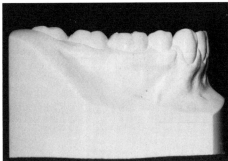

Fig. 14.184

Ortho __11__	Patient __9__	NE ____	E ____
Key	Grade	Key	Grade
I _____	____	IV ___┃___	____
II ___┃___	____	V ___┃___	____
III ___┃___	____	VI _____	

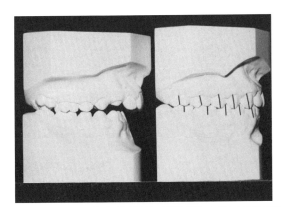
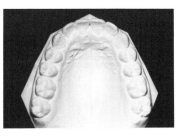
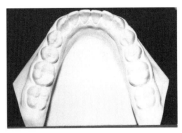

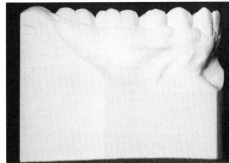

Fig. 14.185

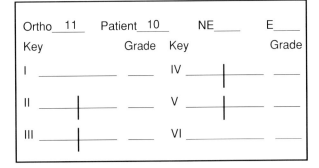

Ortho __11__	Patient __10__	NE ____	E ____
Key	Grade	Key	Grade
I _____	____	IV ___┃___	____
II ___┃___	____	V ___┃___	____
III ___┃___	____	VI _____	

355

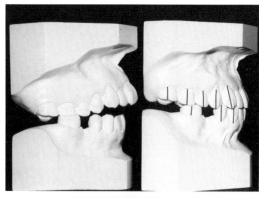
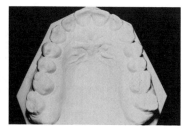
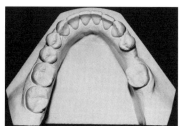

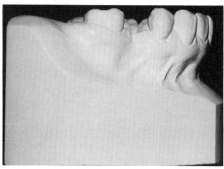

Fig. 14.186

Ortho 11	Patient 11	NE____	E____
Key	Grade	Key	Grade
I		IV	
II		V	
III		VI	

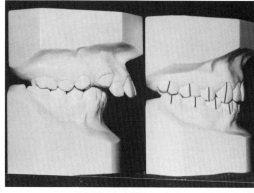
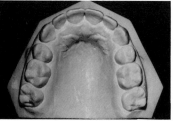
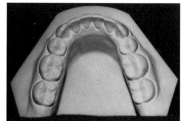

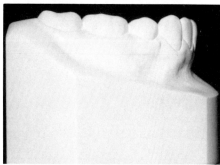

Fig. 14.187

Ortho 11	Patient 12	NE____	E____
Key	Grade	Key	Grade
I		IV	
II		V	
III		VI	

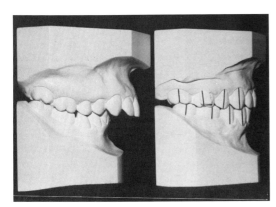
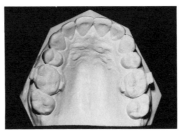
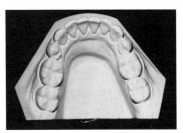

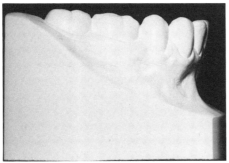

Fig. 14.188

Ortho__11__	Patient__13__	NE____	E____
Key	Grade	Key	Grade
I _____	___	IV __┃___	___
II __┃___	___	V __┃___	___
III __┃___	___	VI _____	___

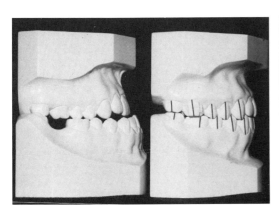
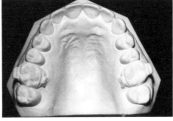
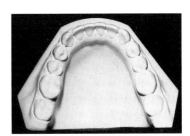

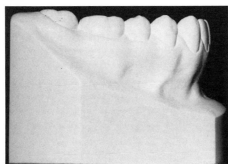

Fig. 14.189

Ortho__11__	Patient__14__	NE____	E____
Key	Grade	Key	Grade
I _____	___	IV __┃___	___
II __┃___	___	V __┃___	___
III __┃___	___	VI _____	___

357

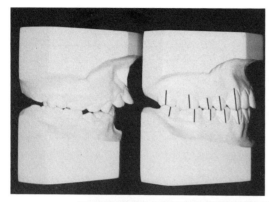
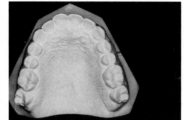
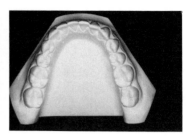
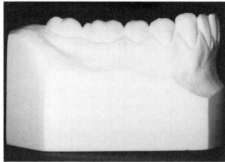

Fig. 14.190

```
Ortho___11___    Patient___15___      NE_____      E_____

Key                        Grade    Key                    Grade

I  _____  _____     IV  _____|_____  _____

II  _____|_____  _____     V  _____|_____  _____

III _____|_____  _____    VI  _____  _____
```

```
Summary for Orthodontist ___11___

Patients ___15___        NE_____            E_____

Keys     50% or more     Less than 50%,     Grade
                         but significant

I    _____  _____  _____

II   _____|_____  _____|_____  _____

III  _____|_____  _____|_____  _____

IV   _____|_____  _____|_____  _____

V    _____  _____  _____

VI   _____  _____  _____
```

ORTHODONTIST #12

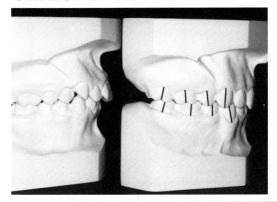
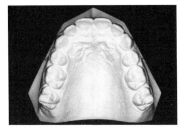
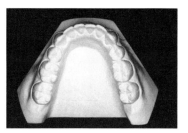

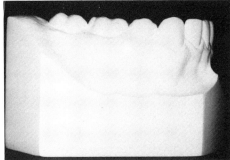

Fig. 14.191

Ortho __12__   Patient __1__   NE____   E____

Key		Grade	Key		Grade
I	_____	____	IV	___|____	____
II	___|____	____	V	___|____	____
III	___|____	____	VI	_____	____

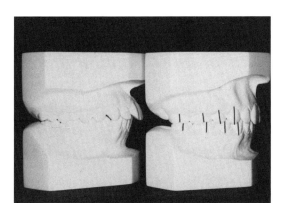
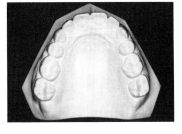
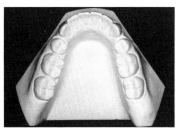

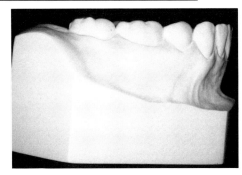

Fig. 14.192

Ortho __12__   Patient __2__   NE____   E____

Key		Grade	Key		Grade
I	_____	____	IV	___|____	____
II	___|____	____	V	___|____	____
III	___|____	____	VI	_____	____

359

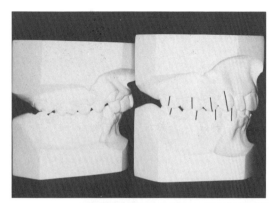
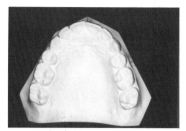
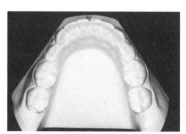

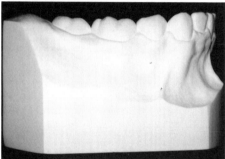

Fig. 14.193

Ortho __12__   Patient __3__   NE____   E____

Key		Grade	Key		Grade
I			IV		
II			V		
III			VI		

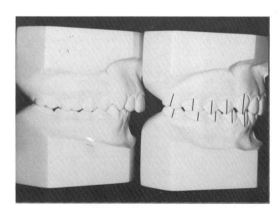
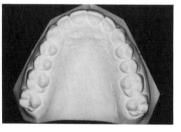
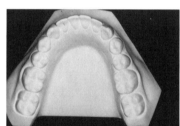

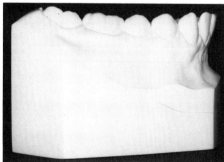

Fig. 14.194

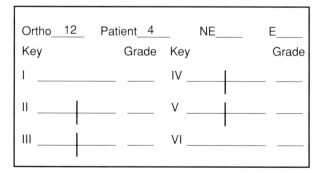

Ortho __12__   Patient __4__   NE____   E____

Key		Grade	Key		Grade
I			IV		
II			V		
III			VI		

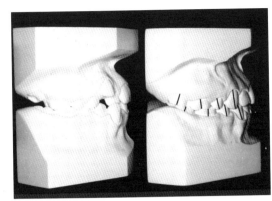
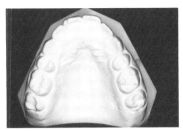
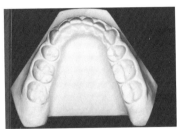

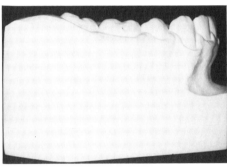

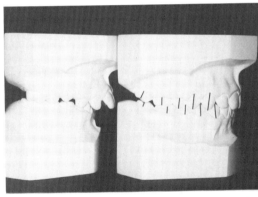

Fig. 14.195

Ortho	12	Patient	5		NE		E	
Key			Grade	Key				Grade
I				IV				
II				V				
III				VI				

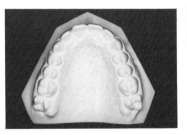
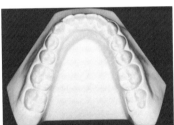

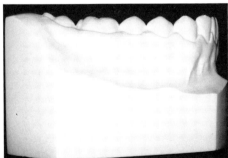

Fig. 14.196

Ortho	12	Patient	6		NE		E	
Key			Grade	Key				Grade
I				IV				
II				V				
III				VI				

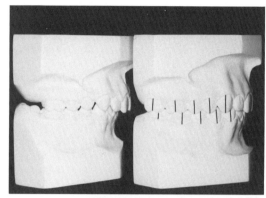
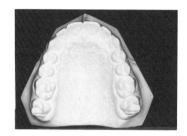
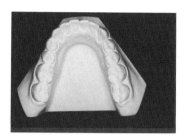

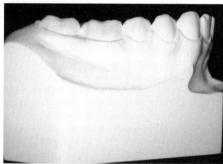

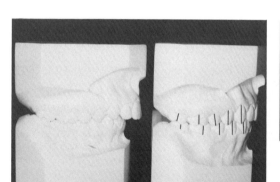

Fig. 14.197

Ortho 12	Patient 7	NE	E
Key	Grade	Key	Grade
I _____	___	IV ___|___	___
II ___|___	___	V ___|___	___
III ___|___	___	VI _____	

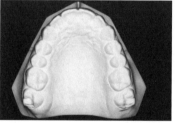
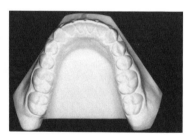

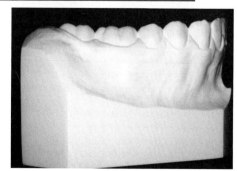

Fig. 14.198

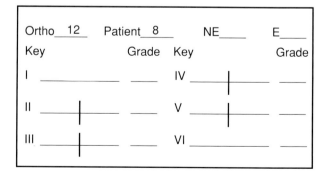

Ortho 12	Patient 8	NE	E
Key	Grade	Key	Grade
I _____	___	IV ___|___	___
II ___|___	___	V ___|___	___
III ___|___	___	VI _____	___

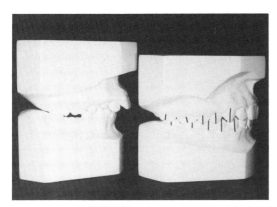
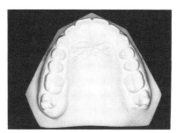
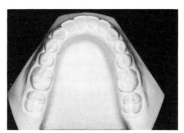

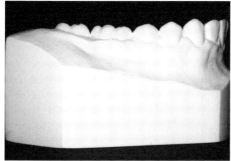

Fig. 14.199

Ortho __12__   Patient __9__   NE____   E____

Key	Grade	Key	Grade
I		IV	
II		V	
III		VI	

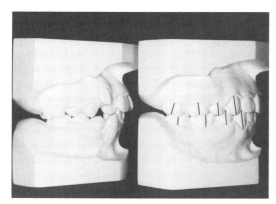
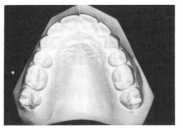
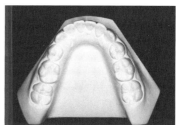

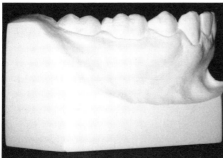

Fig. 14.200

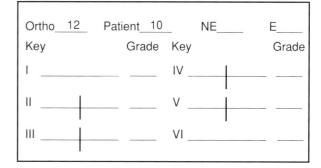

Ortho __12__   Patient __10__   NE____   E____

Key	Grade	Key	Grade
I		IV	
II		V	
III		VI	

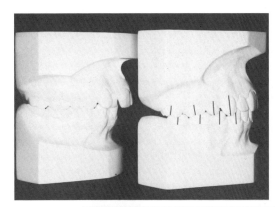
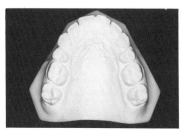
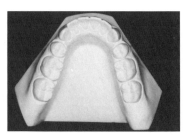

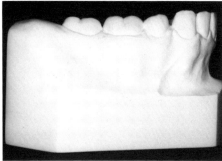

Fig. 14.201

Ortho 12	Patient 11	NE	E
Key	Grade	Key	Grade
I		IV	
II		V	
III		VI	

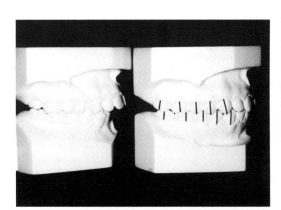
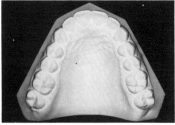
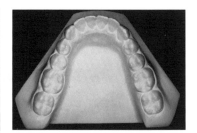

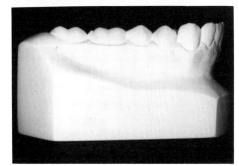

Fig. 14.202

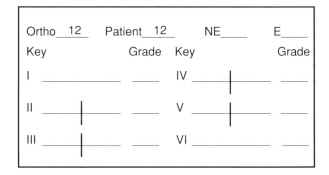

Ortho 12	Patient 12	NE	E
Key	Grade	Key	Grade
I		IV	
II		V	
III		VI	

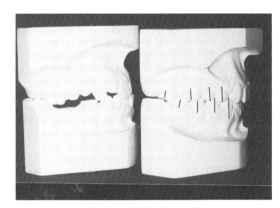

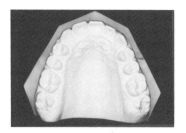

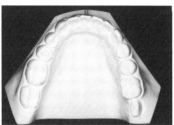

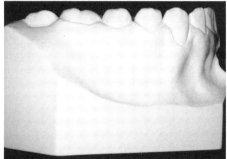

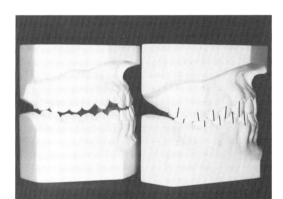

Fig. 14.203

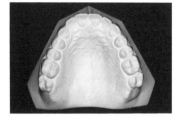

Ortho 12	Patient 13	NE ____	E ____
Key	Grade	Key	Grade
I	_____	IV —|—	____
II —|—	____	V —|—	____
III —|—	____	VI	____

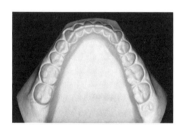

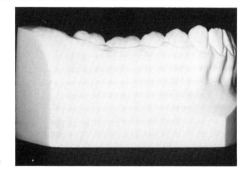

Fig. 14.204

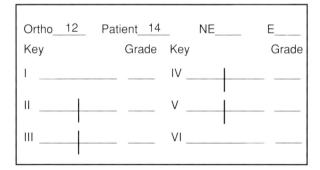

Ortho 12	Patient 14	NE ____	E ____
Key	Grade	Key	Grade
I	_____	IV —|—	____
II —|—	____	V —|—	____
III —|—	____	VI	____

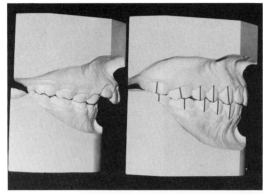

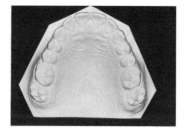

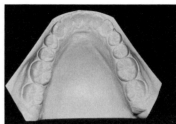

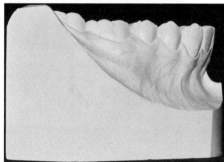

Fig. 14.205

Ortho __12__   Patient __15__   NE____   E____

Key		Grade	Key		Grade
I	_____	____	IV	_____|_____	____
II	____|____	____	V	____|____	____
III	____|____	____	VI	_____	____

Summary for Orthodontist __12__

Patients __15__   NE_____   E____

Keys	50% or more	Less than 50%, but significant	Grade
I	_____	_____	____
II	____|____	____|____	
III	____|____	____|____	
IV	____|____	____|____	
V	_____	_____	
VI	_____	_____	

ORTHODONTIST #13

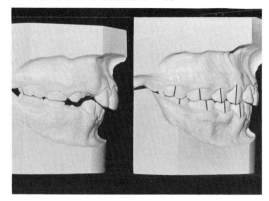

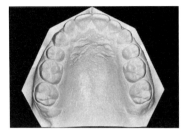

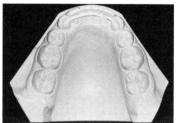

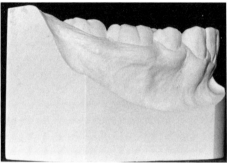

Fig. 14.206

Ortho __13__   Patient __1__   NE____   E____

Key		Grade	Key		Grade
I			IV		
II			V		
III			VI		

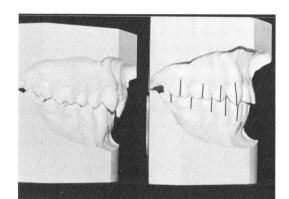

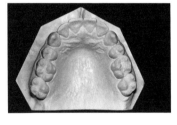

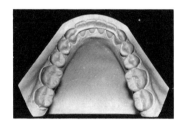

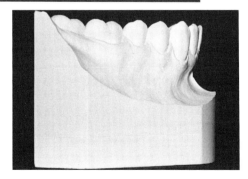

Fig. 14.207

Ortho __13__   Patient __2__   NE____   E____

Key		Grade	Key		Grade
I			IV		
II			V		
III			VI		

367

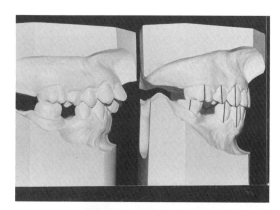

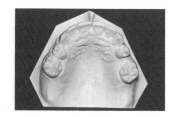

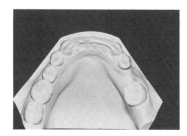

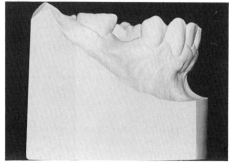

Ortho __13__	Patient __3__	NE____	E____
Key	Grade	Key	Grade
I	____	IV ──┼──	____
II ──┼──	____	V ──┼──	____
III ──┼──	____	VI	

Fig. 14.208

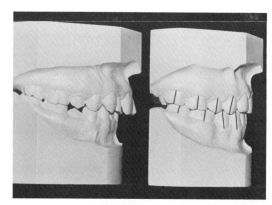

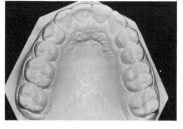

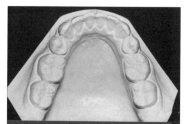

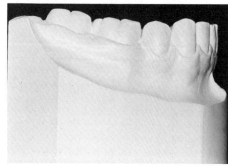

Ortho __13__	Patient __4__	NE____	E____
Key	Grade	Key	Grade
I	____	IV ──┼──	____
II ──┼──	____	V ──┼──	____
III ──┼──	____	VI	

Fig. 14.209

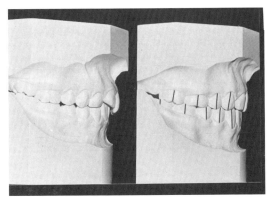
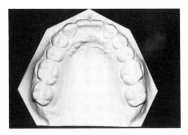
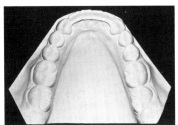

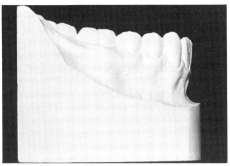

Fig. 14.210

Ortho __13__   Patient __5__   NE____   E____
Key   Grade Key   Grade
I _____ ____   IV _____|_____ ____
II _____|_____ ____   V _____|_____ ____
III _____|_____ ____   VI _____ ____

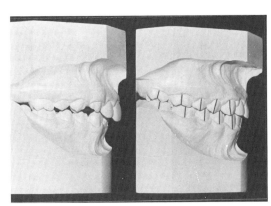
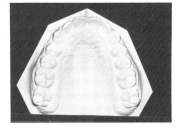
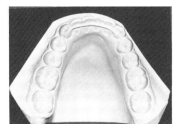

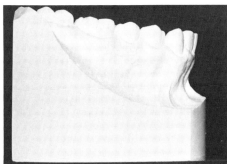

Fig. 14.211

Ortho __13__   Patient __6__   NE____   E____
Key   Grade Key   Grade
I _____ ____   IV _____|_____ ____
II _____|_____ ____   V _____|_____ ____
III _____|_____ ____   VI _____ ____

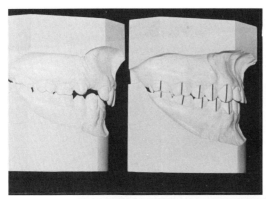
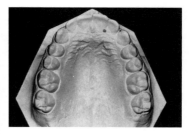
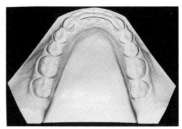

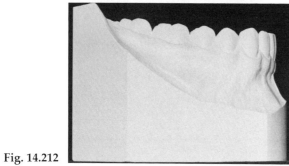

Fig. 14.212

Ortho 13		Patient 7		NE____		E____	
Key		Grade	Key			Grade	
I	_____	____	IV	___|___		____	
II	___|___	____	V	___|___		____	
III	___|___	____	VI	_____		____	

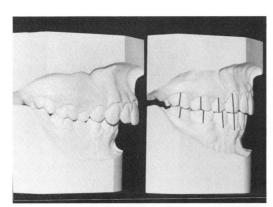
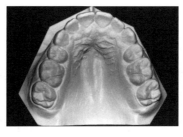
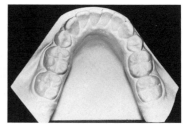

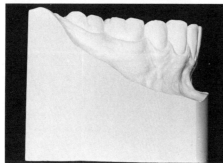

Fig. 14.213

Ortho 13		Patient 8		NE____		E____	
Key		Grade	Key			Grade	
I	_____	____	IV	___|___		____	
II	___|___	____	V	___|___		____	
III	___|___	____	VI	_____		____	

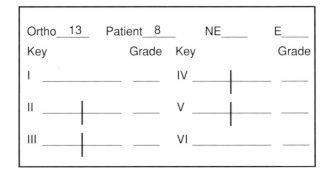

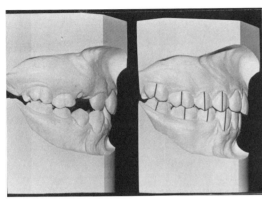
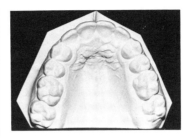
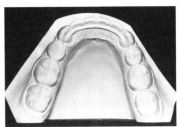

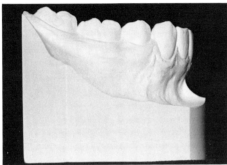

Fig. 14.214

Ortho___13___ Patient__9___   NE____   E____

Key		Grade	Key		Grade
I	_____	__	IV	___|___	__
II	___|___	__	V	___|___	__
III	___|___	__	VI	_____	__

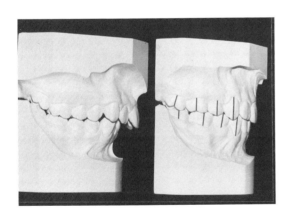
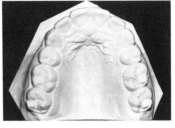
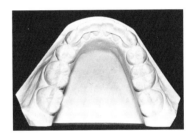

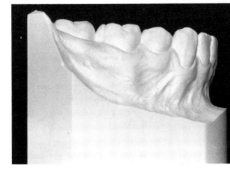

Fig. 14.215

Ortho___13___ Patient__10___   NE____   E____

Key		Grade	Key		Grade
I	_____	__	IV	___|___	__
II	___|___	__	V	___|___	__
III	___|___	__	VI	_____	__

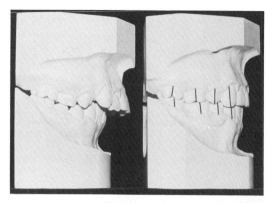
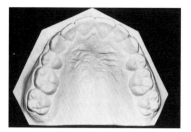
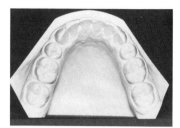

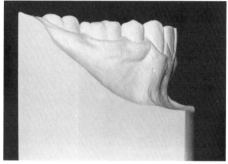

Fig. 14.216

Ortho___13___ Patient___11___   NE_____ E_____

Key		Grade	Key		Grade
I			IV		
II			V		
III			VI		

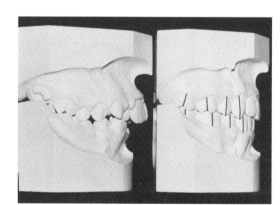
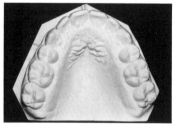
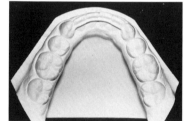

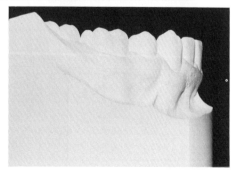

Fig. 14.217

Ortho___13___ Patient___12___   NE_____ E_____

Key		Grade	Key		Grade
I			IV		
II			V		
III			VI		

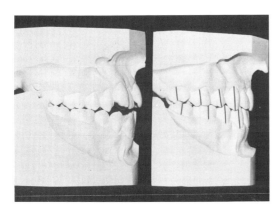
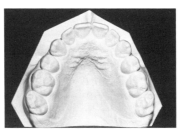
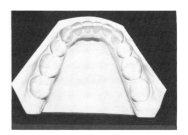

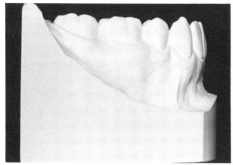

Fig. 14.218

Ortho 13	Patient 13	NE	E
Key	Grade	Key	Grade
I _____ ___		IV ____|____ ___	
II ___|___ ___		V ____|____ ___	
III ___|___ ___		VI _____ ___	

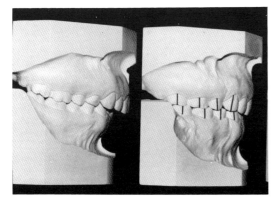
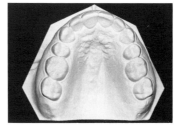
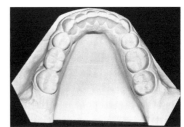

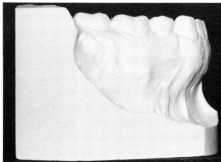

Fig. 14.219

Ortho 13	Patient 14	NE	E
Key	Grade	Key	Grade
I _____ ___		IV ___|____ ___	
II ___|___ ___		V ___|____ ___	
III ___|___ ___		VI _____ ___	

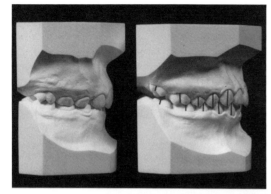
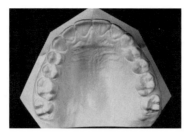
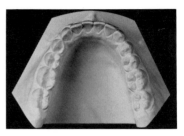
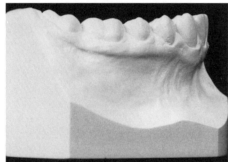

Fig. 14.220

Ortho 13	Patient 15	NE___	E___

Key	Grade	Key	Grade
I	___	IV —+—	___
II —+—	___	V —+—	___
III —+—	___	VI	___

Summary for Orthodontist 13
Patients 15   NE____   E____

Keys	50% or more	Less than 50%, but significant	Grade
I			
II	—+—	—+—	
III	—+—	—+—	
IV	—+—	—+—	
V			
VI			

ORTHODONTIST #14

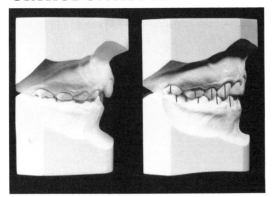
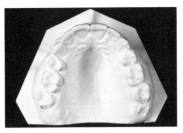
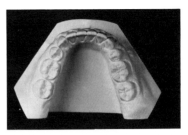

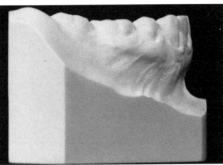

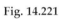

Ortho 14	Patient 1	NE	E
Key	Grade	Key	Grade
I		IV	
II		V	
III		VI	

Fig. 14.221

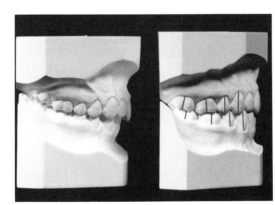
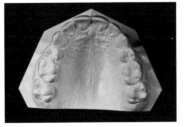
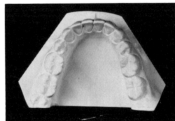

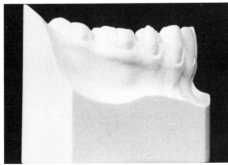

Ortho 14	Patient 2	NE	E
Key	Grade	Key	Grade
I		IV	
II		V	
III		VI	

Fig. 14.222

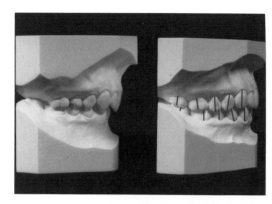
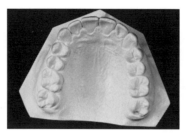
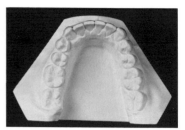

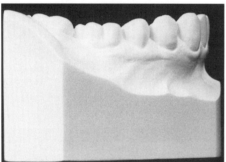

Fig. 14.223

Ortho 14	Patient 3		NE		E
Key		Grade	Key		Grade
I			IV	+	
II	+		V	+	
III	+		VI		

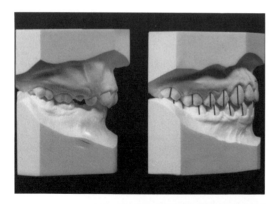
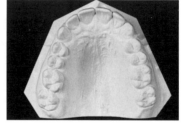
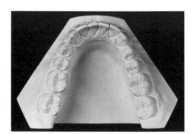

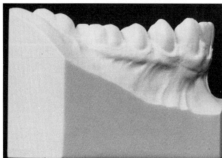

Fig. 14.224

Ortho 14	Patient 4		NE		E
Key		Grade	Key		Grade
I			IV	+	
II	+		V	+	
III	+		VI		

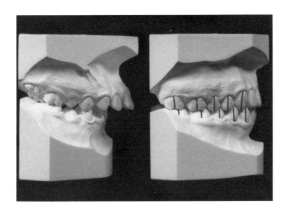
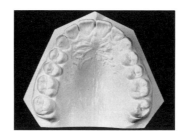
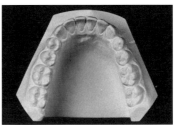

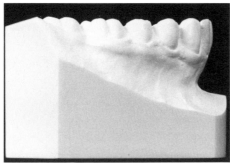

Fig. 14.225

Ortho	14	Patient	5	NE		E	
Key			Grade	Key			Grade
I				IV	†		
II	†			V	†		
III	†			VI			

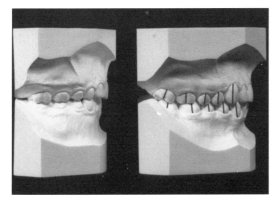
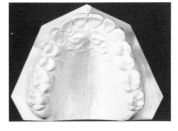
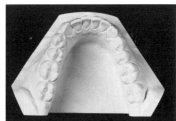

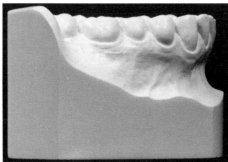

Fig. 14.226

Ortho	14	Patient	6	NE		E	
Key			Grade	Key			Grade
I				IV	†		
II	†			V	†		
III	†			VI			

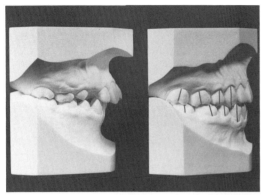
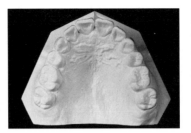
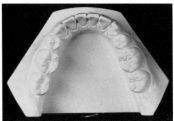

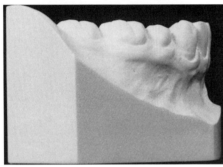

Fig. 14.227

Ortho __14__   Patient __7__   NE____   E____

Key	Grade	Key	Grade
I		IV	
II		V	
III		VI	

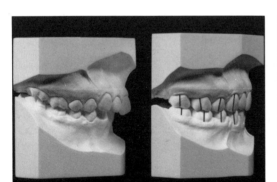
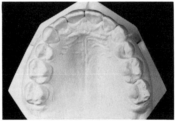
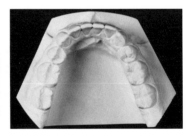

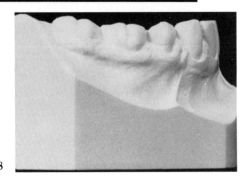

Fig. 14.228

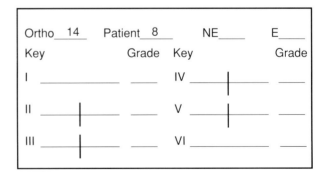

Ortho __14__   Patient __8__   NE____   E____

Key	Grade	Key	Grade
I		IV	
II		V	
III		VI	

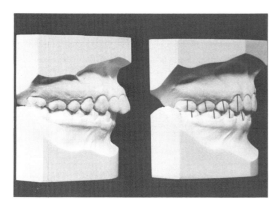
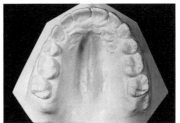
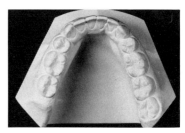

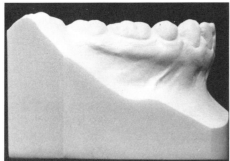

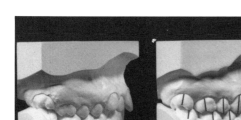

Fig. 14.229

Ortho ___14___   Patient ___9___   NE_____   E_____

Key		Grade	Key		Grade
I			IV		
II			V		
III			VI		

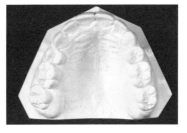
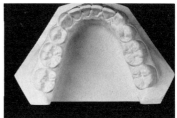

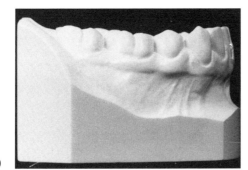

Fig. 14.230

Ortho ___14___   Patient ___10___   NE_____   E_____

Key		Grade	Key		Grade
I			IV		
II			V		
III			VI		

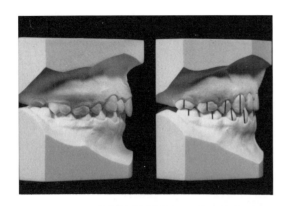
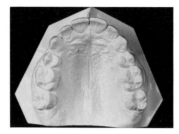
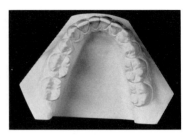

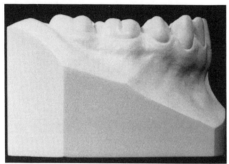

Fig. 14.231

Ortho 14	Patient 11	NE____	E____
Key	Grade	Key	Grade
I _____	____	IV ___|___	____
II ___|___	____	V ___|___	____
III ___|___	____	VI _____	____

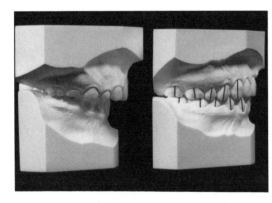
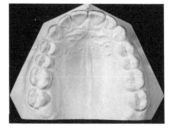
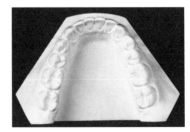

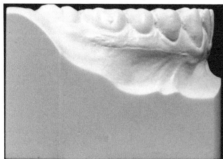

Fig. 14.232

Ortho 14	Patient 12	NE____	E____
Key	Grade	Key	Grade
I _____	____	IV ___|___	____
II ___|___	____	V ___|___	____
III ___|___	____	VI _____	____

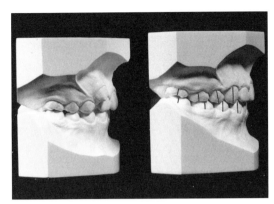
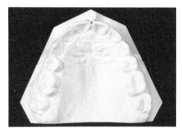
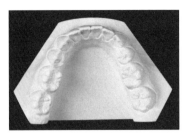
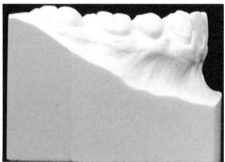

Ortho 14   Patient 13   NE____   E____

Key		Grade	Key		Grade
I	_____	__	IV	―|―	__
II	―|―	__	V	―|―	__
III	―|―	__	VI	_____	__

Fig. 14.233

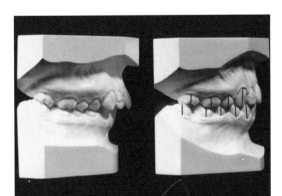
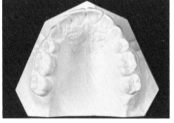
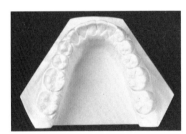
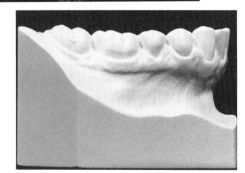
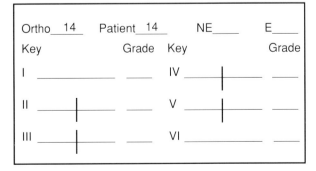

Ortho 14   Patient 14   NE____   E____

Key		Grade	Key		Grade
I	_____	__	IV	―|―	__
II	―|―	__	V	―|―	__
III	―|―	__	VI	_____	__

Fig. 14.234

381

Summary for Orthodontist __14__

Patients __14__   NE_____   E____

Keys	50% or more	Less than 50%, but significant	Grade
I	_____	_____	____
II	_____|_____	_____|_____	____
III	_____|_____	_____|_____	____
IV	_____|_____	_____|_____	____
V	_____	_____	____
VI	_____	_____	____

Appendix

Measurement Data Results for 120 Optimal Occlusions*
(See Chapter 4)

Cast No.		Maxillary Arch Angulation							Mandibular Arch Angulation						
		1	2	3	4	5	6	7	1	2	3	4	5	6	7
1	Left	5	8	9	3	4	6	6	1	2	5	2	3	2	2
	Right	5	7	9	2	2	6	4	2	2	6	2	2	2	2
2	Left	4	6	7	2	2	6	6	2	2	7	4	4	3	3
	Right	0	4	3	2	2	2		-2	-2	4	4	2	6	6
3	Left	2	6	10	2	2	5	2	0	2	5	2	2	2	2
	Right	4	7	10	2	2	5	4	0	2	5	2	2	2	2
4	Left	4	8	6	4	4	5	-4	-2	-2	0	0	2	-1	2
	Right	5	6	6	4	4	7	0	-2	-3	1	2	2	2	3
5	Left	5	9	11	4	4	6	5	1	-2	3	2	2	2	4
	Right	-1	5	10	4	3	7	0	1	-2	2	2	2	2	4
6	Left	4	9	10	4	4	7	4	2	0	5	2	2	2	3
	Right	4	8	8	2	2	6	-6	0	-1	2	2	2	2	2
7	Left	5	11	8	2	2	7	0	1	0	5	2	2	2	3
	Right	5	9	10	2	2	7	-3	0	1	5	2	2	2	2
8	Left	5	6	3	0	0	5	5	2	2	0	1	1	1	2
	Right	4	7	5	2	2	7	0	1	1	3	2	2	4	4
9	Left	5	7	8	3	2	4	4	2	2	-1	2	2	2	2
	Right	5	8	6	0	0	2		1	2	6	2	2	3	3
10	Left	6	9	8	3	3	5	-6	2	0	-3	0	0	2	2
	Right	2	8	5	2	2	6	6	1	0	0	1	1	2	2
11	Left	2	4	9	2	2	5	3	1	1	6	2	2	2	3
	Right	2	5	9	0	1	4	4	0	1	4	2	2	2	4
12	Left	4	8	14	6	6	8	-8	1	1	4	2	1	2	4
	Right	4	6	12	3	3	7	-23	1	1	3	1	3	5	5
13	Left	3	6	4	2	2	6	4	2	2	7	4	3	3	3
	Right	4	7	9	1	2	6	0	2	2	5	1	2	2	2
14	Left	5	9	8	4	4	6	2	1	1	5	2	2	2	2
	Right	4	7	9	2	2	6	4	1	1	7	2	1	2	3
15	Left	3	7	7	2	2	6	2	2	2	2	2	3	3	3
	Right	4	7	8	2	2	6	4	2	1	3	2	2	2	2
16	Left	3	8	8	3	3	6	3	1	0	7	2	2	2	2
	Right	3	8	8	3	3	6	0	1	2	2	2	2	2	3
17	Left	5	7	11	4	4	8	7	0	-2	-2	0	0	2	3
	Right	3	7	4	4	4	7	1	0	1	-1	-1	0	0	2
18	Left	3	8	11	4	4	7	7	2	2	5	2	2	2	2
	Right	4	9	11	4	4	7	5	3	2	7	4	3	2	2
19	Left	4	7	7	2	2	5	5	2	2	4	2	2	2	2
	Right	4	7	9	4	4	6	6	2	2	1	1	2	2	2
20	Left	5	12	10	3	3	7	7	3	1	4	0	2	2	2
	Right	4	8	6	3	3	5	5	-1	-1	3	0	1	2	2
21	Left	4	8	9	2	2	5	5	2	2	5	2	2	2	2
	Right	4	8	10	3	3	5	5	1	2	5	2	2	2	2
22	Left	5	8	7	2	2	5	4	2	2	2	1	1	2	2
	Right	2	7	3	0	0	3	-11	2	2	6	2	2	2	3
23	Left	5	9	10	3	2	5	0	1	1	7	2	2	2	2
	Right	4	8	11	2	2	4	-10	2	2	5	3	3	3	5
24	Left	6	11	12	3	3	5	0	0	1	3	0	0	1	2
	Right	4	7	9	3	2	4	-12	1	1	3	2	2	2	3
25	Left	5	9	10	3	3	5	-2	0	-2	0	0	0	0	0
	Right	3	7	8	2	2	5	-3	1	0	-1	0	2	2	3
26	Left	6	9	6	2	3	5	5	2	2	6	4	4	4	4
	Right	3	7	7	2	2	5	5	1	1	6	3	3	3	3
27	Left	4	8	9	3	3	6	4	1	2	6	2	2	2	3
	Right	4	6	9	1	2	5	0	1	2	5	2	2	2	3
28	Left	3	9	7	2	2	5	0	0	0	4	2	2	3	4
	Right	5	9	9	1	1	6	0	1	0	5	3	3	3	4
29	Left	5	9	9	2	3	7	6	1	2	2	-1	2	2	2
	Right	4	6	9	4	3	5	-6	0	1	1	-1	2	2	2

*Data shown here are from the 120 best samples, as of 1988. The results differ in some instances by several degrees from the 1960 sample. The 1960 data are used throughout the book and remain the values for the Straight-Wire Appliance.

Cast No.		Maxillary Arch Angulation							Mandibular Arch Angulation						
		1	2	3	4	5	6	7	1	2	3	4	5	6	7
30	Left	5	8	8	2	2	5	1	-1	-1	3	3	3	3	30
	Right	3	8	8	2	2	5	-10	2	-1	3	3	4	5	3
31	Left	5	10	11	4	4	7	3	0	-2	3	2	2	2	2
	Right	3	10	9	6	3	7	4	0	1	3	1	1	3	2
32	Left	4	9	12	5	5	10	4	1	-1	6	-1	-1	0	2
	Right	5	8	12	7	7	10	7	1	2	7	3	3	2	3
33	Left	4	11	11	3	2	5	2	-2	-2	-2	-2	-2	-2	2
	Right	2	6	9	2	2	4	-10	1	1	-2	-2	0	2	3
34	Left	5	9	2	2	2	6	0	3	0	4	0	2	2	0
	Right	5	3	7	3	6	-2		1	2	5	0	0	2	3
35	Left	4	12	12	3	3	6	2	-2	-2	-6	-6	-3	-2	2
	Right	4	2	7	2	2	5	-2	0	-1	-2	-2	-2	0	2
36	Left	4	7	7	3	2	5	-2	-2	0	3	2	2	2	2
	Right	2	-2	5	2	2	2	-6	1	1	2	0	0	2	2
37	Left	1	8	3	3	5	4		1	2	-1	-1	1	2	2
	Right	-2	7	9	2	3	5	5	2	2	4	2	2	2	4
38	Left	2	7	9	1	1	7	1	0	0	-3	2	4	4	4
	Right	2	8	11	3	3	6	-7	1	1	4	3	3	3	4
39	Left	3	6	0	4	4	8	7	2	0	-2	0	2	2	2
	Right	4	9	8	4	4	7	0	1	-1	3	2	2	2	3
40	Left	4	8	8	2	3	7	0	1	0	3	1	1	2	4
	Right	3	3	6	0	2	6	-2	-4	-2	3	3	3	3	3
41	Left	4	7	8	4	5	7	1	-1	-1	0	2	2	3	3
	Right	3	5	7	7	7	9	1	1	2	6	2	2	2	2
42	Left	4	12	0	2	3	8	-3	0	2	6	0	1	1	1
	Right	2	6	7	3	3	2	-7	2	2	3	2	2	2	4
43	Left	5	10	11	1	1	6	5	1	-2	-2	-2	-2	-2	1
	Right	4	7	9	0	1	3	2	2	-1	-2	0	2	2	4
44	Left	4	7	7	3	3	5	-3	0	-1	-6	-6	-5	-1	2
	Right	3	6	4	2	2	5	5	1	-2	-2	-1	0	2	4
45	Left	4	9	11	3	3	6	-2	1	0	4	2	2	2	2
	Right	5	10	12	3	3	5	-5	1	2	4	2	2	2	2
46	Left	6	13	12	0	0	-1	-14	0	1	2	2	3	3	4
	Right	9	12	6	6	6	-7	-1	-1	-1	-1	2	3	3	4
47	Left	3	14	7	2	3	9	4	1	0	-4	-3	1	2	4
	Right	3	9	8	-1	5	5	2	0	2	2	0	2	5	7
48	Left	2	10	4	2	2	6	6	1	1	4	2	2	2	3
	Right	2	6	5	2	2	6	-4	1	1	4	2	2	2	3
49	Left	4	8	12	4	4	7	7	0	-2	5	1	1	2	2
	Right	4	15	17	12	12	16	8	1	1	5	3	3	2	3
50	Left	4	9	9	2	2	7	4	1	1	-6	-2	0	2	3
	Right	4	15	1	12	2	5	1	0	1	3	2	0	2	3
51	Left	0	8	9	2	2	6	5	2	2	7	1	-1	2	2
	Right	0	0	8	2	2	6	2	2	2	5	0	0	2	3
52	Left	3	7	6	0	1	6	1	1	1	6	1	1	2	2
	Right	3	8	11	4	4	7	4	1	1	5	3	3	2	3
53	Left	5	15	11	2	3	5	5	1	2	7	10	3	3	3
	Right	4	10	5	3	3	6	-3	1	2	7	6	2	2	3
54	Left	4	12	11	3	3	5	-6	-1	-1	2	2	4	4	5
	Right	4	13	7	2	2	5	2	-2	-1	2	2	4	5	5
55	Left	3	6	7	2	2	3	-4	2	1	2	2	2	2	3
	Right	2	-26	7	2	5	7	-10	-2	-1	3	2	2	2	3
56	Left	3	12	1	4	4	6	3	0	-1	4	2	2	0	2
	Right	4	6	11	6	5	5	5	-1	-1	3	0	0	-1	2
57	Left	5	10	10	2	3	10	5	0	1	2	2	2	2	2
	Right	2	6	5	2	3	8	3	1	1	2	2	2	3	3
58	Left	-1	12	1	12	2	8	5	1	-2	4	2	2	2	2
	Right	2	9	14	3	3	9	5	-1	0	0	0	0	0	2
59	Left	1	7	7	6	5	5	2	1	2	0	2	2	2	2
	Right	0	2	7	2	2	5	-4	0	2	2	2	2	2	3
60	Left	2	6	8	1	1	4	-10	-2	-2	2	4	2	3	4
	Right	2	7	6	2	2	5	1	1	1	3	2	2	3	4
61	Left	6	8	1	12	3	6	6	-2	-2	3	2	0	0	3
	Right	5	8	8	0	2	5	5	0	-1	-1	0	1	2	3
62	Left	5	10	9	6	5	2	4	0	1	3	1	1	1	2
	Right	4	8	8	2	2	5	5	0	0	2	2	2	2	2
63	Left	5	8	8	3	3	7	7	1	1	5	3	3	3	3
	Right	3	4	9	2	2	5	2	0	0	3	0	2	2	2
64	Left	2	7	11	3	3	6	3	1	1	3	-1	2	2	2
	Right	0	0	2	0	2	5	-15	-1	0	4	2	2	3	4
65	Left	3	9	9	3	3	4	4	2	2	2	0	1	1	2
	Right	3	4	4	-2	1	3	0	2	2	1	2	2	2	4
66	Left	4	7	1	2	2	7	3	1	-1	-2	0	0	3	3
	Right	4	7	3	2	2	6	6	1	-1	4	0	2	2	2
67	Left	4	10	10	4	4	6	4	1	1	4	3	2	2	2
	Right	2	2	6	2	2	5	1	1	1	2	2	1	2	2
68	Left	5	6	12	5	5	7	2	0	-1	-1	0	0	2	2
	Right	4	6	6	2	2	6	-3	1	1	2	2	3	3	3
69	Left	3	9	11	3	4	7	5	-1	-1	2	2	2	2	2
	Right	2	6	7	3	3	5	5	0	1	4	2	3	2	3
70	Left	5	11	12	1	2	4	2	0	-1	5	1	2	2	2
	Right	4	7	13	4	4	7	3	1	1	6	3	3	3	3
71	Left	6	15	11	5	5	7	0	1	0	4	4	4	3	3
	Right	3	7	5	3	2	6	0	0	0	4	3	3	3	3
72	Left	-3	6	7	2	2	7	6	-2	0	0	0	0	2	2
	Right	2	5	10	2	2	7	-10	1	0	-2	1	1	1	5
73	Left	3	7	7	5	3	6	5	1	2	10	3	2	2	3
	Right	4	14	12	3	3	6	-2	1	2	10	3	2	2	2
74	Left	4	13	15	5	5	7	2	1	1	2	1	2	2	2
	Right	3	7	10	3	3	4	-8	1	1	4	2	3	3	4
75	Left	3	8	8	2	2	5	1	1	-2	3	3	2	2	2
	Right	3	5	5	2	2	5	-7	-1	-1	4	1	1	2	3
76	Left	2	9	13	4	4	6	3	1	0	4	2	2	2	2
	Right	3	8	6	3	3	8	-3	1	1	0	0	2	2	4

384

Cast No.		Maxillary Arch Angulation							Mandibular Arch Angulation						
		1	2	3	4	5	6	7	1	2	3	4	5	6	7
77	Left	5	9	5	4	4	7	-5	-1	-1	0	0	0	2	4
	Right	4	8	3	2	2	5	-4	-1	0	2	0	2	3	4
78	Left	5	10	1	14	2	5	3	1	-2	0	-2	-2	-2	1
	Right	4	8	11	1	1	5	-2	-2	-5	0	0	1	0	2
79	Left	4	12	12	3	4	11	9	-1	-2	-4	0	1	3	3
	Right	5	10	1	11	4	7	7	-1	2	-2	3	2	2	3
80	Left	4	9	9	4	4	6	6	1	2	3	1	-1	2	4
	Right	3	6	8	2	3	5	-7	2	2	2	2	2	2	4
81	Left	3	8	8	6	8	8	0	-4	-3	3	3	3	3	3
	Right	3	8	8	4	4	5	0	0	2	4	2	2	2	4
82	Left	7	14	13	7	7	9	9	2	2	6	1	0	4	4
	Right	3	7	11	4	4	6	3	-2	-4	4	2	2	2	3
83	Left	5	9	7	4	4	6	6	0	-1	0	0	0	0	0
	Right	2	4	8	3	3	7	-10	1	1	-2	0	0	0	2
84	Left	2	9	9	7	7	9	7	1	-2	3	2	2	2	2
	Right	3	8	7	5	5	7	-12	1	1	4	2	2	3	2
85	Left	5	8	12	6	6	7	-6	0	0	-2	1	1	2	3
	Right	4	9	3	1	3	7	-12	0	0	3	3	2	3	4
86	Left	5	8	9	2	2	5	2	1	1	-2	-1	0	0	2
	Right	4	8	9	3	3	4	2	0	1	1	1	1	1	3
87	Left	3	8	7	3	3	7	5	-1	-1	0	0	0	0	2
	Right	-2	8	6	4	4	6	3	1	1	4	2	2	3	2
88	Left	5	11	5	2	2	5	0	2	2	-3	-3	-3	-1	5
	Right	3	4	10	0	5	5		2	2	-1	2	2	4	3
89	Left	3	10	4	0	0	5	0	1	-2	-1	0	2	2	3
	Right	2	8	5	0	0	5	5	1	-2	0	2	2	3	4
90	Left	3	6	9	2	2	5	-1	2	2	3	2	2	2	2
	Right	3	5	9	2	0	6	-7	2	2	5	2	2	2	3
91	Left	2	12	7	4	2	5	-17	0	-1	-5	0	0	0	
	Right	3	5	5	1	1	4	-17	1	1	-2	1	1	2	
92	Left	4	12	4	0	2	5	5	2	0	-2	-1	-1	1	2
	Right	3	7	7	2	2	5	-3	-2	-4	-2	-2	-2	0	3
93	Left	3	8	2	2	2	5	-2	0	1	-4	2	0	3	3
	Right	0	4	6	0	0	5	-9	-1	0	-2	0	2	2	4
94	Left	2	7	5	2	2	8	3	-1	2	0	3	1	1	1
	Right	4	7	8	2	2	6	5	-2	0	0	0	1	1	1
95	Left	5	10	12	4	4	6	-8	1	1	3	1	1	1	3
	Right	4	9	9	3	2	4	0	0	0	3	1	1	2	4
96	Left	8	1	11	14	3	5	0	3	3	2	2	2	3	
	Right	3	6	6	1	1	4	0	1	0	0	1	2	2	
97	Left	3	6	8	3	2	5	1	1	-1	-1	-1	1	2	2
	Right	2	4	5	-1	2	4	-6	1	0	3	3	3	4	4
98	Left	3	10	12	3	3	7	7	2	2	4	2	2	2	4
	Right	4	7	6	2	2	5	5	-2	0	3	1	1	3	2
99	Left	-1	10	13	6	6	9	9	2	2	7	3	2	2	2
	Right	4	7	5	2	4	7	5	-2	-2	0	-1	0	2	2
100	Left	2	5	5	1	2	3	2	1	-1	-3	3	0	1	1
	Right	2	6	3	1	2	2	-3	1	1	0	0	0	1	2
101	Left	5	12	14	3	3	6	-12	-2	0	0	-1	0	0	0
	Right	3	7	6	3	3	5	-17	-2	1	1	2	3	4	4
102	Left	5	12	14	3	3	5	-2	-1	-2	-3	1	1	0	2
	Right	4	-1	5	1	1	5	-12	2	2	8	7	7	3	4
103	Left	5	8	10	2	2	6	6	-1	-1	-11	-10	2	2	4
	Right	5	7	6	2	2	1	1	0	1	2	2	2	3	5
104	Left	4	12	12	3	3	6	6	0	-1	5	2	2	2	3
	Right	4	8	4	2	2	6	5	1	2	5	1	1	1	2
105	Left	3	9	13	7	6	8	8	1	-2	1	4	4	4	4
	Right	4	9	10	5	4	3	3	1	1	5	2	2	2	2
106	Left	7	9	7	2	2	7	7	1	0	2	0	2	2	5
	Right	5	3	2	0	0	2	-2	1	1	2	0	1	2	4
107	Left	6	10	13	0	3	3	1	3	2	9	2	0	2	4
	Right	3	11	12	0	1	4	-7	1	1	9	0	1	3	4
108	Left	0	8	2	0	0	4	6	1	0	7	3	3	2	3
	Right	5	3	4	3	3	6	-6	0	1	4	4	1	1	2
109	Left	4	10	11	2	3	5	1	-2	1	4	0	0	2	3
	Right	6	9	10	2	3	9	9	0	1	8	2	2	3	3
110	Left	3	11	11	4	3	5	0	1	1	5	1	1	1	2
	Right	4	15	11	2	2	4	-2	0	1	6	2	2	2	3
111	Left	5	12	12	2	2	6	6	0	1	7	3	2	3	4
	Right	5	12	7	4	4	7	2	1	1	6	2	3	3	2
112	Left	1	13	8	1	2	5	5	1	-1	1	-2	1	2	2
	Right	2	10	12	4	3	7	5	1	-1	-7	-5	0	2	5
113	Left	2	7	7	-1	2	4	-2	-2	0	2	2	2	2	4
	Right	3	7	6	3	3	6	2	-2	1	12	2	3	2	3
114	Left	2	8	13	7	7	8	2	2	2	1	1	1	2	4
	Right	4	9	11	4	4	6	-6	2	2	3	2	2	2	4
115	Left	5	8	12	2	2	6	6	1	1	4	1	1	2	3
	Right	4	8	11	3	2	7	6	1	1	4	1	1	4	4
116	Left	3	8	12	2	3	4	2	0	-1	-3	-1	-1	2	3
	Right	4	9	11	2	2	6	-5	-1	0	1	2	3	3	4
117	Left	3	9	11	2	3	6	3	2	1	2	1	2	3	4
	Right	4	8	8	2	2	7	-12	0	-1	6	2	0	2	4
118	Left	7	12	9	3	5	7	5	1	1	5	2	2	2	4
	Right	7	8	7	3	5	7	-2	3	3	5	2	2	2	2
119	Left	6	10	10	3	3	6	-4	0	-2	5	2	2	2	2
	Right	5	10	10	3	3	7	-3	-2	-2	2	2	2	2	2
120	Left	7	13	12	3	2	5	5	1	0	5	2	2	2	4
	Right	6	9	15	2	2	5	-5	2	2	0	2	2	2	4
Count		240	240	240	240	240	240	238	240	240	240	240	240	240	236
Average		3.59	8.04	8.40	2.65	2.82	5.73	0.39	0.53	0.38	2.48	1.28	1.54	2.03	2.94
Std Dev		1.65	2.80	2.97	1.69	1.52	1.90	5.69	1.29	1.47	3.28	1.90	1.35	1.14	2.05
Max Value		9.00	15.00	17.00	12.00	12.00	16.00	9.00	3.00	3.00	12.00	10.00	7.00	6.00	30.00
Min Value		-3.00	-2.00	1.00	-2.00	0.00	-7.00	-23.0	-4.00	-5.00	-11.0	-10.00	-5.00	-2.00	0.00

385

Cast No.		Maxillary Arch Inclination							Mandibular Arch Inclination						
		1	2	3	4	5	6	7	1	2	3	4	5	6	7
1	Left	8	5	-2	-7	-9	-11	0	2	-2	-10	-17	-27	-30	-35
	Right	8	5	4	-7	-8	-10	-4	-2	-4	-11	-17	-22	-28	-35
2	Left	2	0	-11	-11	-8	-10	-10	-7	-6	-13	-27	-30	-32	-40
	Right	1	-1	-6	-6	-6	-15	-15	-4	-7	-15	-22	-28	-35	-40
3	Left	7	5	-7	-7	-7	-12	-8	-10	-10	-14	-22	-22	-25	-30
	Right	6	4	-9	-7	-10	-10	-9	-10	-11	-15	-22	-25	-28	-35
4	Left	7	4	-7	-7	-7	-9	-8	-9			-25	-32	-30	-35
	Right	7	4	-7	-7	-7	-9	-8	-8	-15	-17	-20	-25	-30	-35
5	Left	7	5	-5	-5	-5	-10	2	2	0	-9	-17	-27	-35	-42
	Right	6	6	-2	-3	-3	-12	-4	2	0	-11	-22	-24	-27	-35
6	Left	2	1	-9	-9	-11	-12	-12	0	0	-8	-18	-22	-30	-35
	Right	2	1	-10	-10	-10	-12	-11	0	0	-8	-17	-22	-30	-35
7	Left	12	12	0	-3	-3	-7	-5	-4	-5	-11	-22	-25	-32	-28
	Right	11	11	-5	-2	-7	-10	-4	-4	-4	-10	-20	-22	-30	-34
8	Left	3	-2	-7	-8	-8	-10	-10	0	0	-11	-25	-30	-35	-40
	Right	3	0	-8	-9	-9	-11	-8	0	0	-8	-20	-25	-30	-35
9	Left	10	9	-6	-4	-4	-7	-7	-6	-7	-22	-26	-30	-35	-40
	Right	7	5	-7	-8	-8	-11		-6	-7	-20	-25	-30	-40	-45
10	Left	2	-2	-7	-10	-10	-11	-5	-9	-12	-22	-25	-30	-35	-40
	Right	4	4	-8	-10	-8	-9	-9	-8	-8	-20	-25	-23	-30	-40
11	Left	7	3	-8	-10	-12	-12	-12	-2	-2	-12	-17	-25	-35	-40
	Right	3	-1	-10	-12	-15	-17	-17	-2	-2	-8	-17	-22	-35	-40
12	Left	12	13	-6	-5	-5	-6	0	-1	-2	-11	-17	-22	-30	-35
	Right	12	12	-9	-9	-12	-12	-5	-2	-3	-12	-17	-27	-32	-38
13	Left	10	6	-2	-2	-2	-5	-5	-1	-2	-11	-17	-17	-22	-28
	Right	10	5	-5	-5	-5	-7	0	-2	-2	-7	-10	-10	-20	-26
14	Left	6	3	-12	-11	-11	-12	-2	-7	-7	-15	-20	-25	-30	-40
	Right	7	6	-10	-10	-10	-12	-7	-8	-9	-15	-25	-25	-30	-35
15	Left	8	5	-5	-5	-5	-8	-8	0	-1	-9	-17	-22	-30	-35
	Right	8	7	-5	-6	-7	-8	-8	0	0	-5	-11	-11	-27	-32
16	Left	8	5	-7	-8	-8	-10	-8	0	0	-11	-15	-27	-40	-45
	Right	9	4	-7	-7	-10	-12	-8	0	-2	-16	-18	-28	-38	-43
17	Left	7	7	-5	-4	0	-7	-7	1	1	-8	-15	-20	-26	-35
	Right	8	8	-6	-4	-4	-7	-3	1	-1	-7	-15	-15	-25	-30
18	Left	12	12	-4	-4	-4	-7	-7	6	6	-2	-17	-17	-30	-35
	Right	12	9	-4	-4	-4	-7	-5	6	6	-8	-17	-17	-28	-35
19	Left	1	2	-7	-7	-7	-9	-9	-10	-10	-18	-25	-28	-35	-45
	Right	3	1	-7	-7	-7	-9	-9	-8	-9	-15	-20	-24	-35	-45
20	Left	7	4	-4	-7	-9	-9	-9	-10	-10	-15	-22	-28	-35	-40
	Right	7	4	-4	-7	-7	-9	-9	-10	-12	-17	-25	-30	-35	-45
21	Left	4	0	-7	-7	-7	-9	-9	-2	-2	-15	-20	-22	-25	-30
	Right	4	0	-6	-6	-6	-10	-10	-2	-2	-14	-20	-23	-28	-35
22	Left	7	4	-10	-12	-12	-13	-13	-3	-5	-13	-25	-26	-30	-40
	Right	5	5	-4	-10	-10	-11	-11	-2	-2	-12	-20	-25	-35	-40
23	Left	15	10	-7	-7	-9	-10	-10	10	8	-10	-12	-16	-26	-30
	Right	11	6	-7	-7	-9	-11	-9	10	8	-11	-13	-18	-27	-35
24	Left	12	8	-8	-9	-9	-11	-8	1	0	-12	-20	-25	-30	-35
	Right	12	7	-10	-11	-11	-14	-9	1	0	-15	-20	-23	-25	-30
25	Left	2	0	-12	-8	-8	-15	-15	-9	-10	-18	-28	-30	-38	-40
	Right	2	0	-8	-10	-10	-14	-14	-10	-11	-15	-18	-21	-28	-45
26	Left	7	4	-7	-12	-12	-14	-15	4	0	-13	-18	-22	-20	-22
	Right	5	5	-5	-9	-11	-14	-14	1	-2	-12	-17	-17	-22	-25
27	Left	6	4	-8	-2	-5	-9	-9	5	2	-9	-17	-22	-30	-35
	Right	5	-1	-7	-2	-6	-15	-15	3	3	-12	-17	-20	-30	-35
28	Left	7	7	-7	-2	-2	-8	-5	5	2	-5	-7	-22	-30	-35
	Right	4	2	-4	-4	-5	-10	-7	6	3	-7	-10	-22	-30	-35
29	Left	7	5	-10	-11	-12	-13	-13	-10	-10	-14	-20	-25	-30	-35
	Right	7	5	-7	-9	-9	-11	-10	-9	-7	-11	-17	-22	-27	-36
30	Left	13	6	-9	-12	-12	-17	-14	-2	-3	-12	-25	-29	-40	-45
	Right	9	4	-9	-12	-13	-17	-12	-3	-3	-11	-20	-25	-34	-38
31	Left	11	15	0	-2	-6	-10	-5	5	4	-11	-18	-22	-30	-35
	Right	13	15	-2	-3	-6	-9	5	4	3	-10	-16	-24	-30	-35
32	Left	5	4	-11	-12	-9	-10	-10	0	-2	-12	-17	-20	-25	-33
	Right	6	5	-5	-7	-4	-16	-16	1	0	-10	-15	-22	-25	-32
33	Left	6	0	-9	-9	-9	-12	-10	-12	-12	-16	-24	-32	-38	-42
	Right	4	0	-8	-8	-9	-12	-11	-9	-11	-17	-24	-30	-35	-42
34	Left	8	8	-7	-9	-11	-14	-16	3	0	-10	-20	-22	-27	-35
	Right	8	8	-5	-8	-9	-11	-12	2	0	-14	-22	-28	-33	-46
35	Left	12	8	-12	-16	-16	-16	-16	-17	-19	-23	-29	-32	-35	-40
	Right	12	12	-6	-12	-12	-14	-14	-17	-19	-22	-29	-33	-38	-42
36	Left	4	4	-5	-14	-14	-16	-15	-5	-5	-15	-25	-31	-35	-40
	Right	5	5	-9	-20	-20	-21	-20	-2	-5	-17	-24	-28	-35	-40
37	Left	2	2	-2	-2	-4	-7	-8	-11	-11	-14	-17	-17	-34	-40
	Right	2	2	-5	-5	-5	-9	-9	-12	-12	-14	-14	-12	-27	-36
38	Left	6	2	-9	-10	-6	-10	2	-8	-9	-17	-22	-30	-35	-38
	Right	6	2	-16	-16	-12	-12	2	-6	-6	-13	-21	-27	-29	-32
39	Left	11	7	-7	-11	-11	-13	-13	-10	-12	-22	-28	-34	-38	-38
	Right	7	9	-5	-14	-14	-16	-10	-10	-12	-15	-23	-29	-30	-32
40	Left	5	7	-2	-7	-8	-10	-10	-5	-7	-16	-24	-28	-30	-36
	Right	5	7	5	-5	-12	-15	-10	-6	-8	-9	-16	-20	-28	-32
41	Left	12	12	-3	-6	-6	-9	-9	-1	-1	-9	-14	-14	-23	-27
	Right	6	6	-3	-6	-13	-15	-17	-1	-2	-10	-12	-16	-25	-27
42	Left	2	-1	-12	-15	-16	-16	-8	-2	-3	-15	-27	-32	-39	-39
	Right	-2	-5	-10	-10	-6	-6	2	-2	-2	-17	-27	-30	-36	-41
43	Left	2	2	-6	-6	-6	-8	-8	-9	-9	-15	-20	-22	-30	-33
	Right	1	2	-10	-10	-10	-12	-10	-9	-9	-11	-26	-27	-28	-30
44	Left	3	-1	-11	-11	-11	-14	-14	-4	-6	-19	-22	-30	-35	-38
	Right	0	-3	-8	-9	-12	-15	-14	-5	-7	-13	-20	-27	-33	-40
45	Left	6	5	-14	-15	-15	-15	-5	2	2	-6	-9	-20	-27	-39
	Right	7	4	-8	-8	-9	-11	-5	2	2	-9	-18	-20	-24	-36
46	Left	2	2	-11	-9	-9	-11	0	-2	-4	-14	-22	-28	-32	-30
	Right	-2	-2	-15	-13	-13	-15	-6	-1	-2	-10	-22	-25	-27	-30

386

Cast No.		Maxillary Arch Inclination							Mandibular Arch Inclination						
		1	2	3	4	5	6	7	1	2	3	4	5	6	7
47	Left	7	3	-6	-10	-11	-15	-2	2	1	-9	-9	-13	-36	-42
	Right	2	2	-6	-8	-10	-13	-6	2	0	-10	-13	-18	-32	-37
48	Left	3	3	-3	-12	-10	-16	-16	-2	-4	-10	-23	-30	-34	-23
	Right	0	0	-9	-12	-10	-14	-14	-1	-3	-13	-20	-25	-28	-30
49	Left	12	11	-7	-7	-7	-9	-9	0	0	-9	-17	-17	-24	-30
	Right	10	10	-4	-5	-5	-10	-4	0	0	-10	-12	-12	-22	-30
50	Left	10	8	-9	-9	-9	-12	-12	-8	-9	-16	-22	-27	-32	-39
	Right	10	10	-2	-3	-7	-9	-9	-9	-10	-20	-22	-22	-28	-36
51	Left	2	2	-10	-10	-10	-12	-12	-2	-5	-21	-25	-33	-38	-41
	Right	1	-2	-15	-10	-8	-11	-11	0	-4	-19	-22	-28	-34	-42
52	Left	0	-3	-8	-11	-11	-15	-15	-2	-4	-15	-19	-25	-33	-38
	Right	0	-3	-11	-14	-14	-17	-17	-2	-3	-12	-17	-22	-27	-34
53	Left	5	8	-11	-11	-13	-15	-12	7	4	-15	-20	-25	-30	-35
	Right	6	2	-12	-17	-17	-20	-12	8	8	-10	-12	-20	-26	-30
54	Left	7	6	-11	-4	-4	-7	-7	2	0	-12	-14	-20	-30	-35
	Right	5	2	-12	-4	-6	-11	-6	2	-1	-12	-17	-20	-27	-35
55	Left	6	5	3	-5	-5	-10	-2	-5	-7	-14	-14	-20	-32	-35
	Right	3	3	-4	-4	-3	-5	10	-6	-6	-15	-15	-20	-28	-30
56	Left	6	4	0	-3	-5	-10	-10	3	2	-15	-20	-32	-33	-40
	Right	4	-1	-2	-3	-5	-10	-9	3	-1	-10	-16	-22	-24	-38
57	Left	14	10	-7	-11	-11	-17	-17	5	1	-15	-22	-27	-32	-37
	Right	12	10	-7	-11	-14	-18	-18	1	2	-10	-18	-21	-30	-37
58	Left	7	6	-15	-17	-18	-19	-2	-3	-4	-25	-35	-38	-42	-35
	Right	5	-1	-16	-20	-20	-22	-10	-4	-4	-16	-25	-26	-30	-36
59	Left	3	5	-7	-14	-11	-17	-10	2	-2	-14	-22	-27	-38	-42
	Right	5	2	-10	-10	-8	-16	-3	2	-2	-10	-29	-27	-32	-38
60	Left	-1	-1	-7	-8	-10	-12	-7	-3	-4	-18	-28	-32	-40	-45
	Right	2	0	-7	-7	-9	-12	-12	-2	-4	-11	-22	-28	-33	-40
61	Left	3	1	-11	-11	-12	-14	-10	2	-2	-18	-20	-25	-32	-38
	Right	3	-2	-11	-14	-15	-13	-5	3	-2	-12	-17	-22	-28	-33
62	Left	-2	-6	-10	-16	-16	-14	-14	3	-2	-13	-17	-22	-27	-32
	Right	0	-3	-11	-16	-18	-18	-18	7	-2	-9	-18	-25	-26	-30
63	Left	3	0	-10	-12	-13	-18	-18	0	-2	-14	-19	-28	-42	-45
	Right	4	0	-7	-16	-20	-25	-25	-2	-4	-10	-17	-22	-34	-40
64	Left	2	-3	-10	-16	-13	-16	-5	2	-1	-10	-22	-27	-38	-40
	Right	4	0	-6	-17	-16	-16	-2	5	3	-4	-10	-17	-32	-38
65	Left	7	2	-10	-10	-10	-9	-2	-7	-10	-21	-24	-30	-37	-40
	Right	5	-4	-9	-10	-9	-10	-5	-7	-11	-21	-24	-24	-33	-39
66	Left	8	10	-2	-2	0	-10	5	-2	-4	-10	-17	-22	-34	-42
	Right	3	6	-5	-1	0	-8	-8	-2	-4	-13	-17	-22	-35	-40
67	Left	12	12	-10	-12	-14	-15	-15	6	2	-8	-20	-26	-35	-35
	Right	11	8	-8	-10	-12	-14	-6	6	3	-10	-18	-22	-28	-35
68	Left	7	3	-16	-11	-8	-12	-10	-5	-8	-12	-19	-29	-38	-42
	Right	6	3	-14	-11	-10	-14	-11	-6	-8	-12	-20	-31	-36	-42
69	Left	10	8	-10	-15	-17	-24	-11	-7	-9	-22	-35	-45	-55	-60
	Right	9	6	-8	-9	-12	-22	-10	-7	-12	-15	-25	-35	-50	-52
70	Left	3	3	-8	-8	-8	-10	-7	-6	-6	-12	-22	-31	-36	-39
	Right	3	3	-3	-4	-4	-7	-3	-4	-6	-15	-20	-27	-35	-40
71	Left	12	17	-2	-5	-4	-10	0	-4	-4	-8	-15	-22	-32	-34
	Right	13	12	-4	-2	-2	-8	-2	-2	-2	-5	-15	-22	-30	-40
72	Left	8	7	-5	-7	-7	-9	-7	5	2	-2	-15	-24	-30	-35
	Right	10	8	2	-8	-9	-14	-10	7	2	-4	-9	-14	-18	-34
73	Left	14	13	0	-5	-5	-8	-8	-1	-3	-11	-23	-23	-26	-27
	Right	15	12	-2	-10	-14	-16	-16	2	-3	-11	-22	-22	-24	-29
74	Left	6	6	-6	-6	-7	-9	-9	1	-1	-7	-17	-22	-30	-32
	Right	6	6	-4	-7	-9	-12	-12	-2	-2	-4	-11	-12	-24	-29
75	Left	12	7	-12	-10	-10	-12	2	7	5	-6	-15	-15	-24	-25
	Right	10	7	-3	-2	3	0	12	7	5	-10	-15	-15	-20	-27
76	Left	8	5	-11	-6	-6	-10	5	-5	-6	-12	-16	-22	-30	-35
	Right	8	6	-9	-7	-7	-9	-1	-4	-4	-13	-20	-23	-28	-35
77	Left	3	5	-5	-5	-7	-9	-3	-7	-8	-22	-26	-32	-36	-45
	Right	0	2	-8	-5	-8	-14	-14	-7	-8	-15	-18	-20	-28	-38
78	Left	11	8	-3	-3	-4	-7	-7	-4	-5	-17	-25	-32	-40	-45
	Right	11	8	-5	-5	-8	-10	-6	-4	-5	-17	-22	-31	-35	-42
79	Left	13	12	-10	-10	-11	-13	-13	-6	-8	-18	-22	-23	-27	-31
	Right	12	9	-8	-8	-11	-14	-14	-9	-11	-16	-19	-21	-27	-32
80	Left	2	2	-9	-11	-11	-14	-6	-3	-5	-14	-19	-19	-30	-35
	Right	5	7	-9	-9	-9	-12	-7	-4	-4	-7	-17	-18	-28	-37
81	Left	6	4	-8	-11	-11	-13	-13	1	0	-11	-18	-22	-28	-32
	Right	6	2	-7	-9	-12	-14	-13	1	1	-11	-13	-19	-24	-24
82	Left	5	3	-15	-15	-17	-16	-11	-1	-3	-15	-21	-25	-31	-36
	Right	7	4	-9	-10	-10	-10	-2	-2	-3	-11	-18	-22	-26	-30
83	Left	2	-1	-12	-17	-15	-15	-12	-4	-4	-26	-27	-33	-35	-38
	Right	2	1	-10	-10	-7	-10	-5	-6	-7	-17	-22	-30	-35	-38
84	Left	11	11	-3	-7	-5	-9	-1	9	9	-5	-14	-22	-25	-28
	Right	6	6	-4	-7	-7	-10	2	10	8	-7	-7	-17	-25	-28
85	Left	5	5	-7	-7	-7	-9	-4	-2	-2	-7	-15	-15	-18	-25
	Right	4	2	-6	-5	-5	-9	2	-2	-3	-9	-13	-17	-22	-25
86	Left	6	4	-6	-8	-8	-11	-11	-4	-4	-18	-25	-30	-35	-40
	Right	6	3	-4	-11	-11	-15	-14	-4	-5	-17	-20	-25	-32	-42
87	Left	13	13	1	1	-3	-7	-9	-7	-7	-15	-18	-19	-30	-35
	Right	14	12	6	5	-3	-5	-8	-7	-7	-17	-22	-32	-37	-37
88	Left	4	5	-7	-7	-7	-9	-9	-1	-3	-15	-23	-28	-37	-42
	Right	4	6	-7	-7	-7	-9	-9	-2	-3	-15	-22	-27	-38	-48
89	Left	5	4	-3	-3	-4	-6	-2	-4	-4	-16	-20	-24	-28	-32
	Right	6	6	-8	-8	-8	-8	-8	-3	-4	-12	-10	-12	-16	-23
90	Left	5	3	-9	-5	-5	-8	-3	-1	-1	-10	-15	-27	-25	-27
	Right	4	2	-10	-3	-2	-5	-5	-1	-1	-11	-17	-17	-20	-22
91	Left	4	6	2	-2	-2	-3	-3	-5	-6	-15	-20	-22	-29	-32
	Right	5	6	2	-7	-6	-6	-6	-4	-5	-8	-18	-22	-29	
92	Left	3	4	-7	-2	-2	2	2	-7	-7	-14	-20	-25	-30	-35
	Right	2	0	-3	-6	-6	-5	0	-9	-9	-14	-17	-22	-24	-40
93	Left	7	4	-2	-6	-3	-8	-3	-10	-12	-17	-20	-25	-32	-38
	Right	0	-3	-8	-9	-9	-12	-14	-8	-10	-14	-17	-21	-30	-37

Cast No.		Maxillary Arch Inclination							Mandibular Arch Inclination						
		1	2	3	4	5	6	7	1	2	3	4	5	6	7
94	Left	6	10	-4	0	-4	-10	-5	3	1	-8	-19	-8	-28	-38
	Right	7	10	-2	-2	-8	-12	-5	0	-1	-7	-18	-23	-27	-34
95	Left	8	6	-7	-8	-8	-9	-7	-5	-6	-16	-19	-24	-26	-31
	Right	7	6	-5	-5	-4	-7	-7	-3	-5	-10	-15	-17	-22	-28
96	Left	6	-1	-9	-14	-12	-11	-5	2	0	-14	-20	-25	-29	
	Right	7	0	-7	-12	-10	-11	-1	2	0	-13	-18	-24	-30	
97	Left	8	7	-6	-5	-5	-10	-10	-4	-5	-19	-21	-28	-43	-48
	Right	6	6	-5	-5	-5	-7	-7	-5	-5	-12	-17	-27	-38	-44
98	Left	10	11	-12	-13	-7	-8	-4	8	-1	-15	-17	-22	-20	
	Right	9	12	-11	-13	-8	-14	-12	7	3	-11	-13	-16	-22	-31
99	Left	1	4	-7	-7	-7	-10	-5	-2	-4	-13	-16	-22	-25	-20
	Right	-1	-1	-8	-8	-14	-12	-8	2	0	-4	-7	-11	-16	-23
100	Left	-3	-2	-7	-11	-11	-12	-12	-8	-9	-10	-17	-19	-47	-52
	Right	-7	-4	-10	-10	-10	-11	-11	-12	-13	-15	-20	-20	-31	-35
101	Left	2	2	-17	-17	-17	-17	-6	-12	-13	-22	-23	-30	-44	-44
	Right	-2	-2	-12	-12	-12	-12	-2	-15	-17	-17	-21	-31	-40	-45
102	Left	15	14	-11	-9	-9	-12	-5	15	12	2	-13	-22	-22	-22
	Right	14	14	-14	-8	-8	-10	0	16	15	0	-1	-9	-9	-9
103	Left	8	10	-1	-7	-7	-11	-5	-10	-11	-20	-18	-20	-34	-42
	Right	7	10	3	-4	-5	-6	-6	-9	-11	-15	-14	-17	-30	-32
104	Left	3	3	-10	-10	-11	-15	-12	5	3	-7	-17	-30	-37	-49
	Right	2	-2	-11	-10	-12	-20	-14	5	3	-13	-22	-27	-30	-35
105	Left	6	4	-7	-8	-8	-10	-10	-6	-8	-17	-22	-28	-39	-45
	Right	7	5	-5	-14	-11	-10	-10	-6	-7	-15	-24	-26	-37	-38
106	Left	-3	0	-12	-11	-14	-15	-15	-1	-4	-17	-19	-25	-28	-34
	Right	0	-1	-9	-13	-16	-16	-17	-2	-4	-13	-22	-28	-32	-36
107	Left	7	7	-14	-7	-7	-11	-12	-7	-7	-19	-26	-30	-37	-22
	Right	8	6	-14	-14	-17	-17	-17	-7	-7	-23	-28	-29	-37	-45
108	Left	7	11	-2	-6	0	-3	-3	-2	-2	-15	-17	-22	-32	-38
	Right	7	5	-8	-10	-4	-8	-6	-2	-2	-10	-17	-22	-30	-35
109	Left	2	0	-8	-10	-9	-12	-12	11	8	-6	-15	-20	-30	-40
	Right	2	-2	-12	-12	-12	-17	-17	8	8	-4	-12	-16	-28	-32
110	Left	7	4	-4	-5	-3	-4	2	10	5	-6	-6	-15	-25	-25
	Right	4	1	-5	-6	-6	-8	-3	8	6	-5	-8	-12	-18	-12
111	Left	5	3	-10	-12	-12	-14	-14	12	3	-5	-14	-26	-35	-42
	Right	2	-2	-15	-15	-17	-20	-18	10	5	-10	-16	-25	-30	-38
112	Left	10	5	-12	-10	-10	-12	-12	-10	-10	-16	-22	-26	-35	-45
	Right	10	3	10	-5	-15	-15	-15	-7	-7	-12	-18	-24	-30	-45
113	Left	0	-2	-7	-7	-4	-8	-2	5	1	-18	-20	-22	-27	-35
	Right	0	-2	-7	-9	-6	-13	-7	3	0	-17	-19	-19	-22	-30
114	Left	10	7	-8	-12	-8	-12	-12	-2	-4	-12	-18	-23	-29	-35
	Right	11	10	-2	-8	-8	-11	-9	-1	-4	-15	-17	-20	-31	-41
115	Left	7	3	-8	-7	-12	-12	-12	-2	-2	-7	-15	-20	-30	-40
	Right	7	4	-9	-11	-11	-13	-13	-2	-3	-9	-10	-15	-30	-38
116	Left	7	4	-9	-8	-8	-9	-4	8	6	-10	-11	-13	-19	-22
	Right	7	5	-17	-13	-13	-15	5	7	4	-11	-13	-20	-27	-35
117	Left	6	4	-10	-5	-5	-7	-1	-8	-8	-17	-22	-19	-30	-35
	Right	6	3	-10	-11	-10	-8	5	-8	-10	-24	-27	-28	-35	-40
118	Left	5	2	-8	-6	-8	-17	-5	-2	-3	-11	-18	-24	-35	-40
	Right	6	-2	-15	-14	-17	-17	-14	1	-3	-16	-20	-33	-34	-40
119	Left	14	11	-10	-4	0	-6	-6	7	2	-14	-22	-26	-31	-40
	Right	13	9	-10	-10	-1	-8	-8	5	5	-8	-20	-23	-31	-42
120	Left	8	8	-15	-14	-14	-16	-17	4	2	-12	-17	-22	-35	-40
	Right	7	2	-14	-14	-14	-15	-15	6	4	-21	-21	-29	-41	-44
Count		240	240	240	240	240	240	239	240	239	239	240	240	240	236
Average		6.11	4.42	-7.25	-8.47	-8.78	-11.53	-8.10	-1.71	-3.24	-12.73	-18.95	-23.63	-30.67	-36.03
Std Dev		3.97	4.38	4.21	4.02	4.13	3.91	5.63	5.79	5.37	4.65	4.96	5.58	5.90	6.57
Max Value		15.00	17.00	10.00	5.00	3.00	2.00	12.00	16.00	15.00	2.00	-1.00	-8.00	-9.00	-9.00
Min Value		-7.00	-6.00	-17.00	-20.00	-20.00	-25.00	-25.00	-17.00	-19.00	-26.00	-35.00	-45.00	-55.00	-60.00

Cast No.		Maxillary Arch Prominence							Mandibular Arch Prominence						
		1	2	3	4	5	6	7	1	2	3	4	5	6	7
1	Left	2.0	2.1	2.5	2.9	2.5	2.8	2.4	2.0	1.8	2.4	3.0	2.7	3.1	2.0
	Right	2.0	2.2	2.0	2.4	2.5	2.5	2.5	2.0	1.9	2.5	3.0	2.6	2.8	2.5
2	Left	1.9	2.1	2.7	2.3	2.7	3.0	2.7	1.5	1.5	2.4	2.8	2.5	2.7	2.8
	Right	1.7	2.0	2.8	2.5	2.6	3.0		1.7	1.7	2.4	2.6	2.7	3.0	2.3
3	Left	2.7	2.5	2.7	2.2	2.3	3.0	2.5	2.0	2.0	3.0	2.5	2.4	3.0	2.7
	Right	2.5	2.0	2.6	2.3	2.0	2.7	2.4	2.0	2.1	3.1	3.0	2.7	2.8	3.1
4	Left	1.7	1.8	2.5	2.5	2.4	2.1	3.0	1.3	1.6	2.1	3.0	2.8	2.8	2.8
	Right	1.5	1.7	2.7	2.4	2.5	3.0	2.5	1.4	1.4	1.7	2.5	2.6	2.3	2.5
5	Left	2.2	1.7	2.3	2.3	2.4	3.1	3.0	1.5	1.6	2.7	3.0	3.0	3.0	3.0
	Right	2.0	2.0	2.5	2.8	2.5	3.0	2.5	1.7	1.7	2.4	3.0	2.6	3.0	2.5
6	Left	1.7	2.0	3.0	2.4	3.0	3.0	2.5	1.4	1.5	1.5	2.4	3.0	3.0	2.4
	Right	1.5	1.5	2.4	2.4	2.5	3.0	3.4	1.4	1.5	2.2	3.0	2.5	3.0	2.7
7	Left	2.3	2.0	3.0	3.0	2.7	3.1	3.0	1.5	1.3	2.5	3.1	3.0	3.0	3.0
	Right	2.4	2.0	2.0	2.2	2.5	2.4	2.5	1.5	1.4	2.1	3.0	2.7	3.0	3.1
8	Left	2.1	1.4	2.0	2.2	2.3	2.7	2.9	1.5	1.7	2.0	3.2	2.8	2.5	2.4
	Right	2.0	1.4	1.9	2.6	2.4	2.0	3.0	1.7	1.8	2.5	3.0	2.9	2.6	3.0
9	Left	2.2	1.9	3.0	2.5	2.0	3.0	3.1	1.6	1.7	2.3	2.7	2.5	3.1	2.5
	Right	2.2	1.7	2.5	2.0	2.6	3.1		1.7	2.0	2.6	2.5	2.5	3.0	2.7
10	Left	2.3	2.3	2.8	3.0	2.6	3.0	3.2	1.6	1.7	2.6	3.0	2.7	3.1	2.5
	Right	2.3	2.7	2.8	2.7	2.7	3.0	3.2	1.8	1.8	2.7	3.0	2.5	2.6	2.4
11	Left	2.3	1.7	2.6	2.7	2.4	3.0	2.5	1.3	1.4	2.2	2.5	2.5	3.0	2.2
	Right	2.0	1.8	2.6	2.6	2.5	2.7	3.0	1.2	1.7	2.3	2.2	2.7	3.0	3.0
12	Left	2.0	2.0	2.8	3.0	3.2	3.3	3.0	1.4	1.3	2.4	3.0	2.4	2.8	2.5
	Right	2.0	1.8	2.5	3.0	3.2	2.8	3.0	1.5	1.5	2.2	2.6	2.6	2.8	3.0
13	Left	2.0	1.9	2.4	2.6	2.1	3.0	3.0	1.8	1.8	2.3	3.0	3.3	2.6	3.0
	Right	2.0	2.0	2.7	2.3	2.5	2.3	2.0	2.0	1.7	2.0	2.9	3.0	2.4	3.0

Cast No.		Maxillary Arch Prominence							Mandibular Arch Prominence						
		1	2	3	4	5	6	7	1	2	3	4	5	6	7
14	Left	2.5	1.5	2.4	2.0	2.0	2.5	3.0	1.7	1.4	2.5	3.0	3.2	3.0	2.8
	Right	2.3	1.5	3.0	3.4	2.9	3.3	3.1	1.5	2.0	2.5	2.5	3.0	2.5	3.0
15	Left	2.0	1.4	2.4	2.3	2.0	2.7	2.3	1.4	1.4	2.5	2.3	2.6	2.8	2.5
	Right	1.7	1.8	2.5	2.0	2.0	2.6	2.4	1.3	1.6	2.3	2.3	2.5	3.0	2.4
16	Left	2.0	1.9	3.0	3.0	3.0	3.0	3.4	1.5	2.0	2.6	3.0	3.0	3.2	2.9
	Right	2.0	2.0	2.5	2.6	3.2	2.6	3.0	1.5	1.4	2.4	3.3	2.5	2.5	3.0
17	Left	2.0	1.8	3.0	2.8	2.6	3.1	2.5	1.9	2.0	2.3	2.8	2.5	2.6	3.0
	Right	2.0	1.5	2.3	3.0	2.8	2.5	2.8	1.8	1.7	2.4	2.6	2.7	3.0	2.7
18	Left	2.1	2.3	3.0	2.4	2.8	3.1	2.4	1.8	2.0	3.0	3.0	2.1	3.2	2.5
	Right	2.1	2.0	3.0	2.7	2.7	3.3	2.0	2.0	2.0	3.0	3.0	2.8	2.7	3.0
19	Left	2.0	1.8	2.0	2.4	2.5	2.7	2.8	1.5	1.6	2.3	2.5	2.4	3.0	2.2
	Right	2.0	1.7	2.0	3.0	2.4	2.6	2.4	1.6	1.7	2.0	3.0	2.5	2.5	2.3
20	Left	1.8	1.5	2.7	1.7	1.8	2.2	3.2	1.5	1.3	1.9	2.7	2.3	3.5	2.2
	Right	2.0	2.0	2.8	3.2	3.1	2.9	3.0	2.1	1.3	3.0	2.6	2.9	2.9	2.8
21	Left	1.4	2.0	2.7	1.3	2.2	3.6	2.9	1.4	1.7	2.0	2.3	2.7	3.2	3.0
	Right	1.5	1.6	3.4	2.5	2.4	3.3	4.0	1.7	1.8	2.6	3.2	2.6	2.8	2.8
22	Left	2.6	2.4	2.5	2.3	3.0	3.0	3.0	1.6	1.9	3.0	2.8	2.7	3.4	3.0
	Right	2.5	2.0	2.7	2.5	2.3	3.0	2.7	1.7	2.0	2.6	3.0	2.5	3.0	2.5
23	Left	2.7	1.7	2.9	2.2	1.9	3.2	3.0	2.0	2.1	2.9	3.0	2.7	3.0	2.8
	Right	2.4	2.0	3.7	3.1	2.3	3.6	3.2	1.5	1.6	3.1	3.2	2.8	3.4	3.5
24	Left	2.2	1.7	2.0	2.3	2.7	3.5	3.0	1.8	1.8	2.6	2.2	2.3	2.7	2.4
	Right	2.2	1.9	2.4	1.9	2.0	2.9	2.7	1.6	2.0	2.2	2.8	2.4	3.2	2.8
25	Left	1.5	1.3	2.4	2.7	2.5	3.0	3.4	1.4	1.5	2.5	2.4	2.5	3.1	2.5
	Right	1.9	1.8	2.6	2.7	2.5	3.1	3.9	1.6	1.5	2.2	1.9	2.0	3.0	2.6
26	Left	2.3	1.9	2.3	2.2	2.1	2.4	2.4	1.2	1.2	1.8	2.1	2.3	2.7	2.4
	Right	2.0	2.0	3.0	2.7	2.3	3.2	3.0	1.3	1.7	2.3	2.9	2.3	2.9	2.6
27	Left	1.7	1.7	2.3	2.4	2.0	2.5	2.3	1.2	1.3	2.3	2.6	2.6	2.5	2.4
	Right	1.7	1.5	2.2	3.0	3.3	2.8	2.8	1.2	1.4	2.0	2.2	2.5	3.2	2.4
28	Left	2.0	1.8	2.8	2.5	3.0	2.7	3.1	1.3	1.5	2.3	2.7	2.4	2.9	2.2
	Right	2.0	2.0	2.4	2.5	3.0	3.0	2.5	1.5	1.5	2.0	2.4	2.4	2.6	3.0
29	Left	2.0	2.0	2.7	2.4	2.0	3.0	2.4	1.3	1.6	2.0	2.3	2.2	2.4	2.8
	Right	1.8	2.0	2.5	2.2	2.0	2.8	2.9	1.3	1.7	2.0	2.0	2.4	2.8	2.7
30	Left	2.0	2.1	3.0	3.0	2.1	2.4	2.1	1.9	2.0	2.4	3.0	3.0	2.8	2.4
	Right	2.0	2.0	2.8	2.6	2.7	2.5	2.8	2.0	2.0	3.0	3.0	2.5	3.0	2.3
31	Left	2.1	2.0	2.3	2.4	2.5	2.5	2.0	1.6	1.5	2.5	3.0	2.5	2.3	2.0
	Right	2.0	2.0	2.4	2.8	2.5	2.6	2.1	1.5	1.5	2.0	2.6	2.5	2.6	2.3
32	Left	2.2	1.9	2.5	2.8	3.0	3.0	2.4	1.4	1.4	2.0	2.7	2.5	3.0	2.8
	Right	2.2	1.8	2.0	2.3	2.3	2.9	3.0	1.6	1.8	2.3	2.3	2.0	2.6	2.6
33	Left	1.4	1.5	2.2	2.5	2.5	3.0	3.0	1.4	1.5	2.4	2.5	2.5	2.6	2.4
	Right	1.5	1.6	2.4	2.5	2.6	2.7	2.8	1.4	1.5	2.1	2.9	2.3	3.0	2.6
34	Left	1.6	2.0	3.0	2.2	2.5	2.4	2.4	1.3	1.3	2.0	2.5	2.7	2.8	2.3
	Right	1.8	1.7	2.1	2.8	2.4	3.0	2.8	1.1	1.0	2.4	2.4	2.5	2.5	2.3
35	Left	1.5	1.2	2.0	2.4	2.4	3.0	3.0	1.6	1.5	2.3	2.7	2.7	2.5	2.5
	Right	1.6	1.5	2.5	2.8	2.4	2.7	3.0	1.4	1.5	2.0	2.5	2.7	2.6	2.7
36	Left	2.0	2.0	2.5	2.8	2.4	3.0	3.0	1.0	1.4	2.3	2.5	2.2	2.5	2.0
	Right	2.0	2.0	2.5	2.6	2.8	3.3	3.0	1.3	1.4	1.7	2.3	2.0	2.7	2.5
37	Left	2.0	2.1	3.0	2.4	2.0	2.3	2.0	1.5	1.5	2.0	2.8	2.3	2.4	2.5
	Right	2.0	2.0	2.4	2.5	2.2	3.0	2.7	1.5	1.3	1.5	2.0	2.3	3.0	2.6
38	Left	2.0	1.7	2.8	2.0	2.7	2.8	2.5	1.5	1.7	2.5	2.4	2.4	2.7	1.5
	Right	2.3	2.0	2.0	3.0	2.0	2.4	2.5	1.4	1.4	2.4	2.4	2.0	2.8	3.0
39	Left	2.1	1.7	3.0	2.5	2.7	3.0	2.7	1.3	1.5	2.4	2.6	2.5	3.0	2.0
	Right	2.0	1.5	2.2	2.3	2.5	2.4	2.3	1.0	1.4	2.0	2.8	2.5	2.4	2.0
40	Left	1.3	1.4	2.2	2.3	2.4	2.5	2.8	1.4	1.4	1.8	2.3	2.3	2.6	2.4
	Right	1.2	1.3	2.0	2.0	2.4	2.8	3.0	1.4	1.3	1.7	2.2	2.2	2.4	2.0
41	Left	2.6	2.0	3.4	3.0	2.3	2.3	3.2	2.0	2.2	3.2	3.4	3.0	3.4	2.7
	Right	2.4	2.0	3.3	3.0	3.0	2.8	3.2	2.0	2.3	3.3	3.2	3.0	3.0	2.9
42	Left	3.0	2.2	3.4	3.0	3.5	3.0	3.6	2.0	2.0	2.5	3.0	2.8	3.0	2.4
	Right	2.3	2.3	3.0	3.0	2.7	3.0	3.0	1.9	1.5	2.3	3.0	3.0	3.5	2.7
43	Left	1.8	1.7	3.3	2.3	2.4	2.7	3.2	1.7	1.2	2.5	3.2	2.7	3.1	2.7
	Right	2.3	1.7	3.3	2.8	2.7	3.5	3.5	1.4	1.3	3.0	3.2	2.8	3.8	2.5
44	Left	2.3	2.0	3.2	2.6	3.3	3.4	3.0	1.8	1.7	3.0	3.0	3.1	4.4	3.9
	Right	2.2	1.9	3.1	3.3	3.5	4.1	3.1	1.6	2.1	3.1	3.2	3.0	3.3	3.4
45	Left	2.0	1.7	2.3	2.8	2.3	2.8	3.2	1.2	2.0	2.5	3.0	2.4	3.3	2.6
	Right	1.9	2.0	3.0	2.4	2.3	3.8	2.9	2.0	2.0	2.3	2.7	2.3	2.8	3.2
46	Left	1.8	1.8	2.8	2.6	2.8	2.8	2.4	1.6	1.5	2.3	2.3	2.3	2.9	2.5
	Right	2.6	2.0	2.6	2.9	2.6	2.8	3.5	1.9	2.0	2.7	2.6	2.4	3.2	3.6
47	Left	2.2	2.0	2.9	2.4	2.0	3.4	4.3	1.7	1.7	2.2	2.6	2.4	2.8	2.3
	Right	1.9	2.0	2.9	2.4	2.7	3.0	3.8	1.8	1.5	1.9	2.4	1.8	2.5	2.8
48	Left	1.8	1.3	2.8	3.0	2.8	3.2	4.0	1.7	2.0	2.0	3.2	2.7	3.6	3.0
	Right	1.9	1.8	2.9	2.9	2.5	2.7	3.2	1.7	2.0	2.6	3.0	3.0	3.3	2.9
49	Left	1.6	1.6	3.0	3.0	2.9	3.2	2.6	1.5	1.7	2.5	2.9	2.9	3.0	2.9
	Right	2.0	2.0	3.0	2.4	2.9	3.2	3.7	2.0	1.9	2.4	2.0	2.8	3.0	2.6
50	Left	2.4	1.6	3.0	2.4	2.9	3.2	3.6	1.4	1.9	2.4	2.5	2.8	2.8	3.1
	Right	2.2	2.0	2.9	2.3	2.3	3.0	4.3	1.2	1.7	2.4	2.7	2.9	3.2	3.3
51	Left	1.8	2.0	2.8	2.0	2.4	3.2	3.3	1.7	1.6	2.6	2.7	2.4	3.3	2.3
	Right	2.0	1.8	2.9	2.4	2.6	3.0	4.0	1.8	3.7	3.2	2.8	2.3	3.2	3.2
52	Left	2.1	1.4	2.3	2.7	2.8	3.0	2.9	2.0	2.0	3.2	3.0	2.8	3.2	3.0
	Right	2.5	1.9	3.0	2.5	3.0	2.6	3.3	2.0	1.9	3.4	2.7	3.0	3.4	3.2
53	Left	2.2	2.1	2.7	2.2	2.0	2.7	2.8	1.6	1.4	2.1	2.4	2.4	2.5	2.3
	Right	2.0	1.5	2.4	2.2	2.0	3.0	2.6	1.2	1.4	2.0	2.0	1.9	2.8	2.2
54	Left	2.0	1.9	2.2	1.7	2.0	2.4	3.0	1.2	2.0	2.3	2.7	3.0	3.7	3.3
	Right	2.0	1.8	2.7	2.4	3.0	2.5	3.3	1.3	1.7	2.0	2.6	3.1	2.8	2.8
55	Left	2.0	1.8	2.7	2.7	2.5	3.5	2.7	1.7	1.3	2.6	2.9	2.9	3.1	3.1
	Right	2.0	1.9	2.6	2.6	3.0	2.3	2.7	1.4	1.9	2.3	3.1	3.0	3.3	4.0
56	Left	2.2	2.0	3.1	2.5	2.4	3.0	2.4	2.0	2.0	2.6	3.4	2.7	3.4	2.6
	Right	2.1	2.0	3.1	2.3	2.3	2.8	2.8	1.9	2.0	3.0	3.2	2.8	3.7	3.0
57	Left	2.6	2.1	3.2	2.0	2.1	2.8	3.0	1.6	1.6	3.0	2.5	2.3	3.2	2.6
	Right	2.3	2.0	3.2	3.0	2.7	3.0	3.7	1.2	1.6	2.8	2.5	2.6	2.9	3.0
58	Left	1.5	1.4	2.4	3.0	3.1	2.6	3.3	1.7	1.9	2.2	3.3	3.3	3.0	3.3
	Right	2.2	2.0	2.9	2.9	2.5	2.5	4.2	1.4	1.5	2.7	3.4	3.1	3.3	3.1
59	Left	2.3	2.1	3.3	3.5	2.9	3.1	3.3	1.6	1.6	2.7	2.8	2.8	4.0	3.7
	Right	2.1	2.2	2.9	2.8	2.7	2.5	2.8	1.4	1.9	2.2	2.5	2.4	3.5	2.8
60	Left	1.8	2.0	3.4	2.1	2.0	3.4	3.7	1.2	1.6	2.0	2.6	2.3	3.7	3.0
	Right	1.8	1.3	3.0	2.0	1.8	2.7	3.7	1.2	1.4	1.8	3.1	2.0	3.2	2.8

Cast No.		Maxillary Arch Prominence							Mandibular Arch Prominence						
		1	2	3	4	5	6	7	1	2	3	4	5	6	7
61	Left	2.7	2.0	3.0	3.1	2.7	3.0	2.5	2.0	1.5	2.9	3.2	2.8	3.0	2.8
	Right	2.6	1.4	2.9	2.6	3.0	3.6	3.7	1.7	1.8	2.9	3.0	2.8	3.4	2.7
62	Left	2.0	2.1	3.5	2.8	3.2	2.3	2.8	1.4	1.8	1.8	2.0	3.2	3.3	3.0
	Right	2.0	1.8	3.3	2.4	3.2	2.9	3.6	1.2	2.0	2.4	2.9	3.0	2.5	2.1
63	Left	2.3	2.1	3.3	2.9	2.1	3.5	2.9	1.3	1.4	2.9	3.0	2.1	3.7	3.2
	Right	2.6	2.0	3.3	2.3	2.1	2.6	3.6	1.9	0.9	3.1	3.0	2.6	3.6	3.1
64	Left	2.1	2.0	2.8	2.4	2.4	2.9	2.9	2.0	2.0	2.0	2.5	2.8	3.2	1.7
	Right	2.4	1.4	2.8	2.6	2.7	2.8	2.6	1.5	1.1	3.0	2.8	2.9	3.5	3.2
65	Left	2.0	1.8	3.3	3.2	3.0	3.4	3.1	1.7	1.7	2.8	3.0	3.2	3.3	2.4
	Right	2.3	2.0	3.0	2.6	2.0	3.5	3.7	1.9	1.6	2.7	3.0	3.0	3.7	3.4
66	Left	1.8	2.0	3.0	2.8	2.0	3.3	3.0	1.6	1.9	2.5	3.0	1.7	3.7	2.2
	Right	2.2	1.6	2.9	2.3	2.3	3.0	3.2	1.7	1.9	2.1	2.9	2.0	3.4	2.5
67	Left	2.2	2.0	3.2	3.0	2.7	2.5	3.0	1.5	0.8	3.0	3.2	2.4	2.9	2.8
	Right	2.5	2.1	3.4	3.0	2.5	2.6	3.4	1.7	1.8	2.9	3.5	2.7	2.6	3.4
68	Left	2.3	1.8	3.0	2.2	2.7	3.0	2.7	1.4	1.3	2.1	2.7	2.4	3.0	2.5
	Right	2.3	1.5	2.6	2.5	3.2	3.1	4.6	1.8	1.3	2.6	3.0	2.2	2.6	3.2
69	Left	1.2	1.4	2.3	2.2	2.3	2.3	2.5	1.8	1.8	2.1	2.9	2.7	3.2	2.8
	Right	2.0	1.7	2.7	2.5	2.5	2.6	3.3	1.5	1.7	2.0	2.7	2.5	2.5	2.5
70	Left	1.8	1.7	2.2	2.5	2.7	2.3	2.5	1.8	1.3	2.6	2.5	2.7	2.9	2.4
	Right	1.5	1.3	2.8	2.2	2.2	2.7	3.0	1.5	1.6	2.4	2.1	2.3	2.8	2.4
71	Left	1.8	1.7	2.6	2.3	2.2	2.7	2.6	1.3	1.4	1.7	2.3	2.3	2.7	2.1
	Right	1.7	1.5	2.8	2.1	2.2	2.2	2.0	1.0	1.5	2.2	2.3	2.4	2.4	2.4
72	Left	2.0	2.2	2.1	2.0	2.4	3.0	3.1	1.8	1.1	2.2	2.6	2.8	3.1	1.7
	Right	2.2	2.7	2.3	2.2	2.8	2.8	2.6	1.4	2.0	1.9	2.6	2.4	3.4	2.6
73	Left	1.9	2.0	2.4	2.1	2.2	2.5	4.0	1.5	1.3	2.6	2.2	2.3	2.4	2.0
	Right	1.7	1.7	2.6	2.4	1.8	2.8	3.3	2.0	1.6	2.0	2.6	2.6	3.2	3.2
74	Left	1.8	2.0	2.4	2.2	2.1	2.6	3.8	1.5	1.4	2.7	2.4	2.2	2.6	2.3
	Right	1.7	1.7	2.7	2.5	1.8	2.8	3.3	1.9	1.6	2.0	2.4	2.6	3.2	3.0
75	Left	1.9	2.5	3.3	2.9	2.6	2.9	2.5	1.9	1.6	3.0	3.0	3.2	3.7	3.2
	Right	2.3	2.0	2.7	2.3	2.4	3.0	2.4	1.8	1.4	3.0	2.5	3.0	4.0	3.5
76	Left	3.0	2.2	2.4	2.9	2.4	3.5	3.0	1.6	1.4	3.0	3.0	3.4	3.3	2.5
	Right	2.4	1.8	3.0	3.1	3.0	3.6	3.7	1.3	1.4	2.4	3.4	3.3	4.0	3.7
77	Left	2.3	2.0	2.7	2.8	2.8	2.8	2.5	1.4	1.6	2.4	3.0	2.5	3.0	3.0
	Right	2.5	1.5	2.8	2.8	2.2	3.0	3.0	2.0	1.5	2.3	3.2	3.2	3.5	3.0
78	Left	1.7	1.7	2.7	2.8	2.2	3.6	4.0	1.7	1.8	2.4	2.7	3.0	3.4	2.7
	Right	1.9	2.2	3.0	2.8	2.7	2.7	3.2	1.5	1.4	2.2	2.8	3.0	3.2	3.2
79	Left	2.2	2.0	3.3	2.3	2.5	3.2	3.2	1.5	1.4	2.5	2.4	2.8	3.0	2.4
	Right	2.0	2.0	3.0	2.4	2.4	3.0	3.3	1.6	1.4	2.2	3.1	2.2	3.0	2.3
80	Left	1.7	2.0	2.5	2.3	2.2	2.8	3.2	1.6	1.6	2.5	2.7	2.4	3.2	3.0
	Right	1.8	1.7	2.0	2.3	2.0	2.8	2.4	1.5	1.4	2.5	3.0	2.6	3.4	3.1
81	Left	1.9	1.5	2.4	2.8	2.5	2.2	2.0	2.0	1.7	2.8	2.5	3.0	2.8	2.2
	Right	2.0	2.3	3.4	3.2	2.0	3.4	2.7	2.0	1.5	2.5	2.7	3.0	3.3	3.0
82	Left	1.8	1.9	2.3	3.4	2.2	3.0	3.2	1.4	1.7	2.7	2.4	3.3	3.2	3.2
	Right	1.7	2.2	2.4	2.7	2.5	2.7	3.0	1.3	1.4	2.5	2.5	3.2	3.4	4.0
83	Left	2.1	1.5	2.8	3.2	2.2	3.1	4.1	1.9	2.2	2.8	3.0	3.3	3.8	3.1
	Right	1.6	2.0	3.0	2.4	2.4	3.3	3.8	2.0	2.0	2.4	3.1	2.7	4.2	3.0
84	Left	2.1	1.8	2.6	2.4	2.5	3.2	3.5	1.4	1.3	1.8	2.8	2.2	3.3	2.9
	Right	1.5	1.4	2.4	2.3	2.3	3.2	2.8	1.2	1.5	2.0	2.6	2.0	2.9	2.9
85	Left	3.0	2.3	2.6	2.5	2.5	2.7	2.1	1.9	1.9	2.8	2.9	2.9	4.1	3.6
	Right	2.3	1.8	2.3	2.8	2.2	3.4	3.6	1.6	1.4	2.6	2.9	3.2	3.2	3.2
86	Left	1.8	2.1	1.7	2.3	2.1	3.4	2.3	1.5	1.7	1.4	2.0	2.0	2.9	2.5
	Right	1.7	1.2	2.4	3.0	2.4	3.7	2.9	1.2	1.3	1.7	2.9	2.7	3.9	3.4
87	Left	1.5	1.3	2.4	2.3	1.9	2.8	3.4	1.6	1.4	2.2	3.0	2.3	3.1	2.5
	Right	1.8	1.2	2.2	1.9	2.0	2.9	2.6	1.3	1.2	1.6	2.3	2.0	3.1	3.3
88	Left	2.0	2.0	2.7	2.8	3.0	3.0	3.4	2.1	1.5	2.7	3.2	2.5	3.1	3.3
	Right	2.3	1.6	2.5	3.2	2.8	4.2	3.2	2.3	2.0	2.4	2.9	2.8	3.0	3.4
89	Left	2.0	1.5	2.8	2.2	2.3	2.4	3.6	1.5	1.8	2.0	2.8	3.2	3.3	4.1
	Right	1.6	2.4	2.4	2.5	2.4	3.1	3.5	1.3	1.5	2.4	2.8	2.8	3.0	3.2
90	Left	1.9	1.5	3.0	2.4	2.3	3.0	2.8	1.5	1.7	3.0	2.5	2.3	3.3	2.2
	Right	2.0	1.8	3.0	2.1	2.2	3.0	2.6	1.8	1.5	3.0	2.7	2.5	3.2	3.0
91	Left	2.3	1.9	3.0	2.8	2.5	3.0	3.0	1.7	2.0	2.0	2.5	2.8	3.1	2.5
	Right	2.3	2.0	2.7	2.5	2.4	3.0	4.0	2.0	1.9	2.0	2.7	2.6	3.2	
92	Left	2.0	2.2	3.3	2.9	2.8	2.5	3.9	1.6	1.0	2.3	3.0	3.2	2.8	3.7
	Right	2.3	1.5	2.4	2.8	3.0	2.9	2.9	1.2	1.5	2.8	3.2	3.1	3.2	3.3
93	Left	2.2	1.9	3.1	2.8	2.9	3.9	4.0	1.6	2.0	2.2	3.1	2.3	3.8	4.3
	Right	2.1	2.0	2.6	2.4	2.5	3.8	4.4	1.8	2.1	2.3	2.7	2.8	3.0	3.4
94	Left	1.9	1.4	2.7	2.2	2.3	3.5	3.1	1.2	1.4	2.0	3.0	2.6	3.0	3.5
	Right	1.9	1.8	2.8	2.0	2.3	3.3	2.9	1.3	1.4	2.3	3.0	2.1	3.0	3.1
95	Left	2.2	1.6	2.8	2.5	2.2	2.6	2.9	1.4	2.0	2.8	2.8	2.4	3.0	3.2
	Right	2.1	2.0	2.3	2.4	2.0	2.3	3.0	1.3	1.3	2.1	2.5	2.6	3.0	3.5
96	Left	2.0	1.5	3.0	2.5	2.2	2.8	3.2	1.9	1.8	2.5	2.7	2.6	3.3	
	Right	2.0	1.9	2.7	2.0	2.2	2.6	3.5	1.4	1.7	3.0	2.6	2.7	3.0	
97	Left	1.9	1.5	3.4	2.2	2.5	3.1	3.1	1.8	1.6	2.5	2.6	2.4	2.8	2.3
	Right	2.3	2.6	2.9	2.3	2.4	3.1	3.4	1.5	1.5	3.2	3.4	3.0	3.7	3.7
98	Left	2.0	1.7	2.3	2.3	2.3	2.3	2.8	1.2	1.3	2.0	1.2	2.4	2.5	
	Right	2.0	2.7	2.4	2.3	2.5	2.7	2.9	1.3	1.5	1.4	2.2	2.2	2.6	2.8
99	Left	2.7	2.1	3.1	3.1	3.4	3.3	3.0	1.8	2.0	2.0	3.1	2.8	2.9	3.3
	Right	2.5	2.0	2.2	2.8	3.3	2.8	3.6	2.0	1.9	2.2	3.7	3.9	3.0	3.6
100	Left	2.2	1.9	2.7	2.5	2.6	3.5	2.6	1.5	1.5	2.3	2.3	2.2	2.2	2.2
	Right	1.7	1.7	3.5	2.2	2.1	2.5	2.6	1.4	1.5	2.2	2.6	2.7	2.4	2.1
101	Left	1.6	1.8	2.3	2.3	2.5	3.0	3.1	1.7	1.4	2.0	2.8	2.3	2.9	2.6
	Right	1.6	1.8	2.5	2.3	2.7	2.8	2.9	1.7	1.4	2.3	2.8	2.5	2.5	2.9
102	Left	1.4	1.4	1.9	2.0	2.0	3.0	2.3	1.3	1.4	2.3	2.5	2.5	2.4	2.2
	Right	1.4	1.4	2.0	2.5	2.1	2.3	2.3	1.5	1.5	2.1	2.7	2.4	2.5	2.2
103	Left	2.1	1.6	2.7	2.7	2.7	3.0	3.0	2.0	1.9	2.8	2.7	2.7	3.1	2.7
	Right	1.9	1.9	2.4	2.3	2.6	2.5	2.9	2.1	2.0	2.4	2.6	2.7	3.4	3.4
104	Left	1.7	1.9	2.2	2.3	2.9	2.6	2.8	1.4	1.7	1.6	2.0	2.3	2.4	2.6
	Right	1.5	1.7	2.5	2.3	2.4	2.7	2.9	1.5	1.8	1.7	2.5	2.7	2.2	3.0
105	Left	2.5	2.0	2.8	3.0	2.6	3.5	3.3	2.0	1.7	2.4	3.0	2.8	2.6	2.4
	Right	2.5	2.5	2.5	3.0	2.6	2.7	3.0	1.2	1.8	2.4	3.0	2.8	3.3	3.3
106	Left	1.9	1.5	3.0	2.8	2.8	2.3	3.3	1.5	1.7	1.9	2.6	2.2	2.6	2.2
	Right	2.0	1.7	2.5	2.3	2.5	2.7	2.2	1.4	1.5	2.0	2.8	2.7	3.0	3.0
107	Left	1.8	2.2	2.7	3.3	2.0	3.0	3.5	2.3	2.0	3.0	3.4	2.6	3.2	2.5
	Right	2.2	2.2	2.8	2.5	2.2	3.2	3.0	2.0	2.0	2.7	3.5	2.5	2.2	3.4
108	Left	2.0	2.0	3.1	2.5	2.3	2.6	2.5	1.6	1.5	2.6	2.0	2.0	2.9	2.3
	Right	1.9	1.8	2.4	2.7	2.5	2.9	2.2	1.4	1.6	2.8	2.8	2.6	2.7	2.5

390

Cast No.		Maxillary Arch Prominence							Mandibular Arch Prominence						
		1	2	3	4	5	6	7	1	2	3	4	5	6	7
109	Left	1.9	2.1	2.0	2.3	2.5	2.7	2.5	2.0	2.2	2.4	2.1	2.2	3.4	2.7
	Right	2.0	2.0	2.4	2.0	2.5	2.3	2.7	2.0	1.5	2.2	2.4	2.4	3.0	2.4
110	Left	2.2	1.8	2.3	2.8	2.0	2.8	3.2	1.4	1.8	1.8	0.1	3.1	2.6	3.0
	Right	2.0	1.7	2.6	2.6	2.3	2.5	3.2	1.7	1.3	1.8	1.7	2.6	2.4	3.3
111	Left	1.6	0.9	2.3	2.4	2.6	3.2	2.7	1.1	1.3	1.9	2.3	2.3	3.1	2.2
	Right	1.5	1.4	1.9	1.9	3.3	3.2	3.2	1.4	1.2	2.0	2.5	2.6	2.7	3.3
112	Left	1.4	1.0	2.7	2.6	2.3	2.5	2.7	1.4	1.0	2.3	2.7	2.0	2.9	2.4
	Right	1.5	1.7	2.2	2.8	2.8	2.8	2.9	1.3	1.3	1.8	2.5	2.3	2.5	3.5
113	Left	2.2	1.6	3.2	3.3	2.9	3.9	3.7	1.4	1.9	2.3	4.0	2.5	3.2	2.3
	Right	1.9	2.2	2.5	2.0	2.3	3.2	3.7	1.7	2.5	2.1	3.6	2.9	3.4	3.3
114	Left	2.1	1.9	2.9	2.7	2.4	2.9	3.2	1.5	1.7	2.8	3.3	2.7	3.3	3.3
	Right	1.9	2.4	2.3	2.9	2.3	2.6	3.2	1.7	2.5	2.2	3.3	2.6	3.4	3.3
115	Left	2.1	1.8	2.9	3.0	2.5	2.4	3.9	1.4	2.3	2.1	2.4	2.5	3.9	2.9
	Right	1.5	2.3	2.3	2.3	2.2	0.9	4.0	1.8	1.5	2.2	2.6	2.2	3.0	3.1
116	Left	2.3	1.8	3.0	2.7	2.0	2.7	2.9	1.9	1.8	2.0	2.7	2.2	3.0	2.2
	Right	1.7	1.8	2.1	2.0	1.9	2.5	3.1	1.8	1.8	2.3	2.7	2.8	2.9	2.7
117	Left	1.9	1.7	2.7	2.9	2.3	2.9	3.0	1.5	1.7	2.6	3.5	2.0	3.3	2.4
	Right	1.5	2.0	3.1	2.6	2.2	3.1	3.3	1.7	1.3	3.1	3.4	2.3	2.9	3.3
118	Left	2.2	1.9	2.9	2.8	2.2	2.5	2.7	1.6	1.4	2.0	2.4	2.4	2.6	3.4
	Right	2.3	1.8	2.8	2.4	2.1	2.5	2.4	1.6	1.5	2.8	2.4	2.2	2.7	3.3
119	Left	2.0	1.6	1.9	2.4	2.5	2.0	2.0	1.3	1.4	2.0	1.4	2.2	3.1	2.7
	Right	1.4	1.7	2.2	2.5	2.0	3.0	2.8	1.4	1.0	1.4	2.3	2.5	3.5	3.0
120	Left	1.8	1.6	2.0	2.4	2.4	2.2	3.0	1.2	1.0	1.9	2.3	2.7	3.6	2.1
	Right	1.6	1.4	1.7	2.4	2.7	2.7	3.0	1.4	1.4	2.3	2.8	2.8	3.4	2.6
Count		240	240	240	240	240	240	238	240	240	240	240	240	240	236
Average		2.01	1.84	2.67	2.54	2.48	2.88	3.00	1.59	1.64	2.37	2.72	2.60	3.02	2.79
Std Dev		0.32	0.30	0.39	0.35	0.36	0.40	0.51	0.27	0.32	0.40	0.43	0.34	0.40	0.47
Max Value		3.00	2.70	3.70	3.50	3.50	4.20	4.60	2.30	3.70	3.40	4.00	3.90	4.40	4.30
Min Value		1.20	0.90	1.70	1.30	1.80	0.90	2.00	1.00	0.80	1.40	0.10	1.70	2.20	1.50

391

Glossary

Abnormal malocclusion. A condition in which the occlusion or the anterior limit of the dentition cannot be treated to optimal goals without jaw surgery.

Alternate treatment plan. The less conservative of two treatment possibilities for a specified amount of interim core discrepancy (ICD).

Andrews plane. The surface or plane on which the midtransverse plane of every crown in an arch will fall when the teeth are optimally positioned. If the plane is concave or convex, technically it is a surface; but in all instances it is referred to in this book as the Andrews plane.

Angulated slot. A slot angled more or less than 90° to the bracket's vertical components.

Angulating. Changing the mesiodistal cant of a tooth when the axis of rotation is in the crown.

Angulation. The mesiodistal cant of the facial axis of the clinical crown (FACC) relative to a line perpendicular to the occlusal plane. Angulation is "positive" when the occlusal portion of the FACC is mesial to the gingival portion, "negative" when distal.

Arch core discrepancy (core discrepancy). The difference between the length of the core line and the sum of the mesiodistal diameters of the crowns, measured at their contact points (after allowing for any planned correction of tooth size abnormality).

Another and quicker method of determining core discrepancy is to compute the difference between the sum of the mesiodistal diameters of only the malaligned teeth and the space on the core line available for them.

Arch core line (core line). An imaginary line that best represents the form and length of the arch. It passes mesiodistally through the center of each crown that is in line with the arch form. It can be indirectly represented from the occlusal perspective with a brass wire that is centered over the occlusal surface of each such crown.

Auxiliary feature. A bracket design feature, such as a power arm, that contributes to the biological aspect of treatment but is not involved in targeting the slot.

Base point. The middle of the bracket base. The base point falls on an extension of the faciolingual axis of the bracket stem.

Basic treatment plan. Either the only or the most conservative treatment plan for an arch within a specified range of interim core discrepancy (ICD).

Bracket base. The portion of the bracket stem intended to mate with the surface of the crown.

Bracket siting. Any procedure that affects positioning the bracket.

Bracket stem. The portion of the bracket that includes the bracket base, the lingual half of the slot, and the portions between.

Clinical crown. Normally, the amount of crown that can be seen intraorally or with a study cast. In this book *clinical crown* means the amount visible in late mixed dentitions and adult dentitions with gingiva that is healthy and not recessed. Orban has defined the clinical crown as the anatomical crown height minus 1.8 mm [21]. In young patients or those with hypertrophied or receding gingiva, the clinical-crown height can be found by measuring the distance from the incisal edge or cusp tip of the crown to the cementoenamel junction, and then subtracting 1.8 mm.

Contact area. The portion of the mesial or distal surface of a tooth that will touch an adjacent tooth when both teeth are optimally positioned.

Contact point. The centermost portion of a crown's contact area.

Convenience feature. A bracket design feature that facilitates use by the orthodontist or promotes comfort for the patient but does not contribute to the biologic aspects of treatment or to targeting the slot.

Core discrepancy. The difference between the length of the core line and the sum of the mesiodistal diameters of the crowns, measured at their contact points (after allowing for any planned correction of tooth size abnormality).

Another and quicker method of determining core discrepancy is to compute the difference between the sum of the mesiodistal diameters of only the malaligned teeth and the space on the core line available for them.

Core line. An imaginary line that best represents the form and length of the arch. It passes mesiodistally through the center of each crown that is in line with the arch form. It can be indirectly represented from the occlusal perspective with a brass wire that is centered over the occlusal surface of each such crown.

Counterbuccolingual tip. A slot-siting feature for maxillary molar brackets that counteracts buccolingual tip during translation and then overcorrects.

Countermesiodistal tip. A slot-siting feature that counteracts mesial or distal tipping during translation and then overcorrects.

Counterrotation. A slot-siting feature that counteracts rotation during translation and then overcorrects.

Crown angulation. The angle formed by the facial axis of the clinical crown (viewed from the facial perspective) and a line perpendicular to the occlusal plane. Crown angulation is considered positive when the occlusal portion of the FACC is mesial to the gingival portion, negative when distal.

Crown inclination. The angle between a line perpendicular to the occlusal plane and a line that is parallel and tangent to the FACC at the FA point. Crown inclination is determined from the mesial or distal perspective. It is sometimes incorrectly called torque, which means a twisting force. "Tangent to" means that the line representing the inclination of the FACC should be equidistant from each end of the clinical crown, while touching the FACC. Crown inclination is considered positive if the occlusal portion of the crown, tangent line, or FACC is facial to its gingival portion, negative if lingual.

Customized appliance. An appliance that is designed and fabricated to precisely match the unique morphology and guidance needs of a specific patient.

Edgewise appliance. A set of brackets, each with a rectangular slot. The slot enables three-dimensional tooth movement.

Embrasure line. An imaginary line, at the level of the crown's midtransverse plane, that would connect the most facial portions of the contact areas of a single crown, or of all crowns in an arch when they are optimally positioned.

Facial axis of the clinical crown (FACC). For all teeth except molars, the most prominent portion of the central lobe on each crown's facial surface; for molars, the buccal groove that separates the two large facial cusps.

Facial-axis point (FA point). The point on the facial axis that separates the gingival half of the clinical crown from the occlusal half.

Facial plane of a crown. Any plane that is tangent to a point on the crown's face.

Fully programmed appliance. A set of brackets designed to guide teeth directly to their goal positions with unbent archwires.

Horizontal bracket components. The occlusal and gingival sides of the bracket.

Inclination. The faciolingual cant of the FACC when measured from a line perpendicular to the occlusal plane. Inclination is "positive" when the occlusal portion of the FACC is facial to its gingival portion, "negative" when lingual.

Inclined base. A bracket base that is angled more or less than 90° to the midtransverse plane of the bracket stem.

Inclined slot. A slot whose midtransverse plane is inclined relative to the midtransverse plane of the bracket stem.

Inclining. Changing the faciolingual cant of the FACC when the axis of rotation is in the crown or bracket.

Individualized appliance. An appliance whose design tailors each bracket to morphological and positional norms of its tooth type, and to the most widely used treatment plans.

Interim core discrepancy (ICD). The difference between the sum of the mesiodistal diameters of the crowns at their contact points and the length of the interim core line.

Another and quicker method of determining ICD is to add to the core discrepancy the sum of the effects of changing the core line in all ways proposed other than for its distal boundary.

Interim core line. A proposed core line whose distal ends are those of the arch core line, but whose buccolingual and occlusogingival form and anterior boundary are treatment *goals*. Its length is the core-line length, plus the gain or loss from changing the core line in all ways intended except for distal boundary.

Maxillary molar offset. The angle between the crown's embrasure line and a line connecting the buccal cusps of a maxillary mo-

lar. It is measured along the crown's midtransverse plane.

Maximum translation bracket. A translation bracket for posterior teeth that require more than 4 mm of translation.

Medium translation bracket. A translation bracket for teeth that require more than 2 mm but not more than 4 mm of translation.

Midfrontal plane of the crown. The plane that separates the facial from the lingual half of a clinical crown.

Midsagittal plane of the crown. The plane that separates the mesial and distal portions of a crown at its facial axis.

Midtransverse plane of the crown. The plane that separates the occlusal portion of a clinical crown from its gingival portion.

Minimum translation bracket. A translation bracket for teeth that require 2 mm or less of translation.

Molar offset. The angle between the crown's embrasure line and a line connecting the buccal cusps. It is measured along the crown's midtransverse plane.

Nonprogrammed appliance. A set of brackets designed the same for all tooth types, relying totally on wire bending (except possibly for angulation if the bracket is angulated) to achieve the optimal position for each individual tooth.

Normal arch. Any arch in which each tooth's existing position is within 7 mm of its proposed position. (This range allows a maximum core discrepancy of 14 mm through –14 mm.)

Normal malocclusion. A condition in which the occlusion and the anterior limit of the dentition can be treated to optimal goals without surgery.

Partly programmed appliance. A set of brackets designed with some built-in features, but that always requires some wire bending (though less than is required by nonprogrammed appliances).

Power arm. A lever arm extending gingivally from the bracket, and used for delivering force toward the crown's center of resistance.

Prominence plane of the crown. A plane that is at right angles to each crown's midtransverse and midsagittal planes and is 1 mm farther facially from each crown's embrasure line than is the most facially prominent cusp of the first molar in that arch.

Slot base. The surface of the slot closest to the tooth.

Slot point. The junction of the midtransverse, midsagittal, and midfrontal planes of the bracket slot.

Slot site. The area that the bracket slot must occupy if it is to passively receive a full-size and unbent archwire when a tooth is optimally positioned.

Slot siting. Any procedure that affects positioning the bracket slot. Slot positioning is influenced by bracket design, bracket siting, and crown morphology.

Slot-siting feature. A design feature for positioning the bracket slot.

Slot-target point. The midpoint of the slot site for a tooth. It is located at the junction of a crown's prominence plane and facial extensions of the crown's midtransverse and midsagittal planes.

Standard bracket. A fully programmed bracket designed for teeth that do not require translation.

Stem prominence. Distance from the base point of the bracket to its slot point.

Straight-wire appliance. A set of brackets designed to guide teeth directly to their goal positions with unbent archwires: used synonymously for *fully programmed appliance.*

Straight-Wire Appliance. The registered name of a fully programmed appliance manufactured by a specific orthodontic company.

Subtypes. The eight ranges of interim core discrepancy within a normal arch, each representing where one basic treatment plan begins and ends: (positive discrepancy) 0–4 mm, 5–8 mm, 9–14 mm; (negative discrepancy) 0–6 mm, 7–8 mm, 9–10 mm, 11–13 mm, 14 mm.

Tip. The mesiodistal or faciolingual angle of the long axis of a tooth when measured to a line perpendicular to the occlusal plane. Tip is "positive" when the occlusal portion of the tooth's long axis is either mesial or facial to its apical portion, "negative" when distal or lingual.

Tipping. Changing the mesiodistal or faciolingual angle of the long axis of a tooth when the axis of rotation is in the root.

Tooth class. A group of teeth having similar shape and function. Classes are incisors, canines, premolars, and molars.

Tooth type. A subordinate category within a class of teeth. Premolars are a class of teeth and are similar; a mandibular first premolar is a type and is different from any other tooth type, such as a mandibular second premolar.

Translation bracket. A fully programmed bracket for teeth that require translation. It is designed to promote bodily movement during mesial or distal movement, and to overcorrect in proportion to the distance moved.

Treatment core line. A line that conforms to all treatment goals for the arch core. Its length equals the sum of the mesiodistal diameters of the teeth when measured at their contact points (assuming no tooth size discrepancy).

Types. The three natural divisions of the range of core discrepancy or interim core discrepancy for a normal arch: Spaced (positive discrepancy), Classic (zero discrepancy), and Crowded (negative discrepancy).

Vertical bracket components. The mesial and distal sides of the bracket and tie wings.

References

1] Ackerman, J. L., and W. R. Profitt. Diagnosis and planning treatment in orthodontics. Chap. 1 in *Current orthodontic concepts and techniques*, edited by T. M. Graber and B. F. Swain, vol. 1, 2d ed. Philadelphia: W. B. Saunders Co., 1975.

2] Andrews, L. F. The Andrews straight-wire appliance concept. Thesis presented to Southern California component of the Edward H. Angle Society of Orthodontists, Pasadena, California, November 1968.

3] ———. The diagnostic system: occlusal analysis. *The Dental Clinics of North America* 20(1976): 671–690.

4] ———. The six keys to normal occlusion. *Am. J. Orthod.* 62(1972):296–309.

5] ———. *The straight-wire appliance: syllabus of philosophy and techniques.* 2d ed. 1975.

6] Angle, E. H. Classification of malocclusion. *Dental Cosmos* 41(1899):248–264, 350–357.

7] ———. The latest and best in orthodontic mechanism. *Dental Cosmos* 70(1928):1143–1158.

8] ———. The latest and best in orthodontic mechanism. *Dental Cosmos* 71(1929):260–270.

9] ———. *Treatment of malocclusion of the teeth.* 7th ed. Philadelphia: The S. S. White Dental Mfg. Co., 1907.

10] Björk, A., and V. Skieller. Facial development and tooth eruption. *Am. J. Orthod.* 62 (1972):339–383.

11] Case, C. S. *A practical treatise on the technics and principles of dental orthopedia and prosthetic correction of cleft palate.* 4th ed. Chicago: C.S. Case Co., 1921. Pp. 102–103.

12] Dempster, W. T., W. J. Adams, and R. A. Duddles. Arrangement in the jaws of the roots of the teeth. *J. Am. Dent. Assoc.* 67(1963):779–797.

13] Dewel, B. F. Clinical observations on the axial inclination of teeth. *Am. J. Orthod.* 35(1949):98–115.

14] Gottlieb, E. L., A. H. Nelson, and D. S. Vogels. 1986 JCO study of orthodontic diagnosis and treatment procedures. *J. Clin. Orthod.* 20 (1986):612–625.

15] Holdaway, R. A. Bracket angulation as applied to the edgewise appliance. *Angle Orthod.* 22 (1952):227–236.

16] Jacobson, A. The 'Wits' appraisal of jaw disharmony. *Am. J. Orthod.* 67(1975):125–138.

17] Jarabak, J. R., and J. A. Fizzell. *Technique and treatment with the light-wire appliance.* St. Louis: The C. V. Mosby Co.,1963.

18] Lindquist, J. T. Attachments. In *Current orthodontic concepts and techniques,* edited by T. M. Graber and B. F. Swain, vol. 1, 2d ed. Philadelphia: W. B. Saunders Co., 1975. Pp. 502–514.

19] ———. Orthodontic bands. In *Current orthodontic concepts and techniques,* edited by T. M. Graber and B. F. Swain, vol. 1, 2d ed. Philadelphia: W. B. Saunders Co., 1975. Pp. 475–501.

20] Mayne, W. R. Serial extraction. Chap. 4 in *Current orthodontic concepts and techniques,* edited by T. M. Graber and B. F. Swain, vol. 1, 2d ed. Philadelphia: W. B. Saunders Co.,1975.

21] Orban, B., ed. *Oral histology and embryology.* 4th ed. St.Louis: The C. V. Mosby Co., 1957.

22] Saltzmann, J. A. *Principles of orthodontics.* 2d ed. Philadelphia: J. B. Lippincott Co., 1950.

23] Steiner, C. C. Cephalometrics for you and me. *Am. J. Orthod.* 39(1953):729–755.

24] Strang, R. H. W. *A text-book of orthodontia.* Philadelphia:Lea & Febiger, 1933.

25] Stuart, C. E., and I. B. Golden. *The history of gnathology.* Ventura, California: C. E. Stuart Gnathological Instruments, 1984.

26] Thurow, R. C. *Atlas of orthodontic principles.* St. Louis: The C. V. Mosby Co., 1970.

27] Tweed, C. H. *Clinical orthodontics.* vol. 1. St Louis: The C.V. Mosby Co., 1966.

28] *Webster's ninth new collegiate dictionary.* Springfield, Mass: Merriam-Webster, Inc., 1985.

29] Wheeler, R. C. *A textbook of dental anatomy and physiology.* 4th ed. Philadelphia: W. B. Saunders Co., 1965.

Index

Notes

Notes